BLUEPRINTS IN FAMILY MEDICINE

BLUEPRINTS in
FAMILY MEDICINE

Editors & Lead Authors

Martin S. Lipsky, MD
Professor and Chair
Department of Family Medicine
Northwestern University Medical School
Chicago, Illinois

Mitchell S. King, MD
Attending Physician
Evanston Northwestern Healthcare
Glenview, Illinois
Assistant Professor
Northwestern University Medical School
Chicago, Illinois

Authors

Adam W. Bennett, MD
Co-Chief Resident of Family Practice
Family Practice Residency Program
Saint Joseph Hospital
Chicago, Illinois

Jasmine Chao, DO
Resident of Family Practice
McGaw Medical Center of Northwestern University
Chicago, Illinois

Daria Majzoubi, MD
Resident of Family Practice
McGaw Medical Center of Northwestern University
Chicago, Illinois

Leslie Ann B. Mendoza, MD
Resident of Family Practice
McGaw Medical Center of Northwestern University
Chicago, Illinois

Sanjaya P. Sooriarachchi, MD
Resident of Family Practice
McGaw Medical Center of Northwestern University
Chicago, Illinois

Blackwell
Publishing

Blackwell Publishing, Inc., 350 Main Street, Malden, Massachusetts 02148-5018, USA
Blackwell Science Ltd., Osney Mead, Oxford OX2 0EL, UK
Blackwell Science Asia Pty Ltd, 550 Swanston Street, Carlton, Victoria 3053, Australia
Blackwell Verlag GmbH, Kurfürstendamm 57, 10707 Berlin, Germany

04 05 06 5 4 3 2

ISBN: 0-632-04579-5

Library of Congress Cataloging-in-Publication Data

Blueprints in family medicine / Martin S. Lipsky ... [et al.].
     p. ; cm.—(Blueprint USMLE steps 2 & 3 review series)
   ISBN 0-632-04579-5 (pbk.)
   1. Family medicine—Outlines, syllabi, etc.   2. Primary care (Medicine)—Outlines, syllabi, etc.
   [DNLM: 1. Family Practice—Outlines.   2. Primary Health Care—methods—Outlines. WB 18.2 B6576 2002]
I. Lipsky, Martin S.   II. Blueprints.
   RC59 .B58 2002
   616—dc21
                                                                                      2002001501

A catalogue record for this title is available from the British Library

Acquisitions: Beverly Copland
Development: Amy Nuttbrock
Production: Debra Lally
Cover design: Hannus Design
Typesetter: SNP Best-set Typesetter Ltd., Hong Kong
Printed and bound by Capital City Press in Vermont, USA

For further information on Blackwell Publishing, visit our website:
www.blackwellpublishing.com

Notice: The indications and dosages of all drugs in this book have been recommended in the medical literature
and conform to the practices of the general community. The medications described do not necessarily have specific approval by the Food and Drug Administration for use in the diseases and dosages for which they are recommended. The package insert for each drug should be consulted for use and dosage as approved by the FDA.
Because standards for usage change, it is advisable to keep abreast of revised recommendations, particularly those
concerning new drugs.

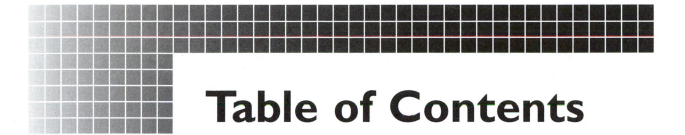

Table of Contents

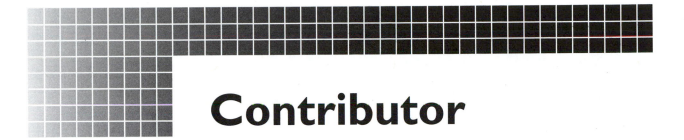

Contributor

Arden Fusman, MD
Resident of Family Practice
Glenbrook and Evanston Hospitals
Glenview, Illinois

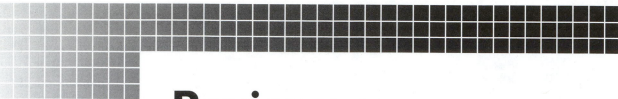

Reviewers

Elissa Gallo, MD
Class of 2001
Northwestern University Medical School
Chicago, Illinois

Alan Ka
Class of 2002
SUNY at Stony Brook School of Medicine
Stony Brook, New York

Sandi Lam
Class of 2002
Northwestern University School of Medicine
Chicago, Illinois

Kate Tulenko, MD, MPH, M.Phil
Resident of Pediatrics
Children's National Medical Center
Washington, DC

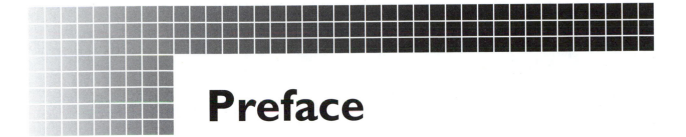

Preface

Medical students, interns, and residents need accurate and to the point core clinical content. The Blueprints series was developed to meet this need.

The original Blueprints series was designed to help prepare students for USMLE Steps 2 and 3. Although there is not a separate Family Medicine section on the Step 2 exam, *Blueprints in Family Medicine is* still a valuable tool for preparing for the USMLE Step 2. The book focuses on common outpatient problems encountered in primary care, conditions that are prominently tested in both USMLE Steps 2 and 3. The material in this book complements the topics covered in the other Blueprints series. The core content in this book should be particularly useful for residents in other disciplines as a broad based study guide for Step 3.

In addition, we believe this book provides a useful review for students rotating on a family medicine or primary care clerkship. For students at schools using a USMLE shelf examination for their Family Medicine final exam this book should also provide a useful study guide.

We hope that you find *Blueprints in Family Medicine* informative and useful. We welcome any feedback and suggestions that you may have about this book. Send it to *blue@blacksci.com*.

The Publisher
Blackwell Publishing, Inc.

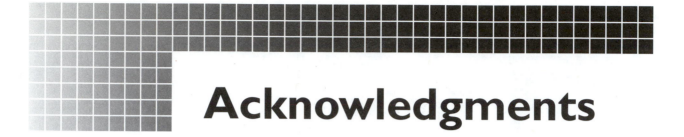

Acknowledgments

We would like to express our appreciation to the many people who made this project possible. To the residents who worked very hard on this project despite the demands of their hectic schedules—we give them our sincere thanks. I would also like to thank Renee Sommers and Olympia Asimacopoulos for their help in organizing this book and for Renee's invaluable contributions in preparing the manuscript. We want to thank Beverly Copland who made this project possible and Amy Nuttbrock. It is hard to imagine working with a better editor than Amy Nuttbrock. We also wish to thank our colleagues and friends in the Department of Family Medicine at Northwestern University Medical School and Evanston Northwestern Healthcare. Finally, we want to thank our family and friends without whom this and other projects would not be possible.

Martin S. Lipsky, MD
Mitchell S. King, MD
December 2001

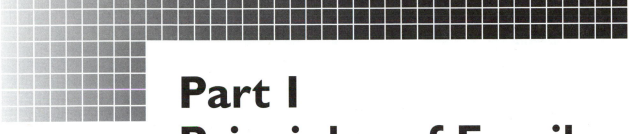

Part I
Principles of Family Medicine

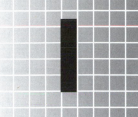

Elements of Primary Care

Primary care is coordinated, comprehensive, and personal care that often serves as a patient's point-of-entry into the health care system. Family medicine emphasizes responsibility for total health care from an initial assessment to continuous care of the individual and the family. Health promotion, wellness, and early detection of disease are important elements of family medicine. A successful primary care physician incorporates several components into caring for the patient including accessibility, medical diagnosis and treatment, comprehensiveness, communication of information, coordination of care, continuity of care, and serving as a patient advocate.

ACCESSIBILITY

A family physician is often the patient's first medical contact and is available if the patient has an urgent or chronic complaint. The majority of encounters with a family physician occur in an office or clinic setting. Accessibility includes being financially affordable and geographically accessible.

MEDICAL DIAGNOSIS

Medical competency is a core value of family medicine. As the patient's first contact, a family practitioner must be knowledgeable about a broad array of diseases and have the skill and judgment to determine the scope, site,

and pace of a medical evaluation. The family physician can care for 90 to 95% of a patient's health care needs. For the remaining problems, the family physician consults the appropriate physician specialist or other health care provider.

COMPREHENSIVENESS

The scope of family practice encompasses all ages, both sexes, and each organ system. A typical family physician provides a broad range of services, including acute and chronic disease management in the office, hospital, nursing home, or via the telephone. Family medicine incorporates both the biological perspective and the social and psychological aspects of care. The large number of office visits to family practitioners for psychosocial and behavioral issues underscores the relationship between emotion and illness.

COMMUNICATION

The need to inform, educate, reassure, and advise patients is an essential part of family medicine. Effective communication depends on understanding what the patient thinks about their illness. Knowing what to say about a medical problem is difficult if the patient's viewpoint has not been determined. For example, many patients visit a family physician with a complaint in order to learn the cause or to get reassurance that the problem is not serious, rather than to cure the problem. A classic example is headache pain, where the primary concern may not be relief but reassurance that there is not a brain tumor present.

COORDINATION OF CARE

The family physician orchestrates a patient's care. This implies maintaining a complete record of the patient's problems and serving as the central source of information about a patient's care. The family physician coordinates patient referrals to specialists and identifies other health care providers needed to assist in a patient's overall health care needs. Coordination mandates that the physician assume responsibility for guiding a patient through what is becoming an increasingly complicated health care system.

CONTINUITY OF CARE

The family physician develops long-term relationships with patients, maintains a longitudinal record of patient problems, and promotes a healthy lifestyle. This involves one physician seeing the patient for acute episodes of illness and for periodic visits for health maintenance. Continuity nourishes a trusting, long-term relationship between the physician and patient. This relationship is a valuable tool for improving patient adherence to treatment recommendations. Assessing disease risk, screening for illness, and promoting health to prevent disease and disability are inherent parts of a successfully continuous relationship. Early intervention

through health education, behavior change, and healthy lifestyles promotion can help prevent morbidity and mortality.

PATIENT ADVOCATE

Once a patient has been accepted into a practice, the family physician must serve as the patient's advocate. In addition, the physician is responsible for educating the patient about treatment outcomes and prognoses, incorporating the patient's preferences into treatment plans, and assuming responsibility for the total care of the individual during times of health and illness. This includes assisting the patient in making health care decisions and helping the patient find the resources necessary for their health care needs.

◆ KEY POINTS ◆

1. The goals of primary care include accessibility, medical diagnoses and treatment, comprehensiveness, communication, coordination of care, and continuity of care.

2. The family physician is often the first contact for patients with the health care system.

3. The family physician view of health care extends beyond the biological model and incorporates social and psychological aspects of care.

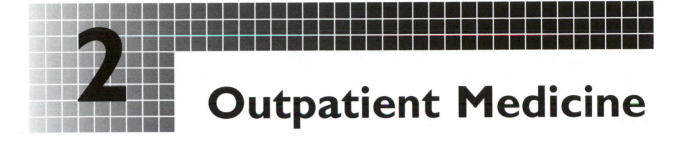

Outpatient Medicine

In the 1980s, as the cost of health care rose exponentially, delivering care in the outpatient setting became more financially appealing. Currently, over 95% of all medical encounters occur in the outpatient setting. Despite the trend to shift more care to ambulatory settings, most medical student and resident training experiences focus on hospitalized patients. In a family medicine setting, it becomes readily apparent that there are many differences between inpatient and outpatient care. Some of the more obvious differences include the environment, communication, type of patient problems encountered, use of time, and increased emphasis on psychosocial needs in the outpatient setting.

DIFFERENT ENVIRONMENT

An obvious difference is that patients look different in ambulatory settings. Instead of lying in a hospital bed in a gown, patients in the ambulatory setting typically walk into the office wearing their usual clothes and incorporating their appointment into their daily lives. Some come from work or school. Tests need to be scheduled to accommodate the patient's daily activities. Tests such as a 24-hour urine collection that can easily be obtained as an inpatient become difficult to arrange. Tests typically cannot be obtained "stat," and results may not be available for several days.

Even when the physician correctly evaluates a patient and gives good advice, many different barriers to adher-

ence to care recommendations exist in the outpatient world. Patients tend to be more concerned about cost. Dietary interventions are controlled in the hospital environment. However, in the outpatient setting dietary interventions such as a low-salt diet require significant change in patient behavior and become more difficult to implement. The successful family physician learns to deal with these practical issues.

COMMUNICATION

In the outpatient family practice setting, giving patients advice, often by providing a prescription medication, is a common task. Unlike the inpatient setting where physician orders are likely to be carried out by staff, in the outpatient setting patients decide whether to adhere to a physician's recommendations. Typically the rule of thirds applies to patients in the outpatient setting. About one-third of patients will follow almost none of their physician's advice, about one-third will follow some of their physician's advice, and about one-third will substantially adhere to their doctor's recommendations. In the primary care setting the alliance formed with patients is critical. Flawless advice does not improve a patient's health if it is not followed. Successful patient partnerships depend on explaining the problem and plan in a clear manner, developing rapport, and inviting patients to ask questions and express concerns.

DIFFERENT DISEASES

It is less common for patients to present with acute life-threatening illness to an outpatient office visit. Acute problems are more likely to be urgent in nature rather than true emergency problems. Management of chronic illnesses commonly takes place in the outpatient setting. The types of illnesses seen are usually common ailments. For example, most hypertensive patients are not in a hypertensive crisis and have essential hypertension rather than hyperaldosteronism.

Many patients may not be ill at all but present for a routine physical or for family planning. The approach for this type of patient will be quite different than for a hospitalized patient. Lifestyle management, cancer screening, smoking cessation, and immunization might be the focus of the encounter rather than treating an illness. In older patients, improving or maintaining function rather than curing disease might be the therapeutic goal.

DIFFERENCES IN TIME

There are several differences between the use of time in the inpatient and outpatient setting. First, the length of time available to see a patient is far shorter in the outpatient setting. Most visits to a family practice office may be scheduled for only 15 minutes and even physical examinations are typically scheduled for 30 to 45 minutes. Unlike the inpatient setting where patients are "captive," outpatients leave the office and are unavailable for the provider to easily go back and take additional history or repeat an examination. Unlike the hospital setting where patients accommodate the physician's schedule and wait patiently, outpatients expect to be seen at their appointment times and are angry if the physician is late. In fact, the most common outpatient complaint is excessive time spent waiting to be seen by the physician.

In the inpatient arena, time is the provider's enemy. Pressure is placed on the physician to diagnose and treat problems expeditiously to reduce the length of stay. In the outpatient setting, time is often an ally to help assess symptoms. Often an exact diagnosis may not be made, but the physician may be convinced that a delay in evaluation will not harm the patient and a follow-up appointment may be scheduled in a week or even more. As time progresses, the diagnosis may become clearer, or as commonly occurs, the symptoms may resolve.

PSYCHOSOCIAL NEEDS

In the inpatient setting, a patient's psychosocial problems are important, but may be overshadowed by his or her acute illness and need for medical intervention. In the ambulatory setting, stress, anxiety, and depression are often the major focuses of the encounter. Almost half of all complaints seen in a family practice setting have a major psychosocial component. Often the patient masks these problems with a somatic complaint. Common complaints that raise suspicions for a contributing psychosocial overlay include headaches, fatigue, backache, abdominal pain, and vague chest discomfort. Picking up clues to identify problems that are functional rather than organic is a key skill for a successful family physician. Diagnosing and effectively treating these problems can be immensely rewarding for the physician and of obvious benefit to the patient.

CONCLUSION

In a successful family medicine practice, the physician adapts successfully to the outpatient setting. This may require a greater reliance on clinical skills and having fewer diagnostic tests immediately available. Although the physician is less likely to encounter an emergent life-threatening problem in the outpatient setting, there are opportunities to dramatically impact patients' lives and improve their health.

◆ KEY POINTS ◆

1. Currently over 95% of all medical encounters occur in the outpatient setting.

2. Successful patient partnerships depend on explaining the problem and plan in a clear manner, developing rapport, and inviting patients to ask questions and express concerns.

3. In the outpatient setting, time is often an ally to help assess symptoms. As time progresses, the diagnosis may become clearer, or as commonly occurs, the symptoms may resolve.

4. Almost half of all complaints seen in a family practice setting have a major psychosocial component.

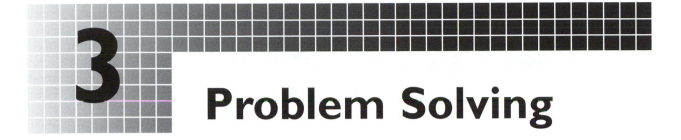

3 Problem Solving

Patients frequently consult their family physicians because of symptoms they experience. These complaints are often undifferentiated, meaning they are non-specific and very general in nature, and can be associated with a number of causes. Common examples of these types of problems include headache, dizziness, and back pain.

The family practitioner must collect information by history and physical examination, interpret test results, arrive at a conclusion, and make a management recommendation. Box 3–1 lists different ways that physicians approach problems. Deductive reasoning is among the most common type of reasoning used by experienced family physicians. The process involves forming a hypothesis, refining the hypothesis, and confirming the hypothesis.

HYPOTHESIS FORMATION

Very early in a patient encounter, the physician develops hypotheses about the patient's complaints based on clues in the history. In some instances, the physician may recognize a pattern of symptoms and quickly limit the tentative diagnosis to one or two diseases. Examples of common conditions that fall into this category include otitis media, tendonitis, and depression. For most complaints, a family physician will consider several possibilities but rarely more than seven or eight.

Considerations in sorting out diagnostic possibilities include the likelihood, potential seriousness, and treata-

bility of various conditions. For example, there are numerous conditions that cause a cough, such as bronchitis, asthma, pneumonia, and lung cancer. In a younger non-smoking individual with a two-day history of a low-grade fever and a productive cough, bronchitis is a likely possibility. However, a more severe and treatable condition such as a bacterial pneumonia might be considered because it is important not to miss this potentially serious and treatable condition.

REFINING THE HYPOTHESIS

Once a differential diagnosis is generated, the physician refines the hypothesis based on additional questions and physical examination. In one example, further questioning of the patient with a cough reveals that the cough produces only a small amount of yellow sputum and there is no associated shortness of breath. Physical examination reveals a temperature of 38.5° centigrade and coarse bronchial sounds in the lungs. In some cases, the history and physical examination are insufficient to make a decision and diagnostic studies such as blood tests or an imaging procedure may be needed to refine the hypothesis. For this patient, the working diagnosis could be either a bronchitis or pneumonia and a chest x-ray might be ordered to distinguish between the two. Often the clinical evaluation provides enough certainty to make a management decision without further testing. The management decision may not always be

---

BOX 3–1

Glossary of Problem Solving Terms

Deductive reasoning—The clinician develops different hypotheses and tests them. Among the most commonly applied reasoning styles in family practice.

Algorithms—Clinical reasoning that proceeds systematically though branching decision points. Most commonly used for mild to moderately complex problems.

Exhaustive—Involves a detailed history and physical and often extensive lab testing. Typically an inefficient and costly means of providing care, it is most useful for complex and unusual problems.

Heuristic—Involves pattern recognition, in which an experienced physician uses previously learned patterns to quickly recognize a diagnosis.

---

based on an exact diagnosis, but on determining whether a condition is serious or not, organic versus functional, or in the case of abdominal pain, surgical versus nonsurgical.

HYPOTHESIS CONFIRMATION

Most decisions in family practice have a degree of uncertainty. The probability of a diagnosis is somewhere between 0 and 100%. Rarely can a family physician assign an exact percentage of probability. Instead, the physician tends to form a qualitative impression based on experience, epidemiology, and the medical literature that allows a management decision to be made. For example, based on their experience a physician might believe that it is rare to have a normal lung examination in patients with pneumonia. However, the presence of coarse lung sounds may increase the likelihood of pneumonia, prompting the physician to order a chest x-ray to determine if the patient has an infiltrate.

A diagnostic test is a maneuver that provides information about the condition. It may be a physical examination maneuver, such as palpation for abdominal tenderness, or it may be an imaging or laboratory test.

There should always be a reason for ordering a test. A good rule of thumb in family medicine is that if the test result will not affect management, then it should not be done. Other considerations include the importance of the condition tested for, the patient's values, concurrent medical problems, and the cost effectiveness and risk of the test.

Ideally, diagnostic testing would be perfectly accurate. Unfortunately all tests have a degree of uncertainty. Some normal people have positive tests (false positives) and some abnormal individuals have negative tests (false negatives). Sensitivity is defined as the probability that a test result will be positive when a person truly has the disease. Specificity is the probability that the test will be negative when administered to a patient without the disease. A perfectly sensitive test can rule out the disease if the test is negative. A perfectly specific test can identify the disease if positive.

The predictive value of a test is related to the pretest likelihood of the disease. That is, the greater the physician's assessment of disease likelihood, the greater the probability that the disease is truly present if the test is positive. Conversely, the less suspicious the clinician is about a diagnosis, the more likely a negative test is truly negative. Ultimately the family physician assembles the information to form a qualitative judgment and plan of action. This plan may range from watchful waiting, to treatment, to further testing, or in some cases to referral to a specialist.

◆ KEY POINTS ◆

1. Deductive reasoning is the most common problem solving style used by family physicians.

2. A negative test that is sensitive is helpful for excluding a disease.

3. A positive test that is very specific is helpful for identifying a disease.

4. Solutions to problems in family medicine include ordering treatment, pursuing a period of observation, ordering further tests, or referring the patient to another health care provider.

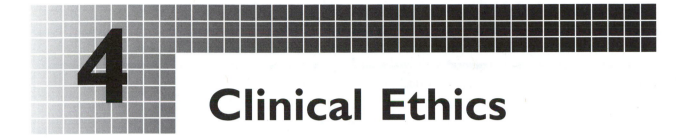

4

Clinical Ethics

Clinical ethics is the discipline that examines and attempts to resolve the moral problems that arise in medicine. Box 4–1 provides definitions of some common ethical terms. Although much attention is given to the dramatic issues encountered in the ICU, family physicians often confront ethical issues in their daily practices.

Traditionally, physicians have the obligation to help patients, avoid harm to patients, maintain confidentiality, and treat all patients fairly. In modern medicine there has been an increased focus on preserving patient autonomy, which is the right for an individual to make his or her own health care decisions. Areas that challenge the primary care physician include confidentiality, informed consent, financial issues, and advanced directives. As knowledge about human genetics grows, undoubtedly these advances may create ethical dilemmas for the future.

CONFIDENTIALITY

Dating back to the Hippocratic oath, the principle of confidentiality has been one of the most widely accepted principles governing the patient-physician relationship. The American Medical Association in 1980 reconfirmed that the "physician shall safeguard patient confidentiality within the constraints of the law." Confidentiality is critical to foster patients' truthfulness in their communications with their physician. It is the requirement for confidentiality that creates some of the most troublesome dilemmas for the primary care physician. Confidentiality may need to be breached to protect a third party from harm. In the precedent-setting Tarsakoff case, a Californian court found that a psychiatrist should have informed a woman that she was at risk from a patient who had homicidal fantasies about her and eventually murdered the woman. The family physician may encounter instances where they must weigh the relative harm in betraying confidentiality. For example, an HIV infected individual may request that their HIV status not be disclosed to their spouse. Although the physician should try to persuade the individual to tell their spouse, the physician may have to make the difficult choice between maintaining the patient's confidentiality and the obligation to prevent harm to the spouse.

Numerous requests may be made for physicians to release confidential information. Insurance companies, employers, and physicians may all request information about outpatient visits. The patient must sign a release for the physicians to release information. In most instances, that physician is not obligated to release information without the patient's approval.

Another common dilemma involves teenage patients, whose parents may also be patients. Unless confidentiality is guaranteed, adolescents may not be open about their behavior. If confidentiality is protected, then teens may not get the support they need from their parents

---

BOX 4–1

Glossary of Clinical Ethics Terms

Autonomy—The principle that individuals have the right to make their own health care decisions.

Benefice—The principle of doing good.

Competency—The presence of decisional capacity. Although an individual may be incompetent for some areas, such as household management, they may still be competent to make health care decisions.

Confidentiality—The principle that a physician will not reveal information without a patient's permission. Exceptions may include legal issues, such as the requirement to report certain diseases, and the potential of harm to others.

Decisional capacity—The ability to make and understand a decision.

Justice—The principle that individuals should be treated equally and fairly.

---

for a difficult problem. By law, teens may be treated in most states without parental consent for sexually transmitted diseases, pregnancy care, contraception, and substance abuse. Minors may also be treated without parental consent if they are married or live independently from their parents.

INFORMED CONSENT

Informed consent involves the receipt and interpretation of information by patients to assist them in arriving at a decision, commonly involving a therapy or diagnostic procedure. It is an important part of an ethically sound physician/patient relationship. The elements of informed consent are listed in Box 4–2.

Each element can be presented to varying degrees of complexity. It is not reasonable to present an exhaustive discussion of each element. The standard most commonly used is to provide the information that a hypothetically "reasonable person" would want to know.

BOX 4–2

Elements of Informed Consent

- Description of condition
- Description of the proposed treatment
- Benefits of the treatment
- Risks of the treatment
- Alternative therapies

Consent also implies that the patient understands the information and that the decision is voluntary.

FINANCIAL ISSUES

Medical ethics dictates that physicians should not exploit their patients financially. Most recently, physicians who work for managed care organizations may find that the needs of the patient may conflict with the patient's insurance company. Alternatively, the physician may have a financial incentive to avoid expensive tests or to create a barrier to hospitalization or consultants. In systems employing incentives, the physician should participate only if they are designed so that they foster good patient care. A useful way to assess the appropriateness of an incentive is to consider if the physician would be hesitant to disclose the relationship to the patient.

Fee splitting arrangements, such as arrangements in which physicians refer patients to facilities in which the physician has a financial interest, refer patients to other physicians who pay a referral fee, or prescribe medications for which the physician receives payment from a drug company are considered unethical. In general, relationships that influence a doctor to act in their own financial benefit rather than the patient's interests are considered unethical.

ADVANCED DIRECTIVES

The term advanced directives refers to provisions that a patient makes to direct their future health care in case their capacity to make decisions is diminished.

Studies show that outpatients are generally receptive to advanced planning, although the physician often needs to take the initiative in asking about preferences. Discussing advanced directives affords the opportunity to explore the patient's values and desires. Involving a family member or close friend is often helpful.

GENETICS

The sequencing of the human genome may present ethical dilemmas in the future. For example, will the primary care physician have to report a genetic finding that places a family member at risk, if the patient tested refuses? Will pregnancies be terminated because a fetus has a genetic disease that may occur later in life? Will cloning be an acceptable alternative for an infertile couple to have a child? These and other perhaps unimagined issues related to genetics will undoubtedly challenge the family physician in the future.

◆ KEY POINTS ◆

1. Clinical ethics is the discipline that examines and attempts to resolve the moral problems that arise in medicine.

2. Confidentiality may need to be breached to protect a third party from harm.

3. Informed consent involves the receipt and interpretation of information by patients to assist them in arriving at a decision, commonly involving a therapy or diagnostic procedure.

4. In general, relationships that influence a doctor to act in their own financial benefit rather than the patient's interests are considered unethical.

5. Discussing advanced directives affords the opportunity to explore the patient's values and desires.

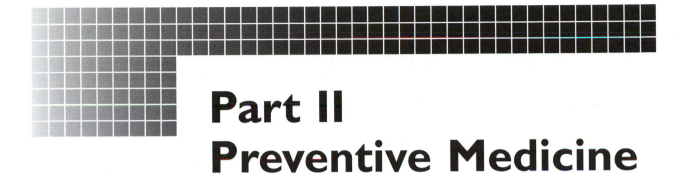

Part II
Preventive Medicine

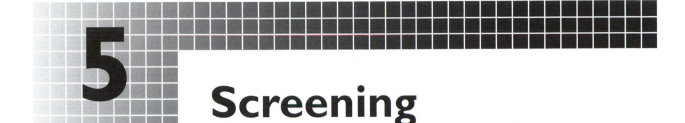

5 Screening

Preventive health care and screening for various diseases are part of routine medical care at all ages. Disease prevention can be primary, secondary, or tertiary. Primary prevention seeks to prevent a disease or condition from developing. An example of primary prevention is vaccination, where many infectious diseases are prevented by immunization. Secondary prevention involves early detection of disease to limit the effects of the disease. Tertiary prevention refers to rehabilitation as well as efforts to limit complications of the disease after the disease has developed.

Screening entails utilizing a test or standardized exam to identify patients who may require special intervention. Examples of screening tests are mammography and hemoccult testing of stool, for early detection of breast and colon cancers, respectively, with hopes of intervention leading to cure. Another example of screening is cholesterol or blood pressure testing in order to lower risks for future cardiovascular disease. Included within the context of primary and secondary prevention are screening and counseling for behaviors, such as smoking or substance abuse, that affect an individual's health.

CRITERIA FOR USE OF SCREENING TESTS

In order for a screening test to be of value for routine use in patient care several criteria should be met. First, the disease or condition screened for must be common and have a sufficient impact on an individual's health to justify the risks and costs associated with the testing. Second, effective prevention or treatment measures must be available for the condition and earlier detection must improve clinical outcomes. The screening and treatment benefits should outweigh any risks associated with testing and therapy. Finally, there must be a screening test that is readily available and accurate. The overall cost effectiveness of a screening program will be a factor in terms of insurers' and individuals' willingness to pay for the test or procedure. Availability and acceptability of the test impacts whether or not patients will actually undergo screening. For example, an individual may refuse sigmoidoscopy because he finds the procedure distasteful. Accuracy determines how many cases are missed or misdiagnosed as a result of the screening.

TEST CHARACTERISTICS

Screening tests should be accurate at detecting the intended disease or condition. Accuracy is a term that considers several different testing measures—namely, sensitivity, specificity, positive predictive value, and negative predictive value (Table 5–1). Sensitivity is a measure of the percentage of cases that a test is able to detect. Specificity measures the percentage of patients testing negative who do not have the disease. These test characteristics are factors in determining the value of screening tests. Desirable characteristics of screening tests include both a high sensitivity and specificity.

Combining disease prevalence with these test characteristics allows the clinician to look at the predictive values of a screening test. The positive predictive value is the percentage likelihood that a patient with a positive test actually has the disease and, conversely, a negative predictive value indicates that a person with a negative test is disease-free. Disease prevalence critically affects the predictive value, as shown by the following example of screening for a disease with a prevalence of 10% in 100,000 patients, using a test that is 95% sensitive and 95% specific. In this instance, the positive and negative predictive values for the test would be 68% and 99.4%, respectively (Table 5–2).

Thus, for every 9500 cases detected, an additional 4500 patients would have to undergo additional testing to determine that they were disease-free. However, a negative test is 99.4% assured of truly being disease-free. For diseases with a potentially fatal outcome and where effective treatments are available, this screening

would be acceptable. However, if the prevalence of the disease was 1% instead of 10%, the positive predictive value would fall to 16% and the vast majority of patients with positive results would actually be disease-free. The health care costs, risks of additional procedures, and patient anxiety may not justify use of this screening test in this instance if the disease prevalence and positive predictive value of the test are low.

CLINICAL IMPLEMENTATION OF SCREENING

For preventive health care measures to be effective, health care providers, patients, and society must all agree that screening and prevention are a priority in providing good health care. Conflicting recommendations by government organizations and professional societies have led to uncertainty on the part of physicians regarding both what the actual guidelines are and the effectiveness of the various screening tools. Reasons for these different recommendations include different methods of assessing evidence, different criteria for defining benefit, and different patient populations. In addition, professional interests may play a role. Some authorities may represent groups that treat high-risk individuals, giving them a different perspective or a financial stake in screening. Time constraints and lack of reimbursement for preventive health care are additional barriers to physicians offering screening tests to patients. It is important that primary care providers keep abreast of the current preventive health care recommendations and prioritize incorporating screening into their everyday practice. To effectively provide primary care to their patients, physicians need to educate their

TABLE 5–1

Determining Sensitivity and Specificity

	Disease present	Disease absent
Positive test	a	b
Negative test	c	d
Sensitivity	a/a + c	
Specificity	d/b + d	

TABLE 5–2

Calculating Predictive Values

	Total number of patients = 100,000			
	Disease present	Disease absent		
Positive test	9,500	4,500		
Negative test	500	85,500		
Sensitivity	9,500/9,500 + 500 = 95%	Positive predictive value	9,500/9,500 + 4,500 = 68%
Specificity	85,500/4,500 + 85,500 = 95%	Negative predictive value	85,500/500 + 85,500 = 99.4%

patients regarding preventive health care and the benefits of different screening tests, as well as healthful behaviors. Subsequent chapters will outline recommendations for health screening at different ages. These recommendations are largely based on recommendations by the United States Preventive Services Task Force, representing input from the various medical specialties, and utilize an evidence-based approach with analysis of disease prevalence, screening and treatment effectiveness, as well as overall cost effectiveness.

◆ KEY POINTS ◆

1. Primary, secondary, and tertiary preventive strategies can limit development and the effects of many diseases.

2. Criteria for use of screening tests include 1) that the disease is common and significantly affects individuals and society, 2) that effective treatments for the disease are available and 3) that the screening tests or procedures are accurate and reasonable in terms of cost, comfort and complications.

3. Characteristics to measure the accuracy of screening tests include sensitivity, specificity, and positive and negative predictive values.

4. Establishing clear standards for preventive health care, along with physician and patient education, may help in improving participation in many effective screening measures.

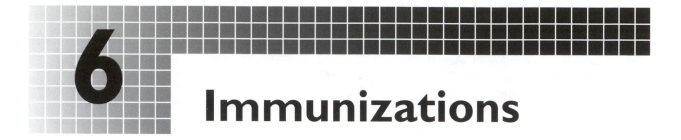

Immunizations

The implementation of routine childhood vaccinations is one of the most successful preventive medicine measures in modern day medicine. Infections causing significant morbidity and mortality were once common in children, but because of routine vaccination, are now rare and reportable diseases. For example, the number of reported cases of polio numbered 20,000 in 1954, but in 1994 there were no reported cases in the United States of polio due to the wild poliovirus. Invasive *H. influenzae* infection in children under the age of five has decreased by 95% since the introduction of the vaccine. Important considerations in deciding whether a vaccine is recommended for routine use are the disease prevalence, disease morbidity and mortality, economic costs to society, vaccine efficacy, and adverse reactions to the vaccine.

SPECIFIC IMMUNIZATIONS

Diphtheria Vaccine

In the 1940s, before vaccination, there were approximately 10,000 reported cases per year of diphtheria. The case fatality rate from diphtheria in unvaccinated individuals is 5% to 10%. In the postvaccination era, this is now a rare disease in the United States, with only two cases being reported in 1994. This vaccine is administered in combination with pertussis and tetanus vaccines in children, and with the tetanus vaccine in adults. Adverse reactions to the diphtheria-tetanus vaccination most commonly include a local inflammatory reaction,

less commonly an Arthrus-type reaction or peripheral neuropathy, and rarely an anaphylactic reaction.

Pertussis Vaccine

Before the introduction of the pertussis vaccine, there were 75,000 pertussis cases per year reported in the United States. This disease most commonly affected infants and caused pneumonia (22%), seizures (3%), encephalopathy (1%), or death (0.3%). Following the introduction of the vaccine, the number of pertussis infections has declined to approximately 4500 per year, and causes less severe disease in vaccinated individuals. Due to adverse reactions associated with the whole-cell vaccine, this vaccine has undergone detailed analysis of efficacy and adverse reactions. The efficacy of the whole-cell vaccine is 59–78% for preventing any disease (including cough), but 96–97% for preventing severe disease. Common adverse reactions to the whole-cell vaccine are local reactions, fever, irritability, and inconsolable crying. More severe and less common reactions include seizures (50/100,000 doses), hypotonic/hyporesponsive episodes (up to 290/100,000 doses), and possibly severe neurologic injury (6.8/1,000,000 doses). These severe reactions led to development of the currently used acellular pertussis vaccine, which has an efficacy of over 90% with fewer adverse reactions.

Tetanus Vaccine

Tetanus cases have decreased from over 600 cases per year prior to vaccination, to 51 cases per year in 1994.

The mortality rate for tetanus is 25%. The vaccine may be administered with diphtheria and pertussis vaccine or alone, and adverse reactions include primarily local reactions, but less commonly may cause Arthrus-type reactions, peripheral neuropathy, or rarely anaphylactic reactions.

Poliovirus Vaccine

Poliovirus infection causes acute neurologic symptoms of paresthesias and paralysis. Up to 1 in 250 affected individuals suffered permanent paralysis. The last reported case of a wild poliovirus infection was 1979. There have been approximately 8 cases per year of vaccine-related infection due to the live attenuated oral vaccine. As a result, as of January 2000, a complete conversion to use of the inactivated injectable form of the vaccine was recommended for the entire poliovirus vaccine series. Adverse reactions to the vaccine include primarily local reactions and in rare instances, allergic reactions may occur in those allergic to the antibiotics present in trace amounts in the vaccine (streptomycin, neomycin, polymyxin B).

Haemophilus Influenzae Vaccine

Haemophilus influenzae was formerly the most common cause for childhood meningitis and epiglottitis, causing significant morbidity and mortality. Since the introduction of the vaccine, the incidence of these invasive diseases has decreased by 95%. The vaccine is well tolerated, with the most common adverse reaction being local reactions of erythema and induration at the injection site.

Hepatitis B Vaccine

Hepatitis B is a viral infection associated with development of chronic liver disease in adults and children. Chronic infection occurs in up to 90% of neonatal infections, 30% of children infected between ages 1 and 5 years and in 2% to 6% of older children and adults. Although over 90% of infections occur in adults, children make up over one-third of those chronically infected. Chronic infection leads to increased risk for cirrhosis and hepatocellular carcinoma. Vaccination is effective in preventing up to 90% of neonatal infections, and when administered with immunoglobulin, prevents 95% of neonatal hepatitis B. Vaccine efficacy in older children and adults is reported to be 95%. Adverse reactions to the vaccine are generally mild and include pain at the injection site and a 1% to 6% incidence of low-grade fever. Uncommon or rare reactions include allergic reactions with anaphylaxis occurring in 1 in 600,000 doses.

Mumps, Measles, and Rubella Vaccine

Mumps is a childhood viral disease associated with orchitis, pancreatitis, myocarditis, and encephalitis. These complications are unusual, and death and long-term sequelae from this disease are rare. Measles is associated with significant sequelae including death. One to three patients per 1000 infections die as a result of respiratory and neurological complications. Rubella is associated with congenital anomalies in the children of infected women. These children are born with ophthalmologic, cardiac, and neurologic defects including mental retardation. The vaccines for these three illnesses have led to a 99% reduction in the incidence of infection. Once administered as a single vaccine dose, outbreaks of measles in the late 1990s led to recommendations for a second booster vaccine. This outbreak was thought to occur due to lack of vaccine administration along with a 5% vaccine failure rate when given as a single dose. Five to fifteen percent of vaccine recipients develop fever up to 103° Fahrenheit in the 6 to 12 days after vaccination. Other adverse vaccine reactions include thrombocytopenia in up to 5% of patients, transient arthropathy in adults receiving the vaccine, and allergic reactions. Patients with allergic reactions after the first dose should undergo allergy evaluation prior to administration of the second dose.

Pneumococcal Vaccine

Streptococcus pneumoniae is a bacterium that causes respiratory tract infections, bacteremia, and meningitis in both adults and children. In patients with severe disease associated with bacteremia, the mortality rate has been reported to be as high as 20% and up to 40% in the elderly. The efficacy of pneumococcal vaccine in adults is disputed and is reported to be between 60% and 92% in preventing invasive disease, with the lower efficacy occurring in immunocompromised patients who fail to develop an immune response. Children younger than age 5 are a higher risk group for invasive disease and do not respond to the 23-valent adult vaccine. Hence, a heptavalent vaccine was developed for use in children and has an efficacy of approximately 93% for preventing invasive disease. High-risk groups targeted for use of the adult vaccine include patients over age 65, and those with cardiac conditions, chronic respiratory

Recommended Childhood Immunization Schedule
United States, January – December 2001

Vaccines[1] are listed under routinely recommended ages. ⬚ Bars indicate range of recommended ages for immunization. Any dose not given at the recommended age should be given as a "catch-up" immunization at any subsequent visit when indicated and feasible. ⬭ Ovals indicate vaccines to be given if previously recommended doses were missed or given earlier than the recommended minimum age.

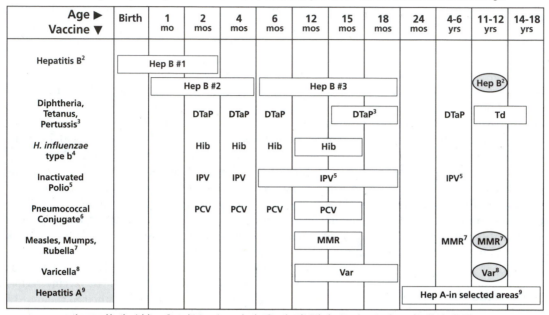

Age ▶ Vaccine ▼	Birth	1 mo	2 mos	4 mos	6 mos	12 mos	15 mos	18 mos	24 mos	4-6 yrs	11-12 yrs	14-18 yrs
Hepatitis B[2]		Hep B #1									Hep B[2]	
			Hep B #2			Hep B #3						
Diphtheria, Tetanus, Pertussis[3]			DTaP	DTaP	DTaP		DTaP[3]			DTaP	Td	
H. influenzae type b[4]			Hib	Hib	Hib	Hib						
Inactivated Polio[5]			IPV	IPV		IPV[5]				IPV[5]		
Pneumococcal Conjugate[6]			PCV	PCV	PCV	PCV						
Measles, Mumps, Rubella[7]						MMR				MMR[7]	MMR[7]	
Varicella[8]						Var					Var[8]	
Hepatitis A[9]									Hep A-in selected areas[9]			

Approved by the Advisory Committee on Immunization Practices (ACIP), the American Academy of Pediatrics (AAP), and the American Academy of Family Physicians (AAFP).

1. This schedule indicates the recommended ages for routine administration of currently licensed childhood vaccines, as of 11/1/00, for children through 18 years of age. Additional vaccines may be licensed and recommended during the year. Licensed combination vaccines may be used whenever any components of the combination are indicated and its other components are not contraindicated. Providers should consult the manufacturers' package inserts for detailed recommendations.

2. **Infants born to HBsAg-negative mothers** should receive the 1st dose of hepatitis B (Hep B) vaccine by age 2 months. The 2nd dose should be at least one month after the 1st dose. The 3rd dose should be administered at least 4 months after the 1st dose and at least 2 months after the 2nd dose, but not before 6 months of age for infants.

Infants born to HBsAg-positive mothers should receive hepatitis B vaccine and 0.5 mL hepatitis B immune globulin (HBIG) within 12 hours of birth at separate sites. The 2nd dose is recommended at 1-2 months of age and the 3rd dose at 6 months of age.

Infants born to mothers whose HBsAg status is unknown should receive hepatitis B vaccine within 12 hours of birth. Maternal blood should be drawn at the time of delivery to determine the mother's HBsAg status; if the HBsAg test is positive, the infant should receive HBIG as soon as possible (no later than 1 week of age).

All children and adolescents who have not been immunized against hepatitis B should begin the series during any visit. Special efforts should be made to immunize children who were born in or whose parents were born in areas of the world with moderate or high endemicity of hepatitis B virus infection.

3. The 4th dose of DTaP (diphtheria and tetanus toxoids and acellular pertussis vaccine) may be administered as early as 12 months of age, provided 6 months have elapsed since the 3rd dose and the child is unlikely to return at age 15-18 months. Td (tetanus and diphtheria toxoids) is recommended at 11-12 years of age if at least 5 years have elapsed since the last dose of DTP, DTaP or DT. Subsequent routine Td boosters are recommended every 10 years.

4. Three *Haemophilus influenzae* type b (Hib) conjugate vaccines are licensed for infant use. If PRP-OMP (PedvaxHIB® or ComVax® [Merck]) is administered at 2 and 4 months of age, a dose at 6 months is not required. Because clinical studies in infants have demonstrated that using some combination products may induce a lower immune response to the Hib vaccine component, DTaP/Hib combination products should not be used for primary immunization in infants at 2, 4 or 6 months of age, unless FDA-approved for these ages.

5. An all-IPV schedule is recommended for routine childhood polio vaccination in the United States. All children should receive four doses of IPV at 2 months, 4 months, 6-18 months, and 4-6 years of age. Oral polio vaccine (OPV) should be used only in selected circumstances. (See MMWR *Morb Mortal Wkly Rep* May 19, 2000/49(RR-5);1-22).

6. The heptavalent conjugate pneumococcal vaccine (PCV) is recommended for all children 2-23 months of age. It also is recommended for certain children 24-59 months of age. (See MMWR *Morb Mortal Wkly Rep* Oct. 6, 2000/49(RR-9);1-35).

7. The 2nd dose of measles, mumps, and rubella (MMR) vaccine is recommended routinely at 4-6 years of age but may be administered during any visit, provided at least 4 weeks have elapsed since receipt of the 1st dose and that both doses are administered beginning at or after 12 months of age. Those who have not previously received the second dose should complete the schedule by the 11-12 year old visit.

8. Varicella (Var) vaccine is recommended at any visit on or after the first birthday for susceptible children, i.e. those who lack a reliable history of chickenpox (as judged by a health care provider) and who have not been immunized. Susceptible persons 13 years of age or older should receive 2 doses, given at least 4 weeks apart.

9. Hepatitis A (Hep A) is shaded to indicate its recommended use in selected states and/or regions, and for certain high risk groups; consult your local public health authority. (See MMWR *Morb Mortal Wkly Rep* Oct. 1, 1999/48(RR-12); 1-37).

For additional information about the vaccines listed above, please visit the National Immunization Program Home Page at www.cdc.gov/nip or call the National Immunization Hotline at 800-232-2522 (English) or 800-232-0233 (Spanish).

Figure 6–1   Recommended Childhood Immunization schedule—United States, January–December 2001. Vaccines[1] are listed under routinely recommended ages. Bars indicate range of recommended ages for immunization. Any dose not given at the recommended age should be given as a "catch-up" immunization at any subsequent visit when indicated and feasible. Ovals indicate vaccines to be given if previously recommended doses were missed or given earlier than the recommended minimum age.
Source: *National Immunization Program Home Page* at www.cdc.gov/nip. Circulation 2001.

disease, asplenia, nephrotic syndrome or chronic renal disease, cirrhosis, and diabetes mellitus. In addition, the heptavalent vaccine is recommended for all children up to 2 years of age. These vaccines are well tolerated with local reactions as the primary adverse vaccine reaction.

Hepatitis A Vaccine

Hepatitis A is a viral infection that causes in children a mild self-limited illness in 30% of patients and is unrecognized in the majority of pediatric patients. Adults suffer gastroenteritis symptoms with an associated elevation in liver enzymes and jaundice, recovering with supportive care. There is no chronic form of this disease. Vaccination is recommended for individuals traveling to areas with high endemic rates of disease. The vaccine may be offered to children attending daycare to prevent infection and exposure of the family to this viral disease that is spread by the fecal-oral route. The vaccine has an efficacy of 94% to 100% and causes local reactions as the primary vaccine adverse reaction.

Influenza Vaccine

The influenza virus generally causes mild respiratory illness in young healthy patients, but in high-risk subgroups of older patients (over age 65), and those with cardiac disease, chronic respiratory illness, renal disease, diabetes mellitus, or cancer, it may lead to severe respiratory illness, pneumonia, and death. The vaccine must be administered annually due to the antigenic variation in the influenza viruses from year-to-year. The vaccine efficacy will vary based upon the accuracy of the antigen match for the particular year with an efficacy of approximately 70% to 80%. The vaccine is recommended in the high-risk groups mentioned above as well as those requiring chronic aspirin therapy (e.g., Kawasaki disease) to help prevent development of Reye's syndrome. Local reactions occur in up to 20% of patients, however serious reactions are rare. Those with severe egg allergies should forego vaccination and use chemoprophylaxis or undergo formal allergy evaluation.

Meningococcal Vaccine

Neisseria meningitidis causes invasive bacterial disease and meningitis in 1 per 100,000 population. Though not a common disease, meningococcal disease is associated with a very high morbidity and mortality and tends to occur in outbreaks. This vaccine is not routinely required, but is being offered and recommended by some groups for college students since it appears that dormitory living represents a potential risk factor for infection.

Varicella Vaccine

Varicella or chickenpox infection is generally a self-limited childhood infection that only rarely leads to more serious illness or death. Complications that can occur secondarily in those with chickenpox include pneumonia, hepatitis, encephalitis, bacterial superinfection, and Reye's syndrome. Serious or complicated illness is more common in adults. Recommendations for chickenpox vaccine differ among practitioners due to the uncertainty as to the duration of vaccine immunity. Experience to date suggests that immunity to the vaccine will last from 10 to 20 years. The vaccine has an 85% efficacy for preventing chickenpox and virtually 100% efficacy for preventing serious disease. The immune response to the vaccine is less in those over age 12, and in this group two doses one month apart are recommended in contrast to the single dose administered to children age 1 to 12 years. Adverse reactions to the vaccine include fever in up to 15% of recipients, local reactions in 20%, and 3% to 5% of recipients develop a varicella-like rash that contain virus and can be spread to others by direct contact with the lesions.

The schedule of recommended ages for routine administration of currently licensed childhood vaccines is shown in Figure 6–1.

◆ KEY POINTS ◆

1. The implementation of routine childhood vaccinations is one of the most successful preventive medicine measures in modern day medicine.

2. Important considerations in deciding whether a vaccine is recommended for routine use are the disease prevalence, disease morbidity and mortality, economic costs to society, vaccine efficacy, and adverse reactions to the vaccine.

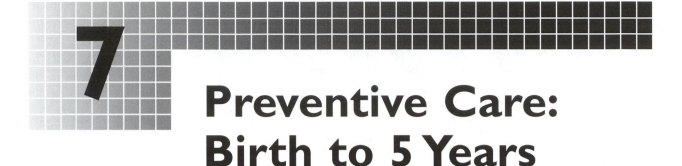

Preventive Care: Birth to 5 Years

The cornerstones of preventive health care include counseling patients about modifiable behaviors, providing vaccines to prevent infectious disease, and early identification of treatable or potentially treatable conditions. The American Academy of Pediatrics recommends a minimum of five visits from birth to 2 years of age and 3 visits for ages 2 to 6. Two factors that determine the content of these visits are the age-related disease prevalence and the psychosocial behaviors or development of that age group. For example, sexually transmitted diseases are more prevalent in the teens and twenties, related to increased risk taking behavior in this age group. Thus, any effort to screen and counsel for sexually transmitted diseases would focus on this age group during their preventive care visits.

During the ages between birth and five years, the most common causes for morbidity and mortality are perinatally acquired disease, congenital disease, sudden infant death syndrome, and accidents. Prior to the introduction of vaccines, infectious disease was also a significant contributor to infant and early childhood morbidity and mortality. The content of preventive health care in children in this age category involves physical examination and assessment of childhood development, provision of vaccines, screening for treatable congenital conditions, and, importantly, counseling about safety issues.

BIRTH

Preventive care for the newborn infant begins after delivery. All infants should receive ocular prophylaxis with erythromycin ointment or silver nitrate to prevent gonococcal and chlamydial conjunctivitis and Vitamin K to prevent hemorrhagic disease of the newborn. Prior to discharge, the infant commonly receives the first hepatitis B immunization and has blood taken to screen for hypothyroidism and phenylketonuria. Depending on the local laws and ethnicity of the child, additional screening tests may be recommended. Many states also require a hearing screening in the neonatal period.

Counseling parents during the hospitalization is an important part of the initial care. Topics to review include bathing, nutrition, and avoiding the prone position for sleep. Breast-feeding should be encouraged since it provides ideal nutrition and protects infants against common respiratory and gastrointestinal infections, decreases the incidence of allergic disease, and promotes mother-child bonding. If the mother elects not to breast feed, the child should receive iron-fortified formula. In addition, other safety issues to cover at this time are infant car seat use, inquiring about the presence of smoke detectors in the home, and advising that the hot water heater be set below 130° Fahrenheit. This may also be a teachable moment for parental smoking cessation when advising parents of the risks to the infant of passive smoke exposure.

ONE TO TWO WEEKS

The first follow-up visit is commonly scheduled at 1 to 2 weeks of age. This visit should reinforce previous counseling and assess the adjustment of the parents and infant to the home environment. Questions regarding infant care and inquiry into infant feeding and elimination patterns should be part of this visit. Review of the perinatal congenital screening laboratories and examination of the infant with a focus on presence of jaundice and weight are important. Newborns should regain their birthweight by 2 weeks of age. Intervention may be required for those with significant elevations in bilirubin levels. Those infants who did not receive hepatitis B vaccine during hospitalization should receive the first of this three-shot series.

ONE TO EIGHTEEN MONTHS

Visits during this period of time will coincide with vaccine administration, with one extra visit at approximately 9 months of age. During this time, in addition to physical examination, the focus of the visits is on addressing parental concerns, reviewing growth and development of the infant, and provision of vaccines. Counseling should also be provided regarding "childproofing" the home, and safety measures such as storage of hazardous or poisonous materials in a locked or out-of-reach cabinet, covering electric outlets and providing the parents with a phone number for poison control.

Growth (height, weight, head circumference) should be plotted on a growth chart in order to follow the growth of the individual child and to assure that the rate of growth is proceeding normally (Figure 7–1a, b, c, d). Generally a child should double their birth weight by 4 months and triple it by 1 year of age. Childhood development can be assessed through use of an instrument, such as the Denver Developmental Screening Tool, or by inquiring and observing behavior in verbal, motor and psychosocial skills of the child (Table 7–1). A lead and hemoglobin level is generally obtained at 9 to 15 months of age. Tuberculosis screening with an intradermal purified protein derivative (PPD) is provided at

12 to 15 months, is required by some preschools, and is recommended for all high-risk children. Fluoride supplementation of infants living in areas with inadequate fluoride in the water supply should begin at 6 months of age. Solid foods should usually be introduced at 4 to 6 months of age. Prevention of bottle caries should be addressed and dental care of newly erupting teeth should also be discussed. Most experts recommend that children be weaned from the bottle by age 12 months to reduce the risk of dental decay.

As the child develops, additional areas for parental counseling will include window and stair guards and gates to prevent falls; storage of firearms, matches and toxic substances in a locked or inaccessible place; and assuring that window shade cords do not pose a risk. Even as a passenger on a bicycle, the infant or toddler should be provided with a helmet to prevent injury. Use of sunscreens and prevention of excessive sun exposure and sunburns to prevent future risk of skin cancer should begin at the infant stage and be reinforced frequently.

TWO TO FIVE YEARS

During this interval, there are usually no vaccinations to administer until the five-year-old visit. Visits during this time are annual check-ups at which time the child will have a physical examination, including blood pressure measurement starting at age 3 years. Review of growth and development and reinforcement of safety measures are a focus of the visits. Prior to school entry, the child should have an assessment of vision and hearing. Tuberculosis screening (PPD) is required for entry into most preschools, schools, and daycare. The National Cholesterol Education Program recommends that children with a positive family history of premature coronary artery disease (<age 50 in men or <age 60 in women) or with parents with elevated cholesterol values undergo cholesterol screening beginning at age 2 years. A lead screening questionnaire can be used to determine which children in this age group need lead screening.

The 5-year visit is important to assess school "readiness." The average child should be able to name 4 to 5 colors, know his age, and draw a person with a head, body, arms, and legs. Parents should make sure their child knows his name, address, telephone, and how to deal with strangers.

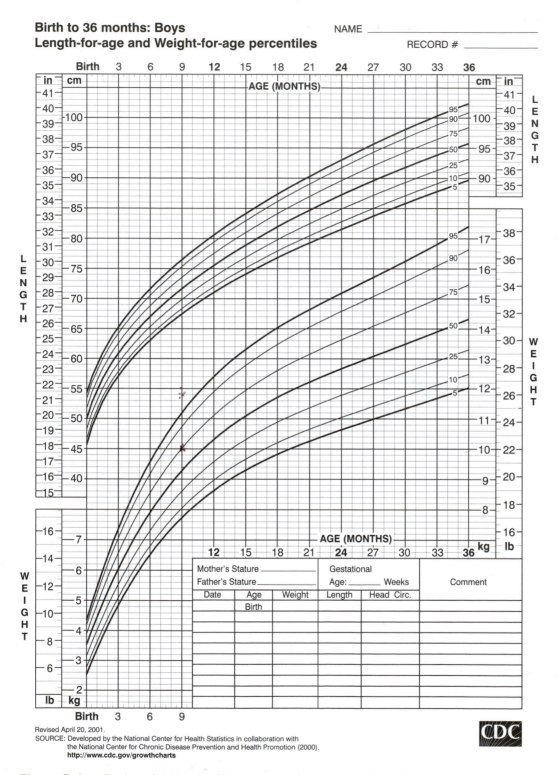

Revised April 20, 2001.
SOURCE: Developed by the National Center for Health Statistics in collaboration with
the National Center for Chronic Disease Prevention and Health Promotion (2000).
http://www.cdc.gov/growthcharts

Figure 7–1a   Birth to 36 Months: Boys—Length-for-age and Weight-for-age Percentiles.
Source: Developed by the National Center for Health Statistics in Collaboration with the National Center for
Chronic Disease Prevention and Health Promotion (2000).
http://www.cdc.gov/growthcharts

Birth to 36 months: Boys
Head circumference-for-age and
Weight-for-length percentiles

NAME _____

RECORD # _____

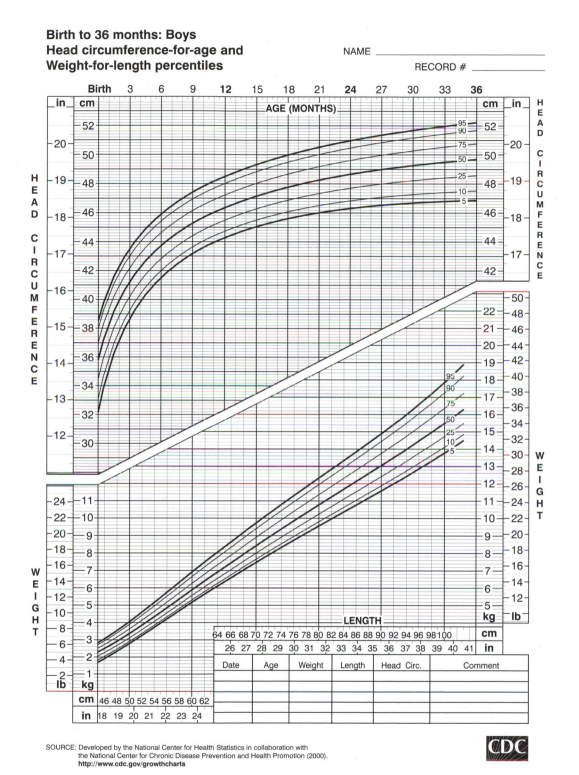

SOURCE: Developed by the National Center for Health Statistics in collaboration with
the National Center for Chronic Disease Prevention and Health Promotion (2000).
http://www.cdc.gov/growthcharts

Figure 7–1b   Birth to 36 Months: Boys—Head Circumference-for-age and Weight-for-length percentiles.
Source: Developed by the National Center for Health Statistics in Collaboration with the National Center for
Chronic Disease Prevention and Health Promotion (2000).
http://www.cdc.gov/growthcharts

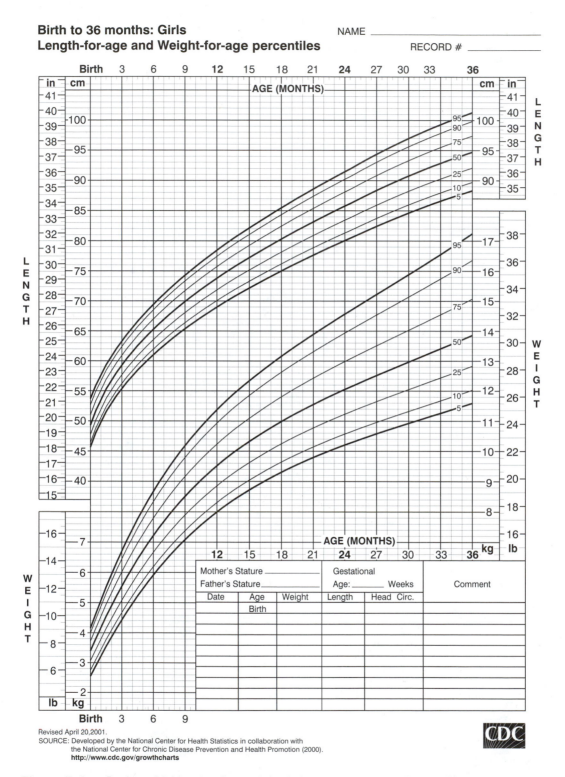

Figure 7–1c Birth to 36 Months: Girls—Length-for-age and Weight-for-age Percentiles.
Source: Developed by the National Center for Health Statistics in Collaboration with the National Center for Chronic Disease Prevention and Health Promotion (2000).
http://www.cdc.gov/growthcharts

**Birth to 36 months: Girls
Head circumference-for-age and
Weight-for-length percentiles**

NAME _____

RECORD # _____

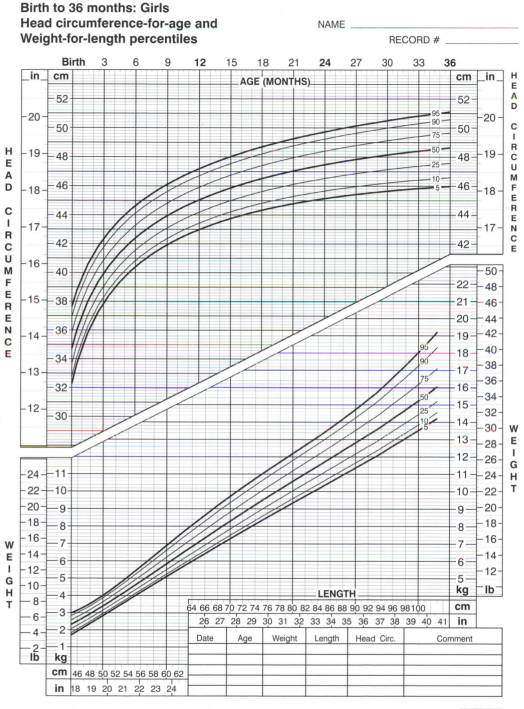

Figure 7–1d   Birth to 36 Months: Girls—Head circumference-for-age and Weight-for-length Percentiles.
Source: Developed by the National Center for Health Statistics in Collaboration with the National Center for
Chronic Disease Prevention and Health Promotion (2000).
http://www.cdc.gov/growthcharts

TABLE 7-1

Developmental Milestones

Age	Gross motor	Visual-motor/problem-solving	Language	Social/adaptive	Age
1 mo	Raises head slightly from prone, makes crawling movements	Birth: visually fixes 1 mo: has tight grasp, follows to midline	Alerts to sound	Regards face	1 mo
2 mo	Holds head in midline, lifts chest off table	No longer clenches fist tightly, follows object past midline	Smiles socially (after being stroked or talked to)	Recognizes parent	2 mo
3 mo	Supports on forearms in prone, holds head up steadily	Holds hands open at rest, follows in circular fashion, responds to visual threat	Coos (produces long vowel sounds in musical fashion)	Reaches for familiar people or objects, anticipates feeding	3 mo
4 mo	Rolls front to back, supports on wrists and shifts weight	Reaches with arms in unison, brings hands to midline	Laughs, orients to voice	Enjoys looking around environment	4 mo
5 mo	Rolls back to front, sits supported	Transfers objects	Says "ah-goo," razzes, orients to bell (localizes laterally)		5 mo
6 mo	Sits unsupported, puts feet in mouth in supine position	Unilateral reach, uses raking grasp	Babbles	Recognizes strangers	6 mo
7 mo	Creeps		Orients to bell (localized indirectly)		7 mo
8 mo	Comes to sit, crawls	Inspects objects	"Dada" indiscriminately	Fingerfeeds	8 mo
9 mo	Pivots when sitting, pulls to stand, cruises	Uses pincer grasp, probes with forefinger, holds bottle, throws objects	"Mama" indiscriminately, gestures, waves bye-bye, understands "no"	Starts to explore environment; plays gesture games (e.g., pat-a-cake)	9 mo
10 mo	Walks when led with both hands held	—	"Dada/mama" discriminately; orients to bell (directly)	—	10 mo
11 mo	Walks when led with one hand held	—	One word other than "dada/mama," follows 1-step command with gesture	—	11 mo
12 mo	Walks alone	Uses mature pincer grasp, releases voluntarily, marks paper with pencil	Uses two words other than "dada/mama," immature jargoning (runs several unintelligible words together)	Imitates actions, comes when called, cooperates with dressing	12 mo
13 mo	—	—	Uses three words	—	13 mo

Age	Personal/Social	Language	Fine Motor	Gross Motor
14mo	—	Follows 1-step command without gesture	—	—
15mo	15–18mo: uses spoon, uses cup independently	Uses 4–6 words	Scribbles in imitation, builds tower of 2 blocks in imitation	Creeps up stairs, walks backwards
17mo	—	Uses 7–20 words, points to 5 body parts, uses mature jargoning (includes intelligible words in jargoning)	—	—
18mo	Copies parent in tasks (sweeping, dusting) plays in company of other children	Uses 2-word combinations	Scribbles spontaneously, builds tower of 3 blocks, turns 2–3 pages at a time	Runs, throws objects from standing without falling
19mo		Knows 8 body parts		
21mo	Asks to have food and to go to toilet	Uses 50 words, 2-word sentences	Builds tower of 5 blocks	Squats in play, goes up steps
24mo	Parallel play	Uses pronouns (I, you, me) inappropriately, follows 2-step commands	Imitates stroke with pencil, builds tower of 7 blocks, turns pages one at a time, removes shoes, pants, etc.	Walks up and down steps without help
30mo	Tells first and last names when asked; gets self drink without help	Uses pronouns appropriately, understands concept of "I", repeats 2 digits forward	Holds pencil in adult fashion, performs horizontal and vertical strokes, unbuttons	Jumps with both feet off floor, throws ball overhand
3yr	Group play, shares toys, takes turns, plays well with others, knows full name, age, sex	Uses minimum 250 words, 3-word sentences; uses plurals, past tense; knows all pronouns; understands concept of "2"	Copies a circle, undresses completely, dresses partially, dries hands if reminded	Can alternate feet when going up steps, pedals tricycle
4yr	Tells "tall tales," plays cooperatively with a group of children	Knows colors, says song or poem from memory, asks questions	Copies a square, buttons clothing, dresses self completely, catches ball	Hops, skips, alternates feet going down steps
5yr	Plays competitive games, abides by rules, likes to help in household tasks	Prints first name, asks what a word means	Copies triangle, ties shoes, spreads with knife	Skips alternating feet, jumps over low obstacles

(Handwritten annotations: "1½ y/o" beside 18mo; "2 y/o" beside 24mo)

From Capute[5–7]. Rounded norms from Capute[8].

◆ KEY POINTS ◆

1. Preventive health care in children begins at birth.

2. In addition to provision of vaccinations and physical examinations, assessment of growth and development should be performed.

3. Counseling regarding infant and childcare along with safety measures is an important part of each health care visit.

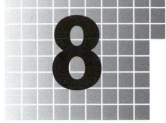

Preventive Care: 5 Years to 18 Years

Health care visits during this time generally occur episodically in association with illness or preparticipation clearance for sporting activities. When children change schools or advance from elementary to middle school or enter high school, they frequently are required to obtain physical examinations prior to entry. Thus, routine health care measures and counseling often need to be incorporated into visits for illness or preparticipation exams.

The leading causes for morbidity and mortality in this age category are accidents, homicide, and suicide. During adolescence, increased risk taking behavior and experimentation frequently leads to use of cigarettes or other substances and high-risk sexual activities. In addition to the physical examination, review of immunization status, growth and development and counseling are important to include with these health care visits (Table 8–1).

5–6 YEARS

The health care visit at this age may be the last required visit until the child enters junior high school or needs a preparticipation sports examination. Accidents continue to be the leading cause for morbidity and mortality at this age. In addition to reviewing the past medical history, including growth and development, preventive services should focus upon updating any necessary vaccinations and providing counseling and anticipatory guidance. For children with chronic diseases, such as asthma, pneumococcal vaccine and annual influenza vaccination is recommended. For children who have not had chickenpox, the varicella vaccine can be offered.

The physical examination should include blood pressure measurement, vision testing and hearing screening. Screening for tuberculosis should be provided to those at risk such as children living in poverty, residing in areas where tuberculosis is prevalent, and those with history of tuberculosis exposure. Lipid screening should be encouraged in children with family history of premature coronary artery disease or with parents with cholesterol over 240 mg/dl. Routine urinalysis is no longer recommended.

Counseling and anticipatory guidance are an important part of health care visits during childhood. Safety issues to discuss include the routine use of seatbelts and bicycle helmets, firearm safety, safe storage of toxic substances (including matches and lighters) and rules regarding encounters with strangers. Parents should be encouraged to provide good role modeling and a healthy environment that is smoke-free, includes a healthy diet and incorporates exercise as part of the family routine. Protection from excess sun exposure should be encouraged for the entire family. Regular teeth brushing, flossing and visits to the dentist should be encouraged. Television viewing should be limited, reading encouraged and exposure to violence monitored. The child should be encouraged to participate in age-appropriate activities and praised liberally for their positive actions.

7–12 YEARS

The child may have no routinely scheduled health care visits during this age range. Preventive care and

TABLE 8–1

Preventive Care Ages 5 Years to 18 Years

Ages	Morbidity and Mortality	Testing/Vaccine	Counseling
5–6	Accidents	Blood pressure Vision Hearing Tuberculosis (high risk) Lipids (high risk) MMR IPV DPT Pneumococcal[a] Influenza[a] Varicella[b]	Seatbelts Bicycle helmets Firearms Water safety Matches/Poisons Exposure to violence Dental care Exercise Sun exposure
7–12	Accidents	Blood pressure Scoliosis Lipids (high risk) Tuberculosis (high risk) Hepatitis B MMR Pneumococcal[a] Influenza[a] Varicella[b]	Seatbelts Bicycle helmets Firearms Water safety Matches/Poisons Exposure to violence Sun exposure Dental care Exercise Diet Tobacco/Drugs/Alcohol
13–18	Accidents Homicide Suicide	Blood pressure Scoliosis Lipids (high risk) Tuberculosis (high risk) STD screen[c] Pap smear[c] DT Hepatitis B Pneumococcal[a] Influenza[a] Varicella[b]	Seatbelts Bicycle helmets Firearms Water safety Violence Sun exposure Dental care Exercise Diet Tobacco/Drugs/Alcohol Sexuality Mental health

[a]at-risk individuals
[b]offer in absence of prior disease
[c]if sexually active

counseling during this time may need to be incorporated into sick visits or preparticipation examinations. The physical examination should include blood pressure measurement, assessment of growth and sexual development, and scoliosis screening. Scoliosis screening can be performed by having the child assume a diving position with the hands together and the trunk forward flexed. Assymetry of the ribcage along the spine may be indicative of an abnormality. Immunization status should be reviewed and updated to ensure that the child is current with regards to MMR and hepatitis B vaccines. Pneumococcal vaccination and annual influenza shots should be administered to at-risk children. Lipid screening can be offered in children with a strong family history of atherosclerosis. Vision and hearing screening should be performed if the history or physical examination suggest concerns about vision or hearing.

Counseling and anticipatory guidance should continue to emphasize accident prevention. Seatbelt and bicycle helmet use should be reinforced. The physician should remind parents about safe storage of poisons, matches and lighters, and firearms. Water safety along with encouraging the child to learn to swim can be discussed during the visit. Parents and their children should be educated regarding the importance of avoiding sunburns as well as use of sunscreens and protective clothing in order to lower future risk for skin cancer. Additional questions to assess violence exposure, mood, potential for engaging in high-risk behaviors should be incorporated into the visit. This portion of the interaction is best performed without the parents in the examination room. Reinforcement of healthful behaviors regarding exercise, sleep, diet and abstinence from sexual activity, tobacco, drugs and alcohol are important messages for the child to receive from the physician and his or her parents. Encouraging the parents to discuss these topics with their children is important, as is role modeling of the positive behaviors desired in the child.

13–18 YEARS

Often when the child changes schools, transitioning from junior high school to high school, they may be required to have a physical examination. In addition to eliciting the medical history, assessment of growth and development and immunization status should be performed. The physical examination should include blood pressure measurement, assessment of growth and development (including sexual maturity), and scoliosis

screening, in addition to the general physical examination. For those with visual or hearing complaints, screening should be performed. A tetanus booster will be necessary between the ages of 14 and 16 years. For those individuals not current on any vaccine or who have not had chickenpox, vaccination should be offered.

Accidents continue to be the leading cause of death in the adolescent population. Other causes that gain increasing importance as the child enters adolescence are homicides and suicides. In addition, increased risk taking behavior occurs during this period leading to experimentation with tobacco, drugs, alcohol and sexual activities. Thus, counseling during this age should include not only emphasis on accident prevention but should include inquiries into these other high-risk behaviors. For example, history of abuse, access to weapons, drug use and exposure to violence are risk factors for the adolescent's participation in violent activities. The incidence of depression increases throughout adolescence to approximately 10% at age 18. Over half of adolescent girls and nearly three-quarters of adolescent boys will have sexual intercourse before they are 18 years of age. Thus, to have an impact on these common issues related to the adolescent period, identification of at-risk individuals, encouraging dialog on these matters between adolescent and parent, and referring those in need of further therapy may be beneficial. In those individuals who are experimenting with alcohol, cigarettes, or other substances, discussion of the risks associated with continued use of the substances should be part of the counseling. In addition, counseling adolescents about abstinence from sexual activity, birth control, sexually transmitted diseases, and about responsible sexual activity is important. For sexually active individuals, examination and screening for sexually transmitted diseases is also recommended. Sexually active women should have a Pap smear performed annually.

◆ KEY POINTS ◆

1. Accidents are a major cause for morbidity and mortality during childhood.
2. During adolescence, accidents, homicides and suicides are leading causes for morbidity and mortality.
3. In addition to accident prevention, counseling should be provided regarding risks associated with substance abuse and sexual activity.

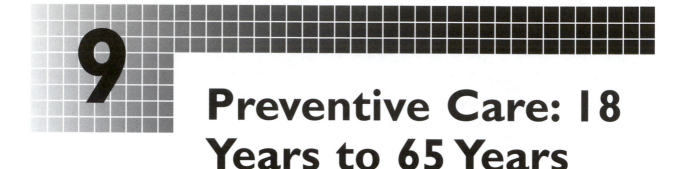

Preventive Care: 18 Years to 65 Years

The focus of preventive care changes as individuals age, reflecting the changes in disease prevalence across different ages. In addition to primary prevention, secondary prevention to prevent or limit future disease is important. For example, hypertension is a significant risk factor for heart disease and stroke. The consequences of hypertension may not be seen for years after a person develops high blood pressure. Thus, blood pressure evaluation and treatment is a preventive measure for future disease that may not manifest until the patient is 70 years of age or beyond.

18 TO 40 YEARS

The most common causes for death in the young adult group are accidents, homicides, and suicides. In addition, diseases that increase in prevalence and contribute to morbidity and mortality in this age range include HIV infection, heart disease, and some forms of cancer. Other conditions and habits that may be acquired at this time may influence risk for future disease. For example, promiscuity may result in sexually transmitted diseases, including HIV. Smoking may lead to a lifelong habit and increased risk for stroke, heart disease, and lung disease. Alcohol and drug abuse may place the individual at risk for hepatitis, liver disease, and accidents or injuries.

Many patients will begin receiving regular preventive care visits after age 30. There is debate as to the value of routine visits in this age group. If patients are not coming to the office for preventive care, then when they are in the office for other reasons, preventive care issues need to be addressed. For example, when a woman comes for an annual Pap smear, she may be instructed to come in fasting in order to check a lipid profile. At each visit, height, weight, and blood pressure can be checked and any issues regarding blood pressure or weight elevation can be addressed. Those presenting with an acute injury may be reminded about injury prevention measures, such as helmet and seatbelt use. Inquiring about domestic violence is important for women seen for acute injuries.

Past medical history may indicate need for vaccination update (e.g., hepatitis B, MMR) or administration. Patients with medical problems such as diabetes or asthma should receive pneumococcal and influenza vaccines. Those who have never had chickenpox may wish to consider the varicella vaccine. In addition to reviewing the past medical history, family history and social history will provide information that may lead to counseling or screening measures. For example, individuals with a family history of premature coronary artery disease or hyperlipidemia should be screened for hyperlipidemia. Patients with a family history of skin cancer and those with fair skin should be counseled about limiting sun exposure. Individuals with a history of substance abuse or smoking should be counseled about the potential consequences associated with these behaviors. Sexually active individuals require counseling about contraception and sexually transmitted disease prevention. Those with firearms should be counseled about their safe storage. Women should be counseled about adequate calcium intake and supplemented if needed and those who desire pregnancy can be counseled about supplementation of folate to prevent birth defects. Patients should be reminded about good dental care and the importance of regular dental visits.

In addition to the annual Pap smear for women, other routine recommended screening measures in this age group include a baseline mammogram for women between the ages of 35 and 40 years, cholesterol screening in men age 35 and older, and periodic screening of blood pressure for men and women over the age of 21 years.

40 TO 65 YEARS

Many physicians recommend starting annual preventive care visits at age 40 years. Screening for cardiovascular risk factors and malignancy become of greater concern as individuals age. Heart disease is the leading cause of death in the United States and is more prevalent in patients over 40 years of age. The prevalence of many different forms of cancer also increase in older populations, making cancer one of the common causes of morbidity and mortality in persons over age 40.

Identification and, if possible, treatment of risk factors for various diseases is a focus of routine health care visits. For some diseases there are no recommendations to screen for the actual disease, but there are recommendations to screen for risk factors. For example, routine screening for heart disease is not recommended, but screening for cardiac risk factors is recommended. Risk factors for heart disease include modifiable factors such as smoking, hypertension, diabetes mellitus, obesity, and hyperlipidemia. For other diseases, such as osteoporosis, screening is recommended only for those with risk factors. Some non-modifiable risk factors for osteoporosis are white race, slight build, and family history of osteoporosis. Modifiable risk factors for osteoporosis include smoking, menopause, sedentary lifestyle, low calcium intake, and high alcohol and coffee consumption. For some diseases, such as breast, cervical, colon, and prostate cancer, screening is recommended for all patients of a certain

age for early disease detection. For other cancers, such as lung, oral, and skin cancers no specific recommendations are made regarding disease detection, but counseling regarding risk factor modification may be beneficial. For example, smoking cessation is advised to prevent lung and oral cancers, and limiting sun exposure to prevent skin cancers.

Blood pressure should be checked every 1 to 2 years to screen for hypertension. Cholesterol screening is recommended in men every five years beginning at age thirty-five years and women every five years beginning at age 45 years. Assessment of substance use can be addressed during the history taking and any concerns should prompt counseling regarding the associated risks. Measurement of height and weight can be performed along with the vital signs and along with a dietary history can screen for obesity as well as risk for osteoporosis. Diabetes screening is recommended with a fasting glucose every 3 years beginning at age 45 years.

Cancer screening assumes a greater role in preventive care after age 40. Cancer screening in women continues to include annual Pap smears and annual mammograms beginning at age 40. There are no recommendations for ovarian or uterine cancer screening. For men, annual prostate exam and prostate-specific antigen testing should begin at age 40 in African-Americans and those with a family history of prostate cancer. In lower risk individuals, prostate cancer screening should begin at age 50. For both men and women, colon cancer screening with annual fecal occult blood testing and sigmoidoscopy every 3 to 5 years is recommended beginning at age 50. In patients with a first degree relative with colon cancer, colonoscopy should be performed every 5 to 10 years beginning at age 40. There are no formal recommendations for routine screening for lung, skin, or oral cancers. Counseling to perform self-exam for testicular and breast cancer may be beneficial.

Immunizations should be updated. During this age, the only routine vaccination is a tetanus booster, which should be provided every 10 years. In patients with underlying medical diseases, such as lung disease, heart disease or diabetes, pneumococcal and influenza vaccines should be considered. Patients at risk, because of occupation or travel, can be provided hepatitis A or B vaccines.

Reinforcement of other healthy behavioral measures should also be incorporated into the visit. These discussions can include topics such as seatbelt use, bicycle helmet use, and firearm and water safety. Healthful eating and exercise should be encouraged. Prevention of unintended pregnancies and sexually transmitted diseases is still an issue that should be discussed with many patients in this age group.

◆ **KEY POINTS** ◆

1. The most common causes for death in adults age 18 to 40 years are accidents, homicides, and suicides.

2. Screening for cardiovascular risk factors and malignancy become a focus of health care visits for individuals over age 40.

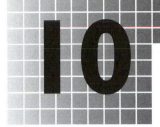

Preventive Care: 65 Years and Older

With increasing age, the effects of years of behaviors and accumulated medical disease result in different states of physiologic health for individuals of the same chronological age. For example, some individuals in their 60s and 70s are debilitated and reside in nursing facilities, while others in their eighties and nineties remain fully independent. The expected lifespan of healthy individuals at 65 is approximately fifteen years. However, the expected lifespan of patients with significant underlying medical conditions, such as severe chronic obstructive pulmonary disease, cancer, or heart disease may be considerably less. The different tests and preventive strategies need to be tailored to individuals' health status and their personal preferences. For example, many patients in their 80s and 90s would no longer consider undergoing aggressive treatments, such as major abdominal or heart surgery and may no longer wish to be screened for diseases that would require such treatment. Involving the patients and the families in the decision about the overall approach to the patient's care can help in deciding what is appropriate for each patient.

The most common causes for morbidity and mortality in the adult over age 65 are cardiovascular disease, cancers, and lung disease. Cardiovascular disease is the leading cause of death in the United States and is more prevalent with increasing age. The prevalence of many different forms of cancer is also increased in older populations. Chronic obstructive pulmonary disease is a smoking related disease with significant morbidity and mortality amongst the elderly. Pulmonary infections in older adults have a higher morbidity and mortality rate than in younger individuals.

CLINICAL MANIFESTATIONS

Most physicians recommend annual preventive care visits in the geriatric age group. In addition to recommendations common to all age groups, the visits should focus on functional issues. For example, falls are a significant cause of injury, and immobility a common cause of decline in function and loss of independence. Thus issues surrounding fall prevention should be incorporated into preventive care discussions.

Reviewing medications is important. Although the elderly comprise 12% of the population, they receive 32% of dispensed medications. Each year, an elderly individual receives an estimated 17 to 20 drugs. Age-related physiologic changes and drug interactions make the elderly adult more susceptible to an adverse reaction. Each visit should afford the opportunity to review diagnoses and the need for medications.

The driving ability of older adults, especially the frail elderly, needs review. Visual problems, hearing difficulty, and cognitive impairment generally occur more frequently in the geriatric population and may compromise driving ability. If there are concerns about driving safety, referral for testing may be warranted. Finally, discussion of the patient's desires for future care should be solicited. The patient should be advised to develop advance directives, assign a health care power of attorney and discuss in advance their wishes for future care.

Blood pressure should be checked every year to screen for hypertension. Orthostatic blood pressure measurements should be checked when considering the use of antihypertensive medications and for those with gait instability. Cholesterol screening is recommended in men and women every five years depending upon the functional status of the patient and the expected longevity. In patients with coronary artery disease, treating hyperlipidemia is of benefit. Measurement of height, weight, and vital signs, along with a dietary history can screen for obesity and malnutrition. Counseling to promote a healthy diet including appropriate amounts of calories, fat, vitamins, and fiber is important. All patients with risk factors for osteoporosis should be counseled about calcium supplementation and weight-bearing exercise. Some groups recommend routine osteoporosis screening for all postmenopausal women and other high-risk groups (chapter 46). Diabetes screening is recommended with a fasting glucose every 3 years. Many clinicians routinely screen for thyroid disease, though no formal recommendations support this at the present time. Routine dental care should not be overlooked.

Substance abuse is a common problem amongst geriatric patients and assessment of substance use should be addressed during history taking. About 10% of patients over 65 have problems with alcohol. Smoking is also an important issue and the benefits of smoking cessation even after years of smoking are still encouraging. If there are concerns about cognition or memory, additional history from family members and screening for dementia with a Mini Mental Status Examination is indicated. Depression is also common in the elderly population and men over age 65 have the highest rate of completed suicide attempts. Screening for mental health and depression can be performed through the patient interview or with use of a screening instrument such as the Yesavage Geriatric Depression Scale. If questions remain regarding a patient's mental functioning, then referral for formal neuropsychiatric testing may be helpful.

CANCER SCREENING

Cancer screening continues to be a major focus of health screening in the geriatric population, but is tempered to some degree by the presence of comorbid disease, the patient's past screening history, and the patient's wishes for continued screening. Cancer screening in women includes annual Pap smears and annual mammograms. Although women with significant comorbid disease and a shortened life expectancy may not benefit from continued breast cancer screening, healthy women who desire mammography should continue to receive screening indefinitely. Women who have had normal prior Pap smears and three consecutive normal results may be given the option of discontinuing cervical cancer screening. There are no recommendations to perform routine ovarian or uterine cancer screening. For men, annual prostate exam and prostate specific antigen testing should be limited to men with a life expectancy of 10 years or more. Colon cancer screening should continue after the age of 65 years. There is no clear-cut age at which to discontinue colon cancer screening. There are no formal recommendations for routine lung, skin, or oral cancers.

IMMUNIZATIONS

Tetanus immunization should be updated every 10 years. All patients over age 65 years should receive pneumococcal and influenza vaccines. Influenza vaccines are administered annually. High-risk individuals are often provided pneumococcal boosters every 5 to 7 years. Tuberculosis screening is routinely recommended for all patients residing in long-term care facilities and others at high risk. Patients at risk because of travel can be provided hepatitis A or B vaccines.

SAFETY ASSESSMENT

Assessment of vision and hearing may be helpful in detecting a correctable deficit that may lead to improved function. Watching the patient walk down the hallway may give clues to neurologic disease or need for assistant devices. Along with assessment of vision and gait, an environmental assessment and education of the family should be included to help with fall prevention. The walkways should be uncluttered, well lit and free of throw rugs. Reinforcement of healthy behavioral measures should also be incorporated into the visit. These discussions can include topics such as seatbelt use, bicycle helmet use, and firearm and water safety.

Healthful eating and exercise should be encouraged. Exercise may be particularly beneficial in the elderly by decreasing fall risk, improving cardiovascular status and mood, and providing some protection against osteoporosis.

◆ KEY POINTS ◆

1. The most common causes for death in adults over age 65 years are cardiovascular disease and cancer.

2. In addition to recommendations common to all age groups, increasing focus in geriatric preventive care on functional issues and future care should be incorporated into the visits.

3. Substance abuse is a common problem amongst geriatric patients.

4. Along with assessment of vision and gait, an environmental assessment and education of the family should be included to help with fall prevention.

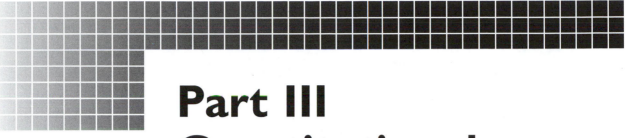

Part III
Constitutional Complaints

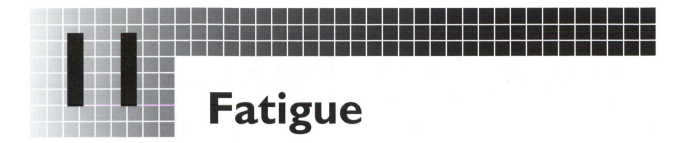

Fatigue

Fatigue is defined as the subjective complaint of tiredness or diminished energy level to the point of interfering with normal or usual activities. It is one of the top ten chief complaints leading to primary care office visits, present in up to 20% of patients presenting to primary care physicians. It is a constitutional symptom with many etiologies, leading to multiple diagnoses, labwork, and repeat office visits. Thus, it is important to narrow down the vast differential diagnosis in which organic causes comprise the minority of cases.

PATHOPHYSIOLOGY

The exact pathophysiology of fatigue is ill defined and will vary depending upon the underlying cause. For example, fatigue associated with psychiatric conditions is part of the symptom complex for many of these diseases and is likely psychogenic in origin. Fatigue associated with conditions such as congestive heart failure, chronic obstructive pulmonary disease, and metabolic abnormalities may be due to altered oxygen and nutrient delivery peripherally. Fatigue associated with inflammatory conditions, such as connective tissue diseases and infectious diseases, may be due to factors released as part of the inflammatory response.

CLINICAL MANIFESTATIONS

The history is crucial in differentiating a patient's source of fatigue. Characterizing the patient's complaint in terms of time course, exacerbating and alleviating factors, stressors, variability in symptoms, and associated symptoms can help in narrowing the potential causes for the fatigue and direct the initial work-up. Pre-existing medical conditions and medication use should be noted. Characteristic features of both psychogenic and organic disease are presented below.

Psychogenic Etiology

Fatigue that has been present for greater than 6 months and that fluctuates in its severity is more likely to be functional. The patient may have identifiable stressors, a stressful and non-supportive family structure, or a primary mood disturbance that points towards psychogenic fatigue. Frequently patients with psychological disease will have disturbance of their sleep with either insomnia or early morning awakening. With psychiatric causes, the fatigue is frequently worse in the morning and activity may alleviate the symptoms. The patient may have multiple and non-specific complaints along with a normal physical examination.

Physiologic Fatigue

Physiologic fatigue results from situations that would cause most people to be fatigued, such as not getting enough sleep. Physiologic fatigue is common in mothers of newborns, individuals who do shift work, athletes who overtrain, and in third-year medical students.

Organic Disease Etiology

In contrast to psychogenic fatigue, fatigue from organic causes will often present more abruptly and show a progressive course. Identifiable stressors are often absent and the family structure may be supportive. Sleep disturbance may be present, but is often related to the underlying disease process. A reactive or secondary depression may result from the patient recognizing that something is wrong. The fatigue will be noted to be less in the morning and worsened with activity. The patient may have fewer and more specific associated symptoms and the physical examination may suggest potential underlying causes.

Physical Examination

In patients presenting with a complaint of fatigue, a complete physical examination should be performed in an attempt to determine the etiology. The general appearance and vital signs of the patient should be noted. A patient with fatigue from physical illness may look pale and sickly with slumping posture and a sagging face. The depressed patient with fatigue may have a characteristic facial expression. Pallor of the skin may suggest anemia, whereas darkening of the skin may point towards Addison's disease as a potential cause. The thyroid gland should be palpated and signs of hyper- and hypothyroidism noted. Careful examination of all lymph nodes is essential along with checking the individual's joints for signs of inflammation. Heart and lung examination may reveal the presence of murmurs, gallops, wheezing, or rales suggesting a cardiopulmonary etiology. Stigmata of alcohol or drug abuse should also be noted. In addition to the complete physical exam, a thorough neurologic exam may identify neuromuscular disease as the cause.

BOX 11–1

Common Conditions Leading to Fatigue, by System and Process

- *Psychogenic:* depression, anxiety, adjustment reactions, situational life stress, sexual dysfunction, physical/sexual abuse, occupational stress, and professional burnout
- *Endocrine:* DM, hypothyroidism, hyperparathyroidism, hypopituitarism, Addison's disease, electrolyte disorders, malnutrition
- *Hematologic:* anemia, lymphoma, and leukemia
- *Renal:* ARF, CRF
- *Liver:* hepatitis, cirrhosis
- *Immunologic/connective tissue:* AIDS or AIDS-related complex, sarcoid, MCTD, polymyalgia rheumatica
- *Neuromuscular:* upper/lower motor neuron disease from stroke, neoplasm, demyelination, ALS, poliomyelitis, disk herniation, myasthenia gravis, muscular dystrophies
- *Pulmonary:* infectious states (TB, pneumonia), COPD, sleep apnea
- *Cardiovascular:* CHF, cardiomyopathy, valvular heart disease
- *Reproductive:* pregnancy
- *Iatrogenic:* medications, alcoholism, drug abuse

DIFFERENTIAL DIAGNOSIS

The differential diagnosis for fatigue is extensive and includes psychiatric, infectious, connective tissue, endocrine, neurologic, oncologic, and cardiopulmonary causes (Box 11–1). By far the most common category of diagnosis in fatigued patients is psychiatric disease, which occurs in 60% to 80% of patients with chronic fatigue. Depression accounts for the majority of cases with a psychiatric cause. Medical causes account for up to 8% of cases. The leading physical causes of fatigue are infections, metabolic disorders, and medications. Of the remainder, 4% meet criteria for chronic fatigue syn-

drome, a disease of unknown etiology often attributed to a persistent mononucleosis infection from the Epstein-Barr virus (Box 11–2). Despite exhaustive work-up, many patients with fatigue remain undiagnosed.

DIAGNOSTIC EVALUATION

The history and physical examination may help in determining the likelihood of an organic versus a psychiatric etiology. In those patients with characteristics suggesting an organic cause, further evaluation should be directed at the suspected underlying cause. For example, in patients with suspected hyperparathyroidism, an elevated serum calcium and parathyroid hormone might confirm the diagnosis.

In patients with suspected organic disease, but without any apparent primary disease, screening labo-

BOX 11–2

Diagnostic Criteria for Chronic Fatigue Syndrome

The diagnosis is established by fulfilling both major criteria plus 6 or more of the minor criteria plus 2 or more of the physical criteria, or 8 or more of the 11 minor symptom criteria.

Major Criteria

1. New onset of persistent or relapsing fatigue not previously present, sufficient to reduce daily activity by 50% or more, lasting at least 6 weeks

2. Exclusion of other conditions which may produce similar symptoms (see Box 11–1)

Minor Criteria

1. Mild fever (37.5–38.6°C) or chills

2. Sore throat

3. Painful cervical or axillary lymph nodes

4. Unexplained generalized muscle weakness

5. Muscle discomfort or myalgias

6. Prolonged (>24 hours) generalized fatigue after previously tolerated exercise

7. Generalized headaches unlike previous cephalalgia

8. Migratory arthralgias without joint swelling or redness

9. Neuropsychiatric complaints, i.e., photophobia, scotomata, forgetfulness, irritability, confusion, inability to concentrate, difficulty in thinking, depression

10. Sleep disturbances

11. Onset of main symptom complex in hours or a few days

Physical Criteria

A physician must document these on at least 2 occasions, at least 1 month apart.

1. Low grade fever

2. Nonexudative pharyngitis

3. Palpable or tender anterior or posterior cervical or axillary nodes (<2 cm in diameter)

ratory tests are recommended. Recommended laboratory screening tests include a complete blood count, erythrocyte sedimentation rate, comprehensive metabolic profile, and thyroid function tests. Pregnancy testing should be considered in females of childbearing age and HIV testing for individuals at risk for this disease. A drug screen can occasionally be productive. Additional laboratory or imaging tests should be ordered based upon findings in the history and physical examination. Examples of tests that are occasionally helpful are a chest x-ray to look for adenopathy, occult CHF, and primary lung tumors or metastatic disease. An EKG may detect a silent infarction or ischemia. In patients at risk, Lyme titers and tuberculosis skin testing might be of help.

TREATMENT

Psychiatric evaluation and treatment may be necessary for patients with persistent fatigue due to anxiety or depression. For patients with an identified medical condition, treatment of the underlying process is the recommended treatment for the fatigue. There is no specific therapy for chronic fatigue syndrome, though data suggest that patients with chronic fatigue syndrome may benefit from psychotherapy and exercise. Additional therapy is targeted towards associated symptoms (e.g., NSAIDs for myalgias).

In individuals with persistent fatigue of unknown causes, therapy may consist of an empirical trial of antidepressants or withdrawal of a medication known to cause fatigue. Some patients also benefit from moderate levels of exercise and reducing the stresses in their life.

◆ KEY POINTS ◆

1. Fatigue occurs in up to 20% of patients seeking primary care.

2. The majority of cases of fatigue have a psychiatric cause.

3. The history can help in determining a psychiatric versus organic cause and thus aid in directing the evaluation of fatigue.

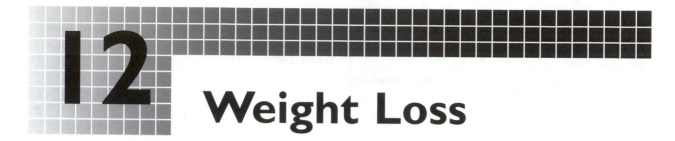

Weight Loss

Unintended weight loss is a worrisome finding that may indicate the presence of a significant underlying illness. A weight loss greater than 5% of total body weight over a period of six months is generally considered abnormal and warrants further investigation. This magnitude of weight loss can occur in people of all ages and has a multitude of potential causes.

PATHOPHYSIOLOGY

Unintended weight loss results when caloric intake is less than caloric expenditure. This may be the result of diminished intake, malabsorption, excessive loss of nutrients, or increased caloric expenditure.

Diminished caloric intake may be the result of decreased interest in food, inability to obtain food, attenuated awareness of hunger, pain associated with the ingestion of food, and early satiety. Malabsorption of calories can occur with hepatic, pancreatic, and intestinal disorders. Loss of nutrients may result in the body being unable to maintain caloric homeostasis. Examples include recurrent vomiting or diarrhea, glycosuria, and significant proteinuria. Increased nutrient demand is the result of any process that increases basal metabolic rate. Chronic infection, hyperthyroidism, excessive exercise, and malignancy are common causes of increased metabolic rate.

CLINICAL MANIFESTATIONS

History

The first step in evaluating a patient with weight loss is to determine the amount and period of time over which the weight loss has occurred. Because many older patients may not recognize a significant weight loss, a decline in serial weight measurements is often the presenting sign. If a previous weight measurement is not available, asking about changes in waist size or how clothing fits may be helpful. Once significant weight loss is confirmed, a thorough review of systems should help direct physical exam and laboratory testing.

Questions about daily food intake, alterations in appetite, pain with swallowing, early satiety, episodes of emesis, and change in bowel habits are important. Foul smelling, greasy, bulky stools suggest malabsorption. Especially in young women, attitudes toward food and body image should be assessed. Distorted body image may be a clue to the presence of an eating disorder.

Patients should be asked about fever, cough, shortness of breath, alterations in patterns of urination, abdominal pain, melena, hematachezia, rash, headaches, and other neurological symptoms. Signs of depression such as difficulty concentrating, change in sleeping patterns, social isolation, and recent losses should be elicited. In cognitively impaired patients, family members and caregivers should be interviewed. The past medical history, previous surgeries, medications, tobacco use, alcohol intake, family history, and HIV risk factors should be reviewed. A social history is important to identify issues such as poverty, isolation, or an inability to shop or cook that may cause weight loss.

Physical Examination

Physical exam should begin with height and weight as well as vital signs to detect the presence of fever or tachycardia. General inspection should note stigmata of systemic disease including hair loss, temporal wasting, pallor, poor hygiene, bruising, jaundice, and diminished orientation. Evaluation of the oropharynx should assess dentition, presence of oral thrush, and petechiae, while the neck examination should note any thyromegaly or lymphadenopathy. The lungs should be examined for decreased breath sounds, crackles, wheezing, and evidence of consolidation while the heart is examined for irregular rhythm, murmurs, gallops, and the presence of a pericardial effusion. Abdominal examination should note any surgical scars, the quality of bowel sounds, and the presence of organomegaly, ascites, tenderness, or masses. The rectal exam is important for evaluating the prostate and to check for occult blood and stool consistency. In women, breast and pelvic exams should be performed to evaluate for malignancy. Neurological examination should assess memory, concentration, posterior column function, and focal abnormalities. Psychiatric evaluation may provide evidence of a mood disorder or anorexia nervosa.

DIFFERENTIAL DIAGNOSIS

Box 12–1 lists some important causes of weight loss. Organizing the differential diagnosis by the categories of decreased intake, impaired absorption, nutrient loss, and increased demand is a useful scheme. For many conditions, such as cancer or endstage CHF, weight loss occurs long after the diagnosis is known. However, anorexia nervosa, pancreatic cancer, early malabsorption, apathetic hyperthyroidism, diabetes, and HIV are examples of illnesses that may cause weight loss early in their presentation. A physical cause for weight loss can be found in about 65% of patients, and a psychiatric cause in another 10%. Depression is the most common psychiatric cause, and along with substance abuse may

---

BOX 12–1

Differential Diagnosis of Weight Loss

I. Decreased Intake

Alcohol/Substance Abuse
Anorexia nervosa
Congestive heart failure
Depression
Dementia

Hepatitis
Medications (e.g., dig toxicity)
Ulcer disease
Uremia
Splenomegaly
Bowel Obstruction
Poverty/Social Isolation

II. Malabsorption

Gastric bypass
Pancreatic insufficiency
Inflammatory bowel disease
Celiac sprue
Cholestasis
Protein wasting enteropathy

III. Nutrient Loss

Significant Proteinuria
Diabetes (uncontrolled)
Chronic emesis
Fistula
Chronic diarrhea

IV. Increased Demand

Chronic infection (e.g., tuberculosis)
Malignancy
Hyperthyroidism
Excessive exercise
Poor dentition
Infection (e.g., parasites)

---

present with profound weight loss. In approximately 25% of individuals, no identifiable cause is found.

DIAGNOSTIC APPROACH

Since weight loss is usually a late symptom of disease, the information gathered through the history and physical exam may identify the cause. However, if no explanation for involuntary weight loss is apparent, then ordering screening tests such as a complete blood count, serum electrolytes, BUN, creatinine, calcium, glucose, liver function tests, lipase, amylase, albumin, and thyroid stimulating hormone (TSH) may be helpful. Urinalysis, chest x-ray, and cancer screening tests such as a mammogram, Pap smear, prostate specific antigen (PSA) stool for occult blood, and sigmoidoscopy may also be appropriate. In patients with gastrointestinal symptoms, upper endoscopy, colonoscopy, abdominal ultrasound, abdominal CT, and stool analysis may be warranted. HIV antibody testing and TB skin testing should be performed in all individuals with risk factors. Although not specific, an erythrocyte sedimentation rate (ESR) may be useful in determining the likelihood of occult malignancy or infection. Serum levels of medications such as quinidine or digoxin should be checked if appropriate. In patients in whom malabsorption is suspected, use of the D-xylose test may further distinguish between pancreatic and small bowel disease. Antigliadin antibodies should be measured if there is concern about celiac sprue. In alcoholics and those with a macrocytic anemia, vitamin B12 and folate levels should be measured.

MANAGEMENT

Patients with an obvious cause for weight loss such as peptic ulcer disease, gallstones, infection, diabetes, hyperthyroidism, or cancer should be treated accordingly. Weight loss associated with depression typically responds well to antidepressant therapy. In patients with

dementia, caregivers providing one-to-one feeding support during each meal along with nutritional supplements such as Ensure™ are often adequate. Patients with anorexia nervosa need psychiatric referral and very close follow-up. In severe cases or if there is no improvement with outpatient treatment, admission to the hospital for bed rest and supervised meals in addition to more intense psychological therapy is indicated. In the setting of pancreatic insufficiency, oral pancreatic enzyme preparations and fat-soluble vitamin supplement (vitamins A, D, E, and K) should be instituted. Alcoholics and those suffering from malabsorption should have vitamin B12 and folate supplementation. Lastly, observation along with frequent follow-up is considered appropriate management in patients with normal history, physical exam, and laboratory evaluation.

◆ KEY POINTS ◆

1. A weight loss greater than 5% of total body weight over a period of 6 months is generally considered abnormal and warrants further investigation.

2. Unintended weight loss may be the result of diminished intake, malabsorption, excessive loss of nutrients, or increased caloric expenditure.

3. A physical cause for weight loss can be found in about 65% of patients, and a psychiatric cause in another 10%.

Part IV
Common ENT and Ophthalmology Problems

13

Red Eye

A red eye is the most common ophthalmological complaint encountered by primary care physicians. Most cases are due to benign and self-limiting conditions, which can be treated by the primary care physician. However, a few conditions that cause red eye are sight threatening, such as corneal ulceration, iritis, and glaucoma. The primary care physician needs to recognize these and if necessary refer the patient to an ophthalmologist.

PATHOPHYSIOLOGY

Redness of the skin around the eye may result from diseases that can affect the skin elsewhere or from inflammation of structures unique to the eye. Infection or occlusion of glandular structures, namely the meibomian glands, glands of Zeis, or the nasolacrimal duct, can cause swelling and redness of the eyelid or periorbital structures. Infection of the meibomian glands is termed internal hordeolum, whereas an external hordeolum or sty is an infection of the gland of Zeis. Sterile inflammation of the meibomian gland due to glandular occlusion is termed a chalazion. Infection, inflammation, and scaling of the eyelid margins is called blepharitis. Occlusion of the nasolacrimal duct with secondary infection is referred to as dacryocystitis. Infection may also spread to the orbital or periorbital region from sinus infections, leading to orbital or periorbital cellulitis.

The conjunctiva is a thin, transparent vascular tissue that lines the inner aspect of the eyelids (palpebral conjunctiva) and extends over the sclera (bulbar conjunctiva) before terminating at the limbus, where it is continuous with the corneal epithelium. Conjunctival tissue contains immune cells (Langerhans' cells, T & B-lymphocytes) in addition to goblet cells that produce the mucus in the precorneal tear film. A healthy conjunctiva is the first barrier to infection from the outside, which makes it understandable that external infections of the eye commonly cause an inflammation or hyperemia of the subconjunctival vessels. This causes the conjunctiva to appear erythematous and injected, hence the term "red eye." Other ocular inflammatory conditions, such as iritis or glaucoma, can also manifest as a red eye due to hyperemia of the ciliary vessels of the sclera through the transparent conjunctiva. Another cause of red eye is a subconjunctival hemorrhage, which is a benign condition that results from bleeding in the small fragile vessels of the conjunctiva, usually in response to minor trauma or straining. However, conjunctivitis is by far the most common cause of red eye.

CLINICAL MANIFESTATIONS

History

A careful history should include a thorough ocular, medical, and medication history. The ocular history should focus on the type of discomfort, changes in vision, presence of discharge, duration of symptoms (acute, subacute or chronic), unilateral or bilateral involvement, contact with anyone having similar ocular symptoms, and any specific environmental or work-related exposure. In addition, particular attention should be given to the following ocular symptoms: *pain*, *visual changes* (blurred vision/photophobia), and the type of *discharge*.

The type of discomfort helps determine the need for urgent referral to an ophthalmologist. Pain suggests a more serious ocular pathology such as acute angle closure glaucoma, iritis, keratitis, scleritis, uveitis, corneal ulceration, or orbital cellulitis. Discomfort associated with conjunctivitis is often described as burning, tearing, or as an irritation. Itching is the hallmark of allergic conjunctivitis, but can also be present in viral or bacterial conjunctivitis. Visual changes also suggest serious ocular disease and are not seen with conjunctivitis. Discharge is a common finding in patients with conjunctivitis and the type of discharge, purulent or mucoid, may help in distinguishing bacterial from viral or allergic causes of conjunctivitis. A history of trauma or a gritty feeling in one eye associated with pain may suggest a foreign body or corneal abrasion.

Physical Examination

The eyelids and periorbital region should be checked for erythema and inflammation. Next, examine the conjunctiva for a pattern of any redness detected. Conjunctival erythema may be due to subconjunctival hemorrhage, conjunctival hyperemia, or to presence of the "ciliary flush." Subconjunctival hemorrhage is a collection of blood under the conjunctiva and has a bright red appearance with distinct borders. Conjunctival hyperemia is diffuse erythema of the conjunctival lining with no borders and involves both the bulbar and palpebral conjunctiva. The ciliary flush refers to a violaceous hyperemia of the vessels surrounding the cornea, and along with photophobia and a sluggishly reactive pupil, are signs of iritis.

Note the presence, quality, and quantity of any discharge. Examine each pupil, looking for any irregularities in shape or size in comparison to the other pupil, and reactivity to light. With the ophthalmoscope, inspect the cornea, looking for opacities, surface irregularities or foreign bodies, as well as the fundus and optic disc, looking for an increase in the cup-disc ratio, which may signify the presence of glaucoma. Next estimate the depth of the anterior chamber (normal or shallow) by shining a light from the temporal side of the head across the front of the eye parallel to the plane of the iris (a shallow chamber will only illuminate the temporal half of the iris). Check extraocular movements. Finally, visual acuity should be checked using a Snellen eye chart.

DIFFERENTIAL DIAGNOSIS

The most common causes for red eye include hordeola, chalazion, blepharitis, corneal abrasion, subconjunctival hemorrhage, and conjunctivitis. One should also be familiar with signs and symptoms of glaucoma and iritis so that prompt referral for therapy can be provided to the patient. These diseases are described in Table 13–1. Other less common causes of red eye include scleritis, episcleritis, anterior uveitis, and keratitis, all of which require ophthalmologic referrals.

DIAGNOSTIC APPROACH

Initial assessment involves a thorough physical examination, including ophthalmoscopic examination. When a patient presents with ocular pain, corneal ulceration or laceration must be ruled out by a *fluorescein dye test*. To perform this test, apply the fluorescein dye to the lower eyelid (drops or impregnated strip) and view the cornea under a cobalt-blue light searching for disruptions of the corneal epithelium (ulcers or lacerations). Additional testing for patients presenting with ocular pain may include measurement of intraocular pressures.

Most cases of conjunctivitis are self-limited and the cost benefit ratio for culturing the eye discharge precludes its routine use. The conjunctiva has a bacterial flora composed of many species, including *Staphylococcus aureus* and, less commonly, *corynebacteria* and *Streptococcus* species. Some healthy patients may also harbor *pseudomonas* and fungi as a part of their normal conjunctival flora. Infectious conjunctivitis is usually due to a viral infection, but about 5% of the time is bacterial. In severe cases, the very young, or in cases that do not respond to therapy, cultures may be useful. Tonometry may be useful in a suspected case of acute glaucoma. Gram staining of the discharge may help identify a bacterial agent. Multinucleated giant cells are suggestive of a herpes infection. In patients with suspected serious orbital or periorbital cellulitis, complete blood counts and imaging studies, such as orbital computed tomography scans, may be indicated.

TABLE 13–1

Differential Diagnosis of Red Eye

Disease	Description	Other
Blepharitis	chronic lid margin erythema, scaling, loss of eyelashes	associated with staphylococcal infection, seborrheic dermatitis
Hordeola/Chalazion	painful nodules on or along lids	hordeola associated with staphylococcal infection; Chalazion-sterile
Conjunctivitis	burning, itching, discharge, lid edema	
—viral	clear, mucoid discharge	associated with upper respiratory infection; very contagious
—hyperacute bacterial	copious purulent discharge	potentially sight threatening; associated with gonorrhea, sexually transmitted diseases (STDs), neonates
—acute bacterial	moderate purulent discharge	*H. influenzae*, staphylococcal, *S. pneumoniae*
—inclusion conjunctivitis	persistent watery discharge	Chlamydia; neonates and young adults, associated with STDs
—allergic	itching, tearing	associated with other allergy symptoms
Subconjunctival Hemorrhage	nonblanching red "spot," painless without visual changes or discharge	associated with trauma, cough, or Valsalva (e.g., straining)
Corneal Abrasion/Foreign Body	pain, "foreign body" sensation	abrupt, associated with incident or work exposure
Iritis	pain, photophobia, pupillary constriction, cloudy cornea and anterior chamber	associated with connective tissue diseases, ocular injury
Acute Angle Closure Glaucoma	pain, tearing, dilated pupil, shallow anterior chamber, halos around lights	ocular emergency, more common over age 50

MANAGEMENT

Therapy for blepharitis generally involves measures aimed at eyelid hygiene. Specifically, use of a mild soap, such as a baby shampoo, diluted with water to scrub the lids is recommended. Additional measures may include use of warm compresses and a topical antibiotic ointment.

The inflammation and pain from a hordeolum or chalazion may respond to use of warm compresses. Hordeolum may also respond to topical antibiotic therapy, and if associated cellulitis is present, systemic

TABLE 13–2

Therapy for Conjunctivitis

Etiology	Treatment
Viral	—Local measures: cool compresses
Herpes	—Oral +/− topical antiviral (e.g., acyclovir) —Ophthalmology referral
Bacterial	—Local measures —Gonococcal conjunctivitis requires systemic antibiotics (e.g., IV or IM ceftriaxone —Chlamydial conjunctivitis requires 2–3 weeks of oral therapy (e.g., erythromycin or doxycycline)
Allergic	—Local measures —Allergen avoidance —Topical or systemic antihistamines (e.g., loratadine, levocabastine)

antibiotics may be used that are active against the most common pathogen, *Staphylococcus aureus.* A chronic chalazion may require intralesional steroid injections or surgical drainage for resolution. Hordeola rarely require incision and drainage for treatment.

Treatment recommendations for conjunctivitis are presented in Table 13–2. For hyperacute bacterial conjunctivitis, prompt aggressive treatment is necessary to avoid sight-threatening complications. Viral conjunctivitis is self-limiting, lasting 7 to 10 days. Ninety-five percent of patients shed the virus for up to 10 days after the onset of symptoms. All patients should receive hygienic advice such as avoiding eye-hand contact, good hand washing, and using their own face cloth and towel in order to limit spread of the infection.

Subconjunctival hemorrhages require no treatment and will usually resolve over several days. Treatment for a foreign body includes removal using a topical anesthetic for the eye and moistened cotton Q-tip. If the foreign body cannot be removed, an ophthalmology referral is indicated.

Patients with iritis and acute glaucoma need urgent referral to an ophthalmologist. After thorough ophthalmological examination, therapy for iritis often involves use of cycloplegic and anti-inflammatory (e.g., topical steroids) medications. Acute medical treatment for glaucoma usually involves acetazolamide 500 mg and topical 4% pilocarpine ophthalmic solution to constrict the pupil.

◆ **KEY POINTS** ◆

1. The most common cause of red eye is conjunctivitis.
2. The most common etiology of conjunctivitis is viral, a self-limited but extremely contagious condition.
3. In conjunctivitis, a purulent discharge usually indicates a bacterial infection while a watery discharge is either allergic or viral.
4. Itching is the hallmark of allergic conjunctivitis.
5. Acute angle closure glaucoma must be considered in patients over 50 with a painful red eye.

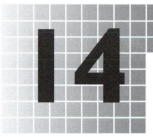

Pharyngitis

Pharyngitis is a common reason for office visits to primary care physicians. There are many potential causes for pharyngitis including viral and bacterial infections, allergies, and irritants. Careful history and physical examination can help determine which patients need further evaluation.

PATHOPHYSIOLOGY

Bacteria and viruses are responsible for causing most infectious pharyngitis and are spread person to person either by inhalation of airborne particles or by exposure to respiratory or oral secretions.

The most common etiologic viral agents are respiratory viruses, such as adenovirus, parainfluenza virus, and rhinovirus. Pharyngitis associated with infections with these agents is usually part of a broader upper respiratory tract infection causing rhinorrhea, cough, and often conjunctivitis. Herpangina, characterized by tonsillar and palatal ulcerations is caused by coxsackie virus. Infectious mononucleosis caused by the Epstein-Barr virus may cause pharyngitis alone or along with systemic illness, with pharyngitis as one of the prominent symptoms. The herpes virus can also cause a pharyngitis or stomatitis.

Streptococcus pyogenes (Group A strep) pharyngitis accounts for about 15% of infectious cases and typically presents with fever and sore throat that is self-limited. Immunologically mediated complications of streptococcal infection include acute rheumatic fever and glomerulonephritis. Rheumatic fever can lead to long-term valvular heart disease, such as mitral stenosis unless treated within 10 days of onset. Acute glomerulonephritis is self-limited and prompt antibiotic therapy does not prevent this complication. Serious local complications include peritonsillar and retropharygeal abscesses that result from tissue invasion by Group A strep. These infections may lead to deeper infections and airway compromise.

Other bacteria that may lead to self-limited pharyngitis, either alone or as part of a respiratory infection include mycoplasma, chlamydia, hemophilus and corynebacterium. Pharyngitis may occur in association with sinusitis. Fungal pharyngitis may occur in immunocompromised patients and gonococcal pharyngitis may occur as a sexually transmitted disease with oral sex.

Non-infectious causes of pharyngitis include sleep apnea, gastroesophageal reflux disease, and cigarette smoke through primary irritant effects. Allergies may cause lymphoid hyperplasia, nasal obstruction, and post-nasal drip, which can lead to pharyngeal irritation.

CLINICAL MANIFESTATIONS

History

Streptococcal infection most commonly occurs in children ages 5 to 15 years and is rare in children less than age 3. Mononucleosis is classically a disease of teenagers. The history should include inquiring about associated symptoms and known exposures to illness. For example, only 25% of patients with positive strep cultures will have rhinorrhea and cough. The presence of these symptoms and a low-grade fever suggests a viral etiology. The classic symptoms for streptococcal infection are fever over 101° F (38.3° C) in association with a sore throat, but few other respiratory symptoms. The chronicity of the disease is also helpful in determining the cause for pharyngitis. Viral and uncomplicated bacterial infections resolve in about 1 week, whereas non-infectious causes are more persistent. Early morning sore throat without fever or other associated symptoms suggests a non-infectious cause such as gastroesophageal reflux disease.

Past medical history may suggest potential causes or may lead to consideration of less common causes for pharyngitis. For example, patients with a history of allergies may be experiencing a sore throat related to the allergies. Immunocompromised patients may develop fungal infection or complications with bacterial infection (e.g., peritonsillar abscess). A past history of rheumatic fever with or without carditis warrants evaluation for recurrence of streptococcal disease.

Physical Examination

Vital signs and an examination of the ears, nose, and throat are an essential part of the evaluation. The throat in classical Group A streptococcus infection is erythematous with tonsillar exudates. There are often palatal petechiae and there may be a "strawberry" tongue with prominent red papillae on a white-coated tongue. Tender cervical lymphadenopathy is often present. Mononucleosis, gonococcal infection, and on occasion other bacterial or viral infections may have a pharyngeal exam indistinguishable from streptococcal pharyngitis. Vesicular lesions suggest either herpes or coxsackie infection, while adenovirus often causes an accompanying conjunctivitis. The physical examination should also include a lung examination since many patients also have respiratory symptoms. About half of patients with mononucleosis have splenic enlargement on abdominal examination.

clude adenovirus, parainfluenza virus, rhinovirus, coxsackie virus, herpes, cytomegalovirus and Epstein-Barr virus. In addition to Group A streptococcus, other streptococcal bacteria (Group C and Group G) may cause pharyngitis but are not associated with the complications of Group A strep. Other bacteria including gonococcus, chlamydia, mycoplasma, corynebacterium, and less commonly pneumococci, staphylococci, fusobacteria, and yersinia can also cause pharyngitis. Fungi may cause infection in immunosuppressed patients.

Non-infectious causes for pharyngitis should be suspected in patients without fever and with persistent or recurring symptoms. Common non-infectious causes for pharyngitis include sleep apnea, gastroesophageal reflux, allergies, and referred pain from primary otologic or dental disease.

DIAGNOSTIC APPROACH

Physical examination alone cannot accurately determine if a bacterial infection is present. Options in testing for Group A strep include rapid antigen detection assays, used in many offices, and throat culture. Throat culture is the gold standard test and is considered definitive. Rapid tests are reported to have a sensitivity of 80% to 90% and a specificity of over 90%. Testing for gonococcal pharyngitis requires a throat swab inoculated in Thayer-Martin media. Fungal infection may be identified by use of KOH slide preparation or may be detected on routine throat cultures.

Testing is also commonly performed for mononucleosis. Heterophile antibody testing, commonly referred to as the *monospot* is available in many offices and may be positive as early as 5 days, but can take up to 3 weeks to convert to positive. Alternatively, Epstein-Barr IgM antibodies may be elevated as early as 2 weeks after infection. In patients presenting with suspected mononucleosis and an initial negative test, repeat testing may be necessary.

DIFFERENTIAL DIAGNOSIS

Most patients with an acute pharyngitis have either a viral or bacterial infection. Common viruses in-

MANAGEMENT

Streptococcal pharyngitis should be treated to prevent rheumatic fever, prevent suppurative complications, and

to decrease person-to-person spread of the infection. The treatment of choice for strep throat is penicillin either as a 10-day oral course or a single intramuscular injection. For those patients allergic to penicillin, erythromycin or a newer macrolide such as azithromycin may be used. For treatment failures, use of amoxicillin-clauvulanic acid or clindamycin are commonly used.

Treatment for viral pharyngitis is largely supportive and symptomatic. Lozenges and warm salt water gargles may provide topical relief. Analgesic drugs such as acetaminophen or ibuprofen can help reduce pain. Treatment for mononucleosis and gonococcal infections is covered in chapters 34 and 37.

◆ KEY POINTS ◆

1. There are many potential causes for pharyngitis including viral and bacterial infections, allergies, and irritants.

2. Evaluation and testing for infectious etiologies is largely targeted towards identification of Group A streptococcal infection due to its association with complications such as rheumatic fever.

3. The treatment of choice for strep throat is penicillin whereas treatment for the other causes of pharyngitis is largely symptomatic.

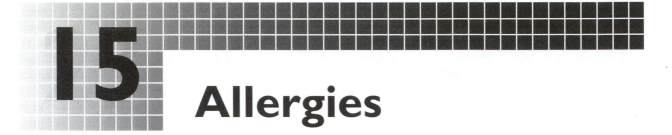

15 Allergies

Allergic diseases encompass a wide range of clinical problems. For example, allergic rhinitis affects up to 20% of the population and 2% to 5% of children suffer from atopic dermatitis. Asthma occurs in 5% to 7% of the population and is associated with significant morbidity and an increasing number of deaths. Food allergies, although less common, occur in a significant number of individuals. The term allergy can be defined as an immunoglobulin E (IgE) mediated hypersensitivity to an antigen. Type I hypersensitivity reactions include allergic rhinitis, conjunctivitis, asthma, food allergies, and systemic anaphylaxis.

PATHOPHYSIOLOGY

In allergic rhinitis, allergens bind to IgE on mast cells on the nasal mucosa of a sensitized individual. This causes mast cells to degranulate, releasing chemical mediators such as histamines, leukotrienes, and bradykinins that cause vasodilatation, fluid transudation, and swelling. Common seasonal allergens include pollens from trees, grasses, and weeds. Perennial rhinitis, which occurs throughout the year, is caused primarily by indoor allergens such as house dust, animal dander, and molds.

IgE mediated reactions can also trigger asthma. Environmentally important allergens leading to asthma include air pollution, dust mites, and cockroaches,

which may explain the increasing prevalence of asthma in the inner city.

Cutaneous, respiratory or gastrointestinal exposure to allergens may cause symptoms in the exposed organ system or may produce more generalized symptoms. Common skin manifestations of allergies include urticaria and eczema. Gastrointestinal symptoms associated with allergen exposure include nausea, vomiting, diarrhea, and abdominal pain. The common foods that are found to be allergenic in children are milk, eggs, peanuts, soy, wheat, tree nuts, fish, and shellfish. In adults, peanuts, tree nuts, shellfish, and fish are the most common.

Severe life-threatening systemic allergic reactions called anaphylaxis can occur from food allergies such as peanuts, during blood transfusions, from medications, or from insect stings of the hymenoptera order (bees, wasps, and ants).

CLINICAL MANIFESTATIONS

History

Symptoms of allergic rhinitis include a runny nose (rhinorrhea), sneezing, nasal congestion, conjunctivitis, and itching of the ears, eyes, nose, and throat. Nonproductive cough, nasal congestion with headaches, plugged or itchy ears, diminished smell and taste, or sleep disturbances may all be symptoms of allergies.

Timing of the symptoms is important. Tree pollens tend to affect people more in the early spring, grasses in mid-May to June, and ragweed from August until the first frost. Those who are allergic to pollens may have the worst symptoms in the morning and gradually improve by night. The common perennial allergens are house dust, feathers, animal dander, or molds. In these patients the symptoms may be worse at night. Continual waxing and waning throughout the year suggest a combination of perennial and seasonal allergies. Genetic factors appear to play a role and patients with allergies often have a family history of atopy.

Food allergies often affect the skin and the gastrointestinal system. Food allergies may present with urticaria, usually within an hour of ingesting the offending agent. Patients should be asked if they have ever experienced symptoms suggestive of more severe or anaphylactic reactions. Manifestations of anaphylaxis include agitation, palpitations, paresthesias, pruritus, difficulty swallowing, cough, and wheezing. Patients with these symptoms need emergency care since the initial symptoms may progress rapidly and even lead to cardiovascular collapse.

Physical Examination

The physical exam should focus on the eyes, nose, throat, lungs, and skin. Patient may have conjunctivitis and increased lacrimation. The nasal mucosa may appear swollen and pale. The turbinates should be inspected to rule out any nasal polyps, which is common in patients with allergies. *Allergic shiners* is a term used to describe the darkening of the infraorbital skin in people with chronic allergies. Some patients may have a nasal crease across the bridge of the nose due to the frequent nose rubbing ("allergic salute") to relieve itching. The sinuses should be examined for tenderness and the lungs for wheezing.

Skin reactions such as eczema and urticaria are common in children with food allergies. An abdominal examination should be performed in patients presenting with gastrointestinal symptoms to exclude other causes for their symptoms.

DIFFERENTIAL DIAGNOSIS

The differential diagnosis depends on the presenting complaint. In allergic conjunctivitis, it is important to differentiate between viral, bacteria, allergic, or irritant causes of conjunctivitis. Viral and bacterial conjunctivitis are discussed in chapter 13. Allergic conjunctivitis is often seasonal and occurs during periods of high exposure. Patients may also get red eyes due to irritants such as dust and smoke.

Rhinorrhea can occur due to a common cold, vasomotor rhinitis, atrophic rhinitis, rhinitis medicamentosa, or sinusitis. In the common cold, the mucosa is usually red with thickened discharge, whereas with allergies the nasal mucosa appears pale and boggy or bluish. In nonallergic rhinitis, there is no pruritus. Patients with vasomotor rhinitis present with chronic nasal congestion with watery rhinorrhea, which may be intensified by sudden changes in temperature, humidity, or odors. Atrophic rhinitis is a condition seen in elderly patients and is characterized by marked atrophy of the nasal mucosa, chronic nasal congestion, and a bad odor. Rhinitis medicamentosa is caused by chronic use of cocaine or topical nasal decongestants. In sinusitis, the nasal discharge may be purulent and accompanied by headaches, nasal congestion, facial pain, and tenderness over the sinuses. Other causes of rhinitis include foreign bodies, nasal polyps, tumors, and nasal congestion associated with hormonal causes such pregnancy, birth control pill use, and hypothyroidism. Wegener's granulomatosis, midline granuloma, and sarcoidosis are rare but serious causes of nasal discharge.

The symptoms of food allergies include skin reactions and gastrointestinal symptoms. Urticarial lesions, or hives, are characterized as pruritic erythematous raised lesions, which may be migratory. Atopic dermatitis is an eczematous rash that is flat erythematous and scaly and can be confused with contact dermatitis or lichen simplex chronicus. Evaluating the gastrointestinal symptoms requires a thorough history and physical as well as an association of symptoms with the suspected allergen.

DIAGNOSTIC APPROACH

The diagnosis of allergic disease is usually made on the basis of the history and physical exam. In most patients treatment may be started without any diagnostic tests and if the patient responds to therapy, no further testing is needed.

Esosinophils found on microscopic examination of nasal smears are characteristic of allergic rhinitis. However, this test is not commonly performed because of poor sensitivity and specificity. In patients who do not respond to empiric therapy, allergy testing is helpful. Radioabsorbant allergen testing (RAST) tests the blood for the presence of IgE to different allergens. The test is sensitive but not specific, thus many individuals may be positive on RAST testing but may not be having clinical symptoms from the allergen identified by RAST tests. Skin prick testing involves injecting a small amount of allergen into the skin and observing for local responses. This test is more specific but less sensitive than RAST testing and is usually performed by an allergist. Identifying offending allergens is useful for directing avoidance therapy. If no allergens are identified and the patient continues to have symptoms, flexible nasolaryngoscopy may be performed to rule out any anatomic or pathologic abnormalities. In patients with food allergies, the history should help formulate a possible list of allergenic foods. Avoidance and challenge testing can assess for different food allergies.

TREATMENT

The first treatment for any allergic disorder is allergen avoidance. Examples include staying indoors during a high pollen day or reducing household dust by frequent cleaning, vacuuming, and removing dust collecting items such as book shelves or shag rugs. Pharmacological therapy includes antihistamines, oral and topical decongestants, intranasal and oral corticosteroids, and intranasal cromolyn sodium. Antihistamines are the first line therapy for allergic rhinitis and are also helpful for other forms of allergy. They block the H-1 receptors, preventing the release of histamine and help reduce sneezing, rhinorrhea, and itching. The main side effect of these drugs is sedation. However newer non-sedating antihistamines are now available. Recently a topical antihistamine nasal spray (azelastine) was developed. Topical nasal decongestant sprays have a very limited role in allergic rhinitis because of the risks of tachyphylaxis and rebound nasal congestion. Oral decongestants, such as pseudoephedrine can relieve nasal congestion, but should be used with caution in patients with hypertension, thyroid disease, diabetes, and difficulty in urination.

Intranasal steroids are the treatment of choice for most patients with allergic rhinitis because of their effectiveness and minimal side effects. Oral corticosteroids are potent medications but have significant long-term side effects and as a result should be used only for 3 to 7 days. Cromolyn is a mast cell stabilizer that is available as an over-the-counter nasal spray. Cromolyn is only moderately effective but is very safe and well tolerated. It is often the first line of treatment in children and pregnant women. Topical therapies or oral antihistamines may provide relief for allergic conjunctivitis.

For patients with skin manifestations, oral antihistamines, topical steroids, and cool colloid baths may be helpful. Oral steroids can be used for acute urticaria, but should not be used chronically. Moisturizing lotions and creams may improve symptoms. As with other forms of allergy, avoidance of any known triggers should be advised. Patients with food allergies should avoid the foods that bring about the symptoms.

Therapy for patients with asthma is outlined in chapter 19. In cases of anaphylaxis, the treatment of choice is epinephrine. Patients who have a history of anaphylaxis should carry injectable epinephrine. They should wear an alert bracelet and have an emergency action plan that describes the signs and symptoms of anaphylaxis and emergency instructions.

In recalcitrant cases immunotherapy may be tried. In this process, patients are exposed to the allergen by subcutaneous injections of increasing concentrations of allergens. The goal of immunotherapy is to induce a tolerance within the patient for the specific allergen triggering their symptoms.

◆ KEY POINTS ◆

1. Allergies are common diseases in the population and the prevalence is increasing.

2. Type I hypersensitivity reactions are mediated by antigen binding to IgE on mast cells and basophils that causes the mast cell or the basophil to degranulate and release mediators of the symptoms of allergy.

3. Inquiry into known triggers for the symptoms should be elicited.

4. The first and definitive treatment for any allergic disorder is avoidance of the allergens.

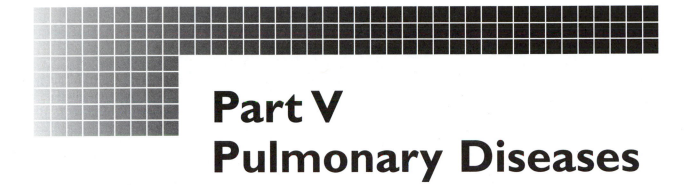

Part V
Pulmonary Diseases

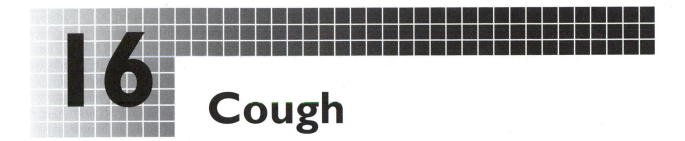

16 Cough

Cough is one of the most common complaints seen in family practice. Cough is defined as a sudden reflex expulsion of air from the glottis in an attempt to clear the airways of secretions and inhaled particles. This maneuver helps to protect the lungs against aspiration and harmful irritants. Common causes of cough include viral or bacterial infections of the upper respiratory tract, irritant exposure, allergies, chronic obstructive pulmonary disease (COPD), cancer, cardiac diseases, or psychological factors.

PATHOPHYSIOLOGY

Ciliated pseudostratified columnar epithelium and mucous-producing goblet cells line the trachea and bronchi. These two types of cells are responsible for filtering particles in inspired air. Certain irritants (e.g., smoke) and viral infections can damage the cilia lining the airways, impairing the filtering process and allowing microscopic particles to reach the lungs. These particles and thermal or chemical stimulants may irritate afferent receptors in the airways and trigger the cough reflex. The cough reflex is a complex interaction mediated peripherally by the vagus, trigeminal, glossopharyngeal, and phrenic nerves. Centrally, the cough center is located in the medulla.

With upper respiratory tract infections, inflammation and increased mucous secretions stimulate the cough receptors found in the upper airway. Common viral causes of infection include influenza, parainfluenza, adenovirus, respiratory syncytial virus, and rhinovirus. Bacterial causes include *Streptococcus pneumoniae*, *Mycoplasma pneumoniae*, and *Haemophilus influenzae*. Cough is also a common presenting complaint in tuberculosis (TB). The most common irritant associated with cough is cigarette smoke. Cancers and foreign bodies elicit the cough reflex by direct stimulation.

CLINICAL MANIFESTATIONS

History

A complete history of cough should include the timing, quality, associated symptoms, past medical history, and medications. The timing of when the cough started is essential. This helps to classify the cough as acute or chronic. Patients who have a seasonal pattern may have a cough secondary to allergic rhinitis. Nocturnal coughing may indicate asthma, gastroesophageal reflux disease (GERD), postnasal drip, or congestive heart failure. If symptoms occur with meals, aspiration should be considered. Exercise- or cold-induced cough points to asthma. Cough and dyspnea on exertion suggest a cardiac etiology.

The quality of the cough is also very important. A productive cough can be seen in infections such as bronchitis and pneumonia. A dry cough is common in postnasal drip and asthma. Furthermore, patients with postnasal drip feel an itching sensation in the throat and as a result cough in an attempt to clear the throat. Hemoptysis is often seen in tuberculosis and cancers.

Patients also should be asked about other symptoms such as fever, chills, night sweats, weight loss, and hoarseness. Patients with weight loss should be investigated for cancers.

Patients who present with cough and a past medical history of congestive heart failure (CHF) may have worsening CHF. Weight gain may be an associated symptom. Postnasal drip is a common cause of cough in patients with allergies or a recent upper respiratory tract infection.

Certain medications such as an angiotensin converting enzyme (ACE) inhibitor may cause a chronic nonproductive cough. For patients with asthma, B-blockers may exacerbate the asthma and cause a cough. Chronic use of nitrofurantoin can cause a cough secondary to interstitial fibrosis.

Physical Examination

The physical exam should focus on the ears, nose, throat, neck, and chest. Ears plugged with cerumen can result in a reflex cough (Arnold's reflex). Patients with allergies often have a pale, boggy nasal mucosa with swollen turbinates. A purulent discharge from the nose may indicate sinusitis. In pharyngitis, the tonsils appear swollen and hyperemic. The posterior pharynx should be checked for increased secretions, which are often seen in patients with postnasal drip. Palpable lymph nodes in the neck support the diagnosis of an infectious cause. During the chest examination, close attention should be paid to the lung and heart sounds. Murmurs and gallops suggest a possible cardiac cause. Crackles may indicate an inflammatory process or worsening CHF. Diminished or bronchial breath sounds can occur with pneumonia. Wheezing may be heard with foreign body aspiration, COPD, or asthma.

DIFFERENTIAL DIAGNOSIS

The common causes of cough include viral and bacterial infections of the respiratory tract, irritants, allergies, asthma, COPD, cancer, GERD, and psychogenic cough. Viral causes of cough are more common in the winter months. Following a viral infection of the respiratory tract, a cough may persist for up to 8 weeks. Bacterial infections of the respiratory tract are common causes of acute cough and include sinusitis, pharyngitis, bronchitis, and pneumonia. Cigarette smokers often have a chronic cough due to chronic irritant exposure. Allergies may present with a chronic cough usually due to a postnasal drip. A child who presents with a chronic cough lasting more than 8 weeks should be suspected of having asthma and/or allergies. Typically the cough seen in asthma is dry and may worsen at night or after exercise. Cold air may also exacerbate a cough due to asthma. Patients with COPD or bronchiectasis may present with a chronic cough.

In those individuals presenting with weight loss, night sweats, hemoptysis, and chronic cough, lung cancer and tuberculosis (TB) should be considered. Gastroesophageal reflux can cause a cough that is worsened by lying down and may be associated with substernal burning or a sour taste in the mouth. Patients who cough when eating should be evaluated for aspiration. Individuals with an acute cough, dyspnea, and a swollen leg should be evaluated for possible pulmonary embolism. Certain medications such as ACE inhibitors, amiodarone, and nitrofurantoin can cause a dry cough. Finally, psychogenic cough may be a possibility. However all the organic causes should be ruled out before this disorder can be diagnosed.

DIAGNOSTIC APPROACH

The diagnostic approach to cough begins with a good history and physical exam. When viral infections of the respiratory tract are suspected, no further work-up is necessary as long as the cough resolves over a period of up to 6 to 8 weeks. If sinusitis is suspected, a patient may be started on antibiotics and monitored for resolution of the symptoms. If a cough is from an ACE inhibitor, discontinuing it should result in improvement in a few days.

A chest x-ray (CXR) is necessary in most patients without an upper airway abnormality who have a new cough, persistent cough, or hemoptysis. The chest x-ray can detect pulmonary infections, masses, pleural effusion, congestive heart failure, interstitial lung disease, bronchiectasis, hilar lymphadenopathy, and may show changes consistent with COPD. The CXR may be normal in some patients with neoplasm, pulmonary embolus, sinus disease, and pulmonary hypertension. If these diseases are suspected, further testing with CT scanning, bronchoscopy, V/Q scan, or an echocardiogram is indicated.

In patients with a persistent cough and a normal CXR, occult bronchospasm should be considered. Spirometry or an empiric trial of bronchodilator therapy is helpful. Rarely, patients may require a methacholine challenge or post exercise spirometry to confirm the diagnosis. In patients with symptoms of reflux, empiric treatment for GERD or an UGI may be helpful.

TREATMENT

Cough is a symptom and as a result treatment should focus on the underlying disease process as outlined in the respective chapters in this book. For example, patients with GERD should respond to a course of antireflux therapy with antacids and histamine-2 blockers. However, if the cough is significant enough to seek medical attention, patients may warrant symptomatic treatment with an antitussive. For example, the postinfectious cough of some viral illnesses may last up to 8 weeks and cough suppression may provide significant symptom relief. Antitussive medications may be classified as either centrally acting or peripherally acting medications. Centrally acting drugs include codeine and dextromethorphan. Codeine is a narcotic that binds to the opiate receptors and suppresses the medullary cough center. Sedation is a common side effect. Dextromethorphan also suppresses the cough center in the medulla. This non-narcotic agent is available in many over-the-counter preparations. It lacks the addiction potential of codeine and the narcotic antitussive medications but is not as effective. Peripherally acting drugs such as benzonatate anesthetize the respiratory passage, lungs, and the pleural stretch receptors but are of questionable value. Mucolytic agents (guaifenesin) increase the volume and decrease the viscosity of secretions, which may help to clear secretions from the respiratory tract more easily.

◆ KEY POINTS ◆

1. Cough is defined as a sudden reflexive expulsion of air from the glottis in an attempt to clear the airways of secretions and inhaled particles.

2. The cough reflex is associated with the vagus, trigeminal, glossopharyngeal, and phrenic nerves.

3. The cough center is located in the medulla.

4. Postnasal drip is a common cause of cough in patients with allergies or a recent viral infection of the upper respiratory tract.

5. Centrally acting antitussive medications include codeine and dextromethorphan.

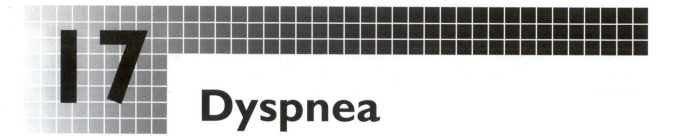

17

Dyspnea

Dyspnea, defined as a sensation of difficult or uncomfortable breathing, is a common complaint associated with a variety of different underlying causes. The range of different causes and presentations may vary from acute dyspnea, associated with myocardial infarction or pulmonary embolus, to a chronic dyspnea, associated with congestive heart failure or chronic obstructive pulmonary disease. The manner and location in which a patient may present will likewise vary. For example, the patient with acute dyspnea is more likely to present to an acute care setting, such as the emergency room. Patients with chronic dyspnea will more likely present to an office setting for evaluation and care. This chapter will briefly discuss acute dyspnea and focus more on chronic causes.

PATHOPHYSIOLOGY

Dyspnea may be caused by one of several different mechanisms. In general, dyspnea occurs when the perceived demand for oxygen or respiration is not being met or when the work of breathing is increased. For example, with a pneumonia or pulmonary embolus the ability of the lungs to provide sufficient oxygen to the peripheral and central chemoreceptors for oxygen is diminished and the patient experiences the sensation of dyspnea. Other causes associated with limitations in respiration or oxygen delivery include congestive heart failure, interstitial lung disease, pulmonary hypertension, and severe anemia. With obstructive lung disease, such as asthma, the patient may have a normal or near normal pO_2 and decreased pCO_2, yet experience dyspnea due to the increased work of breathing. Other mechanical causes for patients experiencing dyspnea include obesity, pleural effusion, ascites, and kyphoscoliosis. Finally, anxiety may cause the patient to hyperventilate and perceive this increased respiratory effort as dyspnea.

CLINICAL MANIFESTATIONS

History

The onset, progression, associated diseases, and symptoms direct the evaluation of the patient with dyspnea. Patients presenting with acute and rapidly progressive symptoms should be questioned about chest pain, history of cardiopulmonary disease, fever, and recent surgery or travel. These patients should, in general, be directed or sent to the emergency room setting where they can be monitored and promptly evaluated for cardiopulmonary causes such as pneumonia, myocardial infarction, and pulmonary embolism.

Patients with chronic dyspnea, a gradually developing course, or episodic dyspnea may be evaluated in the outpatient setting. The history should focus on a past history of cardiac or respiratory disease. Patients with a history of asthma, COPD, or congestive heart failure may be experiencing exacerbation of their underlying disease. Associated symptoms should be noted. For example, substernal chest pressure in association with dyspnea occurs with angina. A patient who complains of a swollen leg in association with dyspnea may be experiencing a pulmonary embolus. Patients with a history of melena or dysfunctional uterine bleeding may be experiencing dyspnea due to severe anemia. Inquiring about stress and eliciting symptoms of perioral numbness and paresthesias help assess whether anxiety is the cause of symptoms.

Physical Examination

The history and physical examination should focus on the heart and lungs. Heart examination should note the rate and rhythm of the heart in search of arrhythmias, such as atrial fibrillation that may trigger dyspneic symptoms. Presence of murmurs along with an S3 may indicate congestive heart failure as the cause. Peripheral edema may be a sign of fluid overload contributing to the patient's symptoms.

The lung exam should note respiratory rate and effort as indicated by use of the accessory muscles. Inspection should note the chest and abdominal contours looking for the barrel-chested appearance of chronic obstructive pulmonary disease or the stigmata of cirrhosis and ascites. Percussion should be performed to assess for possible pleural effusions. Auscultation for presence of rales, wheezing, rubs or diminished breath sounds should be performed in the assessment for cardiopulmonary causes.

DIFFERENTIAL DIAGNOSIS

The differential diagnosis can be divided into acute and chronic dyspnea. Box 17–1 presents some of the common causes for dyspnea. Anxiety or cardiopulmonary causes account for the majority of patients with dyspnea, with asthma, chronic obstructive pulmonary disease, pneumonia and congestive heart failure the most frequently occurring cardiopulmonary causes.

DIAGNOSTIC APPROACH

Initial assessment of the patient presenting with dyspnea can include pulse oximetry to assess oxygenation. This

---

BOX 17–1

Common Causes for Dyspnea

Acute Dyspnea
  Bronchospasm
  Pulmonary Edema
  Pulmonary Embolism
  Pneumothorax
  Pneumonia
  Myocardial Infarction
  Acute Anxiety Attack/Panic Disorder
  Anemia

Chronic Dyspnea
  Congestive Heart Failure
  Chronic Obstructive Pulmonary Disease
  Asthma
  Interstitial Lung Disease
  Pulmonary Hypertension
  Pleural Effusion
  Obesity
  Ascites
  Kyphoscoliosis
  Anemia
  Anxiety

---

test is available in many offices and along with the history and physical examination will help in determining where and how to further evaluate the patient. A chest x-ray should be obtained for most patients with a complaint of dyspnea. Chest x-ray findings may show an infiltrate characteristic of pneumonia, vascular engorgement, or pulmonary edema characteristic of congestive heart failure, or the hyperinflation characteristic of obstructive lung disease. A chest x-ray can also demonstrate pleural effusions, a pneumothorax, or may show increased interstitial lung markings and the characteristic honeycomb appearance of interstitial lung disease. Patients with myocardial infarction, pulmonary embolism and acute anxiety may have normal chest x-rays.

For patients with suspected pulmonary disease, pulmonary function testing may be helpful in diagnosing obstructive or restrictive lung disease as the cause. In addition, arterial blood gases may be indicated to document respiratory status.

An electrocardiogram can help in assessing those with acute presentations of dyspnea. In addition to detecting arrhythmia, acute ST segment changes may suggest angina or myocardial infarction and the need for hospitalization. An echocardiogram can assess systolic function and detect diastolic dysfunction that may underlie pulmonary congestion and congestive heart failure. The echocardiogram can also be helpful in detection of pulmonary hypertension. Exercise stress testing may be helpful in the evaluation of cardiac abnormalities as well as exercise-induced asthma.

A complete blood count is indicated to determine the white blood count and hemoglobin. An elevated white blood cell count may suggest an underlying infectious process, such as pneumonia, as the cause for dyspnea. Anemia, especially acute anemia, may be a cause for dyspnea. If detected, further work-up to determine the cause for the anemia is indicated (see chapter 50).

In patients with episodic symptoms and a normal cardiopulmonary evaluation, gastroesophageal reflux disease (GERD) with secondary bronchospasm should be considered. Empiric therapy may be diagnostic if symptoms are relieved. For still undiagnosed patients, pulmonary referral should be considered. Finally, consideration of psychiatric causes such as anxiety and panic disorder is warranted for those patients with a normal cardiopulmonary evaluation.

MANAGEMENT

Management of dyspnea depends upon the underlying cause. For example, patients with pulmonary embolism require hospitalization and anticoagulation. Patients diagnosed with pneumonia may be treated with antibiotics as an inpatient or outpatient depending upon the severity of the disease. Those with bronchospasm require bronchodilators. Congestive heart failure should be treated acutely with diuretics and long-term as outlined in chapter 23. Therapies for chronic obstructive pulmonary disease, asthma, obesity, anxiety, anemia, and pneumonia are outlined in chapters within the remainder of this book.

◆ KEY POINTS ◆

1. The most common causes for dyspnea are cardiopulmonary diseases.
2. Chest x-ray should be obtained in most patients with dyspnea.
3. Anemia, anxiety, obesity, ascites, and kyphoscoliosis are other potential causes for dyspnea.

18 Chronic Obstructive Pulmonary Disease

The obstructive lung diseases include asthma, cystic fibrosis, bronchiectasis, and chronic obstructive pulmonary disease. Chronic obstructive pulmonary disease (COPD) is a collective term used to describe emphysema, chronic bronchitis, or both diseases. Chronic bronchitis is defined as a productive cough that occurs for at least 3 months a year for more than 2 consecutive years. Emphysema is defined as an abnormal dilatation of the terminal airspaces with destruction of alveolar septa. Thus, chronic bronchitis is defined clinically, while emphysema is defined pathologically. It is estimated that 16 million Americans are diagnosed with COPD and an equal number have the disease but are as yet undiagnosed. COPD is the fourth leading cause of death in the United States for individuals 65 to 85 years of age. Cigarette smoking is the most common cause of COPD, accounting for up to 90% of cases of COPD.

PATHOPHYSIOLOGY

The pathophysiology of COPD is not completely understood, but is thought to result from chronic inflammation. Smoking and other inhaled irritants may promote an inflammatory response in the airways resulting in mucosal edema, increased mucous production and reactive airways, characteristic of chronic bronchitis. Bronchospasm may result in airway narrowing, which along with impaired cilia function results in difficulty clearing secretions, air trapping, and alterations in gas exchange.

Similar changes may occur in patients with emphysema; however, the inflammatory response may predominantly affect the smaller airways leading to tissue destruction and loss of the normal elastic recoil of the lung. This results in increased dead space and air trapping, in essence creating functionless lung tissue where there is minimal to no air exchange.

There is great overlap between these two categories of COPD and many patients will have features of both chronic bronchitis and emphysema. In addition to cough and increased mucous production, changes that occur as a result of COPD include decreased concentration of oxygen in the blood and decreased clearance of carbon dioxide from the blood. This results in lower oxygen delivery to the various organs and can lead to compromised organ function. For example, decreased oxygen delivery to the lung tissue will result in elevation of pulmonary artery blood pressure, which can cause right-sided heart failure or cor pulmonale.

CLINICAL MANIFESTATIONS

History

The typical patient with COPD has been smoking for 10 or more years. Early in the course of the disease, COPD patients will have minimal or no symptoms. Subsequently, a productive chronic cough will develop.

With continued smoking, patients may begin to note shortness of breath with exertion. The cough and shortness of breath progress over time and ultimately the cough may become disabling and patients may have shortness of breath in the recumbent position, thus requiring them to sleep in the upright position.

Other important historical factors include smoking history, defined in pack-years (packs per day times number of years smoking), personal or family history of respiratory disorders, and exposure to second-hand smoke or environmental irritants. An assessment of the limitations in their activities may help in assessing the disease severity prior to pulmonary function testing.

Physical Examination

Physical examination will focus on the lung examination; however, chronic hypoxia may also lead to changes in other organs. The patient with COPD may appear overweight and cyanotic as typified by the "blue bloater" associated with chronic bronchitis. Alternatively, they may appear thin and barrel chested typical of the "pink puffer" associated with emphysema. Use of accessory muscles of respiration should be noted. On percussion, there is hyperresonance associated with the air trapping that is present. Auscultation may reveal diminished peripheral breath sounds due to the limited air movement. Many patients with chronic bronchitis or those with an acute exacerbation of chronic bronchitis may have rhonchi or wheezing. Skin examination may reveal the presence of cyanosis as well as clubbing of the digits. Heart sounds may be more distant due to altered chest configuration and increased air between the chest wall and the heart. In addition, presence of rhonchi and wheezing may obscure the heart sounds. With cor pulmonale and right-sided heart failure, peripheral edema, jugular venous distention, and hepatojugular reflux may be present.

DIFFERENTIAL DIAGNOSIS

Respiratory symptoms and cough may occur due to several different etiologies. In addition to COPD, upper respiratory infections, bronchitis, or pneumonia may cause shortness of breath and cough. Allergies, asthma, and cystic fibrosis are chronic conditions that typically present in childhood and may include increased cough, mucous production, shortness of breath and wheezing. Patients with decompensated congestive heart failure commonly have shortness of breath and on examination may have wheezing, rales, and peripheral edema.

Alpha-1 antitrypsin deficiency should be considered in patients less than age 45 with a family history of respiratory disease who present with features of COPD, particularly in the absence of smoking. Up to 10% of these patients will also have serious liver disease and may have findings consistent with hepatitis or cirrhosis.

DIAGNOSTIC APPROACH

Evaluation of the patient suspected of having COPD should include a detailed history and physical examination, which will provide the diagnosis in most cases. Other tests that may be performed to confirm the diagnosis and exclude other disease include chest x-ray and pulmonary function testing. In patients with a diagnosis of COPD, arterial blood gases, pulse oximetry, and an electrocardiogram may be obtained to assess disease severity and to detect cor pulmonale.

Chest x-ray findings in patients with COPD may vary depending upon the predominant component (bronchitis or emphysema). The classic findings in patients with chronic bronchitis are increased lung markings, termed *dirty-chest appearance*. In patients with predominantly emphysema, there are decreased lung markings, hyperlucency of the lung fields and flattening of the diaphragms, all consistent with the hyperinflation of the lungs that is present.

Pulmonary function testing can measure the movement of air into and out of the lungs as well as lung volumes. With COPD, there is difficulty and delay in movement of air out of the lungs, thus resulting in prolonged expiration on both physical examination and pulmonary function testing. In addition, due to the air trapping that occurs from incomplete emptying of the lungs, residual volumes are increased. The forced expiratory volume in one second (FEV1) is the measure of the maximum air that can be expired from the lung in one second after a full inspiration. The FEV1 is the most accurate and reproducible measure of outflow obstruction. This measure is significantly decreased in patients with COPD and is one of the primary measures used to assess disease severity. The FEV1 also correlates with patient symptoms and disease severity. Patients with stage 1 disease will have minimal limitations in activities and an FEV1 50% or more of their predicted FEV1 (based upon age, gender, height, and weight). Stage 2 disease occurs when patients are limited in their activities because of the COPD and they have FEV1 measures of 35% to 49% of their predicted FEV1. Patients with stage 3 disease are severely limited in activity and their FEV1 is less than 35% predicted. In patients with stage 2 or 3 disease, arterial blood gases, pulse oximetry, or electrocardiograms can be obtained and may help in management of the disease, particularly as it relates to need for supplemental oxygen use.

MANAGEMENT

Preventing the progression of disease through early identification and aggressive smoking cessation programs should be the primary goal in approaching patients with COPD. Pulmonary function testing to detect a decrease in lung function and education of the patient regarding the continued expected accelerated decline in lung function that is associated with smoking needs to be communicated to the patient. With smoking cessation, lung function will show a modest improvement initially and then follow the normal age-related decline as with non-smokers.

For patients with established COPD, goals of therapy are improvement in lung function, avoiding or reducing hospitalizations, early treatment or prevention of acute exacerbations, and minimizing disability. Smoking cessation is an important part of treatment for any smoker with COPD. In addition to smoking cessation, pulmonary rehabilitation programs can be of benefit. Although these programs do not actually improve pulmonary function testing, they enhance physical endurance and thus overall function.

Other treatments include bronchodilators, steroids, antibiotics, and oxygen. Bronchodilators, in the form of anticholinergics (e.g., ipratropium), which cause bronchodilation thorough inhibition of vagal stimulation, or beta2-agonists (e.g., albuterol) are used to treat acute exacerbations of COPD and can be used in patients who have daily symptoms. When used together, anticholinergics and beta2-agonists have a synergistic effect. For patients with daily symptoms, a long-acting beta2-agonist, salmeterol, is available for twice-daily use. Short-acting bronchodilators then can be used for breakthrough symptoms. Theophylline also has a bronchodilating effect and may increase respiratory drive.

Serum levels need to be monitored since nausea, palpitations, and seizures can result from toxic levels.

Oral steroids are used to treat acute exacerbations of COPD in a 2-week tapering dose. Long-term use of oral steroids has the potential for significant side effects and their use is not well defined. Inhaled corticosteroids may be helpful in limiting inflammation and improving airway reactivity, however, as with oral steroids their use in COPD is not clearly defined.

Antibiotics are useful for treating acute exacerbations of COPD, particularly those patients with an increase in cough and mucous production. Antibiotics commonly used include tetracyclines, sulfonamides, penicillins (e.g., amoxicillin with or without clavulanic acid), fluoroquinolones, macrolides and cephalosporins. Antibiotics should include coverage for the most common organisms associated with COPD exacerbations, namely, *S. pneumoniae*, *H. influenzae*, and *M. catarrhalis*. For those individuals requiring frequent antibiotics or with severe underlying disease, many experts recommend using fluoroquinolones for an acute exacerbation.

Patients with severe disease will often need supplemental oxygen. Candidates for oxygen supplementation are those with pO2 less than 55, pulse oximetry less than 88% and those with cor pulmonale. Continuous positive airway pressure (CPAP) use, either daily or nocturnal use, can improve the patient's functional status, oxygenation, and arterial blood gases. Use of CPAP is generally reserved for those patients with COPD who are hypercapneic. For patients with cor pulmonale and right-sided heart failure, treatment of the heart failure and diuretics may be beneficial. Immunizations, including pneumococcal and influenza vaccines, should be provided to patients with COPD.

◆ KEY POINTS ◆

1. Chronic obstructive pulmonary disease is smoking related in over 90% of cases.

2. Pulmonary function testing (FEV1) can help with assessing disease severity.

3. Smoking cessation is an important aspect of therapy for COPD.

4. Bronchodilators, steroids, antibiotics, and oxygen are the mainstays of therapy.

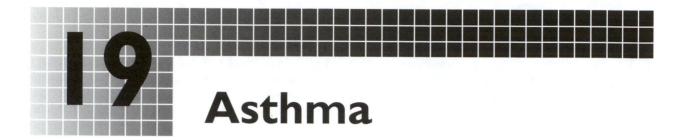

19 Asthma

Asthma is a chronic inflammatory disease of the airways that affects 5% to 7% of the U.S. population. Approximately 5 million children have asthma, which makes it the most common chronic disease of childhood, with the greatest prevalence and mortality among inner-city residents. Death rates for asthma are highest among African-American youth ages 15 to 24 years. Risk factors for mortality include a previous history of intubation, admission to the intensive care unit, two or more hospitalizations, or more than two emergency room visits in a single year. Other risk factors include the use of two canisters of short-acting B_2-agonists in a single month, an inability to perceive airway obstruction, and the use of systemic steroids.

Recognition of the importance of the underlying inflammatory process of asthma has made anti-inflammatory therapeutic agents the cornerstone of asthma management. Effective outpatient treatment of asthma can prevent exacerbations and reduce emergency room visits and hospitalizations.

PATHOPHYSIOLOGY

Asthma is caused by airway inflammation triggered by exposure to airborne allergens, irritants, cold air, or exercise. The initial event involves the degranulation of presensitized mast cells as a result of re-exposure to the triggering agents and release of inflammatory mediators (histamine, cytokines, leukotrienes, Platelet Activating Factor, etc.) that result in increased bronchiolar vascular permeability and edema, increased glandular and mucus secretions, and induction of bronchospasm and bronchoconstriction. All of this decreases the airway diameter and increases airway resistance, making it difficult to "breathe-in" air and even more difficult to "breathe-out" air. These events result in the *early-phase asthmatic response*, producing classical symptoms of wheezing, cough, and dyspnea. Degranulation of mast cells also stimulates alveolar macrophages, helper T lymphocytes (TH2) and bronchial epithelial cells to release chemotactic factors for the recruitment and activation of additional mediator-releasing leukocytes (eosinophils and neutrophils). This migration and activation of eosinophils and neutrophils occurs several hours (6–12 hours) after the mast cell degranulation phase (acute-phase reaction) and constitutes the *late-phase asthmatic response* that can last for up to 48 hours if left untreated. During this phase, the release of mediators from eosinophils causes epithelial damage, mucus hypersecretion, hyperresponsiveness of bronchial smooth muscles, as well as further airway edema, bronchiolar constriction, and mast cell degranulation. Therefore, the recruited eosinophils amplify and sustain the initial inflammatory response without additional exposure to the triggering agent.

Over time, chronic inflammation can change the morphology of the bronchioles resulting in an increase in the number of mucous-producing goblet cells at the epithelial surface, hypertrophy of submucosal mucous glands (more mucus production), thickening of basement membrane (decrease in airway compliance), edema and inflammatory infiltrates in the bronchial walls with prominence of eosinophils and hypertrophy of bronchial wall muscle. These changes in bronchiole morphology are referred to as airway *remodeling*, and are a sign of chronic long-standing airway inflammation.

CLINICAL MANIFESTATIONS

History

Patients with asthma present with symptoms of *wheezing*, *dyspnea*, *cough* and *sputum* production. In the classification of a patient's asthma, the asthma is described as being either intermittent or persistent. As outlined in Table 19–1, persistent asthma is further classified as mild, moderate, or severe. These classifications are important in determining the recommendations for the appropriate therapy.

The frequency of symptoms and presence of nocturnal symptoms are important elements of the history. In addition, identification of the triggers for the patient's asthma, their current symptoms and attempts at treatment should be determined. The past medical history should cover the onset of the disease, prescribed and over-the-counter medications, history of allergies, past hospitalizations, and the use of steroids. A history of intubation for treatment of asthma is a significant predictor of the severity and need for aggressive therapy. The family history may be significant for atopy or asthma. Assessment of the home environment, including exposure to smoke, pets, and other irritants or potential triggers is important in attempting to properly treat a patient with asthma.

Physical Examination

Vital signs may reveal tachypnea and tachycardia during acute episodes. Fever suggests an underlying viral or bacterial illness as a trigger. The physical examination focuses on the lung examination, listening for the wheezing, rhonchi, and prolonged expiration characteristic of asthma. With severe exacerbations and limited air movement, the lung fields may be deceptively quiet.

DIFFERENTIAL DIAGNOSIS

In children, conditions that can also present with wheezing, cough, and increased sputum production include

TABLE 19–1

Asthma Classifications

Classification	Symptoms	Nighttime Sx	Lung Function
Intermittent	Sx ≤2 times per week Brief exacerbations Asymptomatic between attacks	≤2 times per month	FEV_1 or PEF ≥80% predicted PEF variability <20%
Mild Persistent	Sx >2 times per *week* But <1 time a day Attacks *may* affect activity	>2 times per month	FEV_1 or PEF ≥80% predicted PEF variability 20–30%
Moderate Persistent	*Daily* Symptoms Daily use of B_2-agonists Attacks *affect* activity Exacerbations may last for days	>1 time a week	FEV_1 or PEF **60–80%** predicted PEF variability >30%
Severe Persistent	*Continual* Symptoms Limited physical activity *Frequent* attacks	Frequent	FEV_1 or PEF ≤**60%** predicted PEF variability >30%

bronchiolitis, cystic fibrosis, croup, epiglottitis, bronchitis, and foreign body aspiration. Bronchiolitis has many similarities to asthma, but presents as an acute illness and is not a chronic disease. Cystic fibrosis is a chronic disease that initially may be confused with asthma, but patients also develop gastrointestinal symptoms, growth disturbance, and recurrent sinus infections and pneumonia. Croup, epiglottitis, bronchitis and foreign body aspiration are discrete episodes and not chronic diseases. In adults, the primary diseases confused with asthma are chronic obstructive pulmonary disease and congestive heart failure. Both of these diseases have their onset in adulthood. Chronic obstructive pulmonary disease is smoking related. A chest x-ray, echocardiogram, and other testing can help to distinguish between congestive heart failure and pulmonary disease.

DIAGNOSTIC APPROACH

The history and physical examination often lead to the diagnosis of asthma. Peak flow testing can also provide additional evidence of airway obstruction and support the clinical diagnosis. Airway obstruction exists when the peak flow is less than 80% of the predicted value based upon the patient's age, height, and gender. In cases where the diagnosis is still uncertain, complete pulmonary function testing can also be obtained. A chest x-ray is recommended during the initial evaluation of the wheezing patient to detect pneumonia, a foreign body, CHF, or other non-asthmatic causes for wheezing. The chest x-ray in the asthmatic patient typically shows hyperinflation due to air trapping. In patients with suspected allergic triggers, allergy testing may be helpful. For patients with suspected cystic fibrosis, sweat testing can be a useful screen.

TREATMENT

For appropriate management, asthma can be divided into 4 categories (see Table 19–1). The goals of asthma therapy are to prevent symptoms, maintain normal pulmonary function and activity level, prevent emergency room visits and hospitalizations, and minimize the adverse effects of medications.

There are four components of effective asthma treatment:

1. Objectively assessing and monitoring lung function. This is achieved using the *Peak Expiratory Flow (PEF)* meter. PEF monitoring is advocated for patients with *moderate-to-severe persistent asthma*. Patients should first establish their personal best and then their response to PEF measurement should be based on a "color zone" system. The *green zone*, defined as more than 80% of personal best PEF, indicates good control. The *yellow zone*, between 50% and 80% of personal best, indicates the need for prompt inhaled short-acting B_2-agonists and contact with a physician about adjustments in current medication. The *red zone*, 50% or less of personal best, indicates immediate use of inhaled B_2-agonists and emergency assessment by a physician.

2. Environmental control of asthma triggers to limit exacerbations. It is imperative that patients be made aware of not only the basic facts about their disease, but also the things that trigger their asthma (i.e., "respiratory infections," pollen, change of weather, tobacco smoke, animal dander, mold, dust) so that they can take appropriate environmental control measures to limit their exposure to them.

3. Treatment for long-term management.

4. Thorough and detailed patient education. This includes basic facts about the disease and the role of medication, proper use of inhalers, establishing a plan of action for episodes of exacerbation and recognizing signs of airway obstruction.

Asthma medication is classified into *long-term control medication* (anti-inflammatory meds) to *prevent* exacerbations and the development of symptoms, and *quick-relief medication* (bronchodilators) to *treat* symptoms and exacerbations. All patients with persistent asthma need both types of medication.

Inhaled corticosteroids are the most potent and effective anti-inflammatory agents used for the long-term treatment of persistent asthma. They prevent irreversible airway injury, improve lung function, and reduce asthma deaths. Most patients can be adequately maintained on twice-daily doses. Patients should be advised to rinse their mouths with water after inhaled steroid use in order to prevent oral candidiasis. As the severity of asthma increases so does the strength of the inhaled corticosteroids. High-dose inhaled steroids used for severe asthma have been shown to interfere with the normal vertical growth of children. For this reason oral ***leukotriene inhibitors***, which have an additive effect

TABLE 19–2

Stepwise Approach to Asthma Management

		Long-term Control	Quick Relief of Sx
Step 1: Intermittent	→	No daily medication	—Short acting inhaled **B₂-agonist** (If use >2 times/wk, may need to initiate long-term treatment)
Step 2: Mild Persistent	→	One daily medication: — **Inhaled corticosteroids** (Low dose) or — **Cromolyn** or **Nedocromil** (recomm. as initial therapy in children) or — **Leukotriene** modifiers (for children >12 yo)	—Short acting inhaled **B₂-agonist** (Increasing use or Daily use may indicate the need for additional long-term control therapy.)
Step 3: Moderate Persistent	→ →	One daily medication: — **Inhaled corticosteroids** (Moderate Dose) or Two daily Medications: — **Inhaled corticosteroids** (Low-moderate dose) and **Long acting Bronchodilators** (salmeterol, leukotriene modifier, sustained-release theophylline)	—Short acting inhaled **B₂-agonist** (Increasing use or Daily use may indicate the need for additional long-term control therapy.)
Step 4: Severe Persistent	→	Daily medications: — **Inhaled corticosteroids** (High-dose) and **Long acting Bronchodilators** (salmeterol, leukotriene modifier, sustained-release theophylline) and **Oral corticosteroids** (daily dose of 2 mg/kg) (**max dose 60 mg/day**)	— Short acting inhaled B₂-agonist (Increasing use or Daily use may indicate the need for additional long-term control therapy.)

when given in conjunction with inhaled steroids, can be added to low-moderate dose inhaled corticosteroids, in order to reduce the need for high-dose steroids.

Cromolyn Sodium and *Nedocromil* are mast cell stabilizers, preventing mast cell degranulation, in addition to inhibiting bronchoconstriction. They have mild to moderate anti-inflammatory effects and are relatively safe to use in children and pregnant women with mild persistent asthma. They are also effective agents against exercise-induced asthma in a single inhaled dose taken 15 to 30 minutes before exercise.

Salmeterol is a long-acting B_2-agonist and useful in the management of nocturnal symptoms and exercise-induced asthma. It is more effective than nedocromil in the treatment of exercise-induced asthma since its duration of action is 9 hours as opposed to 2 to 3 hours for Nedocromil. It is also useful as additive therapy to low-dose inhaled corticosteroids to avoid high-dose steroids. Studies have shown that salmeterol combined with low-dose steroids is more efficacious in improving symptoms and reducing the use of rescue medication than simply doubling the dose of inhaled steroids.

Oral (systemic) corticosteroids are recommended and effective as "burst" therapy for gaining initial control of asthma when initiating therapy or during an acute exacerbation. One method of burst therapy is to give prednisone (adults 40–60 mg/day, children 1–2 mg/kg/day) for 3 to 10 days or until PEF improves to 80% of personal best. Long-term use of oral steroids should only be considered for patients refractory to all other therapies due to their potential for side effects and growth retardation.

Anticholinergics for asthma include inhaled Ipratropium (Atrovent), which inhibits vagally mediated bronchoconstriction and mucous production. It is effective when used in conjunction with short-acting B_2-agonist for treatment of severe asthma exacerbations.

Non-adherence and poor asthma control are usually related to either inadequate understanding of the disease and its treatment, improper use of inhaled medication, lack of environmental control of asthma triggers (i.e., outdoor allergens, tobacco smoke, animal dander, dust, cockroaches, molds) or lack of continuity of care. Patient education remains the cornerstone of a successful asthma management strategy; increasing patient involvement and fostering a strong partnership between the patient, their families and the physician. This relationship is imperative for the adherence of the patient not only to the treatment regimen but also to the continuous follow-up with his or her primary care physician.

For step-wise approach for managing asthma refer to Table 19–2.

◆ KEY POINTS ◆

1. Asthma is a chronic inflammatory respiratory condition (*Type-I hypersensitivity reaction*).
2. Asthma can be classified into intermittent, mild-persistent, moderate-persistent, and severe-persistent.
3. Short-term control includes short-acting inhaled bronchodilators (B_2-agonists), and long-term control includes inhaled corticosteroids.
4. The early-phase inflammatory process is mediated by mast cells and the late-phase mediated by eosinophils.
5. The symptoms of asthma include cough, wheezing, and dyspnea.
6. Pathophysiology of asthma includes airway edema, increase in mucus production, and bronchospasm.
7. Intermittent asthma does not need daily medication.
8. Persistent asthma is controlled by inhaled corticosteroids as well as short-acting inhaled bronchodilators.

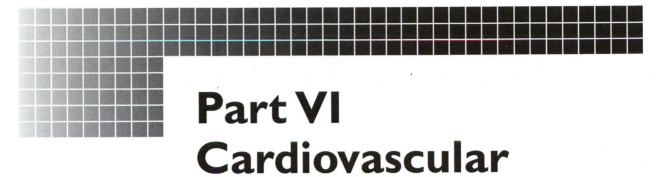

Part VI
Cardiovascular
Diseases

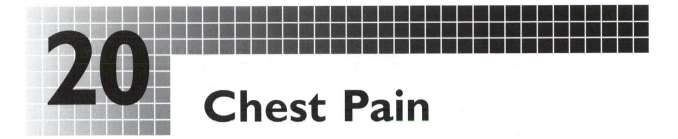

20 Chest Pain

The primary concern for patients with chest pain is whether or not the pain is of cardiac origin. In addition to cardiac disease, chest pain may be due to pulmonary, gastrointestinal (GI), musculoskeletal, or psychological diseases. Emergent causes of chest pain include myocardial infarction (MI), aortic dissection, pulmonary embolus, and pneumothorax. Patients with these diagnoses usually present to the emergency room, but may on occasion present in the outpatient setting. Chest pain in the office setting is most commonly due to musculoskeletal, gastrointestinal, and cardiac causes. Approximately 13% of patients with chest pain do not fit into any diagnostic category and remain undiagnosed, despite evaluation.

PATHOPHYSIOLOGY

Chest pain may emanate from inflammation or injury to the structures in and around the thoracic cavity. Muscular chest pain is common and may occur when there is inflammation from overuse or injury to the muscles of the chest wall. The costochondral joints may also become inflamed from overuse, injury, or in association with viral illnesses. Rib fractures may produce significant pain and generally result from trauma, but may also occur as a result of metastatic cancer.

Gastroesophageal reflux disease and esophageal motility disorders are common causes of chest pain. The reflux of acidic gastric contents into the lower esopha-gus may produce esophagitis and chest pain indistinguishable from cardiac chest pain. The symptoms of gastritis and peptic ulcer disease may also be perceived by some patients as a substernal pain. Cholelithiasis and cholecystitis, which usually cause right upper quadrant pain, may also produce substernal pain.

Cardiac chest pain results from an insufficient oxygen supply to myocardial tissue, usually from coronary artery disease. The initial step in the development of atherosclerotic heart disease is the fatty streak. Over time, the fatty streak can enlarge into a calcified plaque, eventually narrowing the vessel lumen and impairing blood flow. If the plaque ruptures, lipids and tissue factors are released from the plaque triggering a series of events that ultimately result in intravascular thrombosis and myocardial infarction. If the plaque doesn't rupture, a gradual narrowing of the lumen can cause anginal chest pain. This chest pain is typically brought on by exertion as the myocardial oxygen demand exceeds the supply.

Since lung tissue does not have pain fibers, inflammation or irritation of the parietal pleura is responsible for the chest pain from pulmonary diseases such as pneumonia or pulmonary embolus.

Other causes for chest pain include psychological disease and neurologic diseases, such as herpes zoster or cervical or thoracic radiculopathies. Patients with herpes zoster may experience pain before the rash appears. Disc herniation or osteoarthritic narrowing of cervical or thoracic foramen may result in nerve compression and chest pain following a radicular pattern. Patients with psychological disease, such as anxiety and panic disorder, may present with a variety of chest symptoms including palpitations, dyspnea, and chest pain as part of their symptom complex.

CLINICAL PRESENTATION

History

Patients with chest pain should be asked about the severity, quality, location, duration, aggravating factors, relieving factors, radiation of pain, and other associated symptoms. Myocardial pain is often described as substernal chest tightness or pressure that radiates to the left arm, shoulders, or the jaw. Patients may also complain of diaphoresis, shortness of breath, nausea, and vomiting. Anginal pain is typically brought on by exercise, eating, or emotional excitement. The pain usually lasts from 5 to 15 minutes and disappears with rest or nitroglycerin. Pain that lasts less than 1 minute or longer than 30 minutes should not be considered anginal. Pericardial pain is often persistent, sharp, severe, and relieved by sitting up. Breathing, lying back, or coughing may aggravate the pain. The pain of aortic dissection is anterior, severe, and often has a ripping or tearing quality with radiation to the back or abdomen.

Tracheobronchitis may cause a burning pain in the upper sternal area associated with a productive cough. Pain with pneumonia commonly occurs in the overlying chest wall and is aggravated by breathing and coughing. In pneumothorax, the pain is of sudden onset, sharp, unilateral, pleuritic and is associated with shortness of breath. Pleurisy is a sharp pleuritic chest pain, often in association with a preceding viral illness.

GERD causes a burning pain that radiates up the sternum. It is worsened by large meals and lying down. Antacids may relieve the pain. The pain of esophageal spasm, which is usually associated with swallowing, may be indistinguishable from cardiac pain. Since nitroglycerin relaxes smooth muscle, nitroglycerin may relieve the pain.

Musculoskeletal pain from costochondritis can often be reproduced on palpation. Patients are also reluctant to take a deep breath since this aggravates the pain.

Patients with generalized anxiety will often complain of chest pain. However, this pain is non-specific. Associated symptoms include overwhelming fear, palpitations, breathlessness, and tachypnea.

Physical Examination

Vital signs can provide clues to the urgency of the patient's complaints. Hypotension can occur with myocardial ischemia, pericardial tamponade, pulmonary embolus, and gastrointestinal bleeding. Tachycardia may indicate severe illness and arrhythmias can occur with cardiac or pulmonary causes for chest pain. The presence of fever suggests an infectious cause, such as pneumonia. Inspection and palpation may reveal ecchymosis from an injury, the rash of shingles, crepitus associated with rib fractures, and the tenderness of musculoskeletal chest pain.

A thorough cardiopulmonary exam is warranted for all patients with chest pain. Patients with myocardial ischemia may have an audible S4 or signs of congestive heart failure, such as an S3 and pulmonary rales. Pericarditis may cause a friction rub and pulsus paradoxus. In severe cases, pericarditis may cause an effusion resulting in cardiac tamponade. Beck's triad, consisting of jugular venous distention, muffled heart sounds, and decreased blood pressure suggests cardiac tamponade. In aortic dissection patients may have hypotension, absence of peripheral pulses, and a murmur of aortic insufficiency. Patients with pneumonia will have crackles on inspiration, dullness to percussion, and egophony indicating consolidation. Signs of pneumothorax include hyperresonance to percussion, tracheal deviation, decreased breath sounds, and decreased tactile and vocal fremitus. Patients with pulmonary embolism will likely have normal auscultatory findings, but may be tachycardic, tachypneic, and have lower extremity edema.

Patients with acute cholecystitis may have right upper quadrant abdominal tenderness. GERD and gastritis will often have epigastric pain on deep palpation. Esophageal spasm and psychogenic chest pain typically do not produce abnormal physical findings.

DIFFERENTIAL DIAGNOSIS

Common causes for chest pain are presented in Box 20–1. In the outpatient setting, musculoskeletal disease is present in over one-third of patients with chest pain. Gastrointestinal disease occurs in approximately

BOX 20–1

Causes of Chest Pain

Cardiac chest pain
    Myocardial infarction
    Angina pectoris
    Pericarditis
    Aortic dissection
Pulmonary causes of chest pain
    Pulmonary embolus
    Pneumothorax
    Pneumonia
    Tracheobronchitis
Musculoskeletal causes
    Costochondritis

Muscular strain
Gastrointestinal causes
    GERD
    Esophageal spasm
    Cholelithiasis
Psychogenic causes
    Somatization disorders
    Anxiety disorders (including panic disorder)
Neurogenic causes
    Herpes zoster
    Cervical or thoracic disease

20% of patients seen in the office with chest pain, followed in frequency by cardiac, psychogenic, and pulmonary causes. Cardiac and pulmonary disease, though not the most common in the outpatient setting, need to be considered in any patient presenting with chest pain due to the potentially life-threatening diseases they represent.

DIAGNOSTIC APPROACH

The history and physical helps classify the chest pain into cardiac, pulmonary, GI, musculoskeletal, or psychogenic causes. An EKG is a critical element for evaluating anyone with possible cardiac chest pain. Although an EKG can be normal in patients with heart disease, ST elevation or depression is indicative of myocardial ischemia. Diffuse ST elevation is consistent with pericarditis while Q waves can indicate an old or recent myocardial infarction. Serial cardiac markers are useful for determining if a myocardial infarction is present. Creatine phosphokinase (CPK) level is a sensitive test for MI. CPK levels begin to rise within 4 hours and peak at 24 hours. Other markers of cardiac injury include troponin and myoglobin. Troponins are the first enzymes to rise and remain elevated for 5 to 14 days. They are the most sensitive and specific for myocardial infarction. Any patient with suspected myocardial infarction, unstable angina or pulmonary embolism should be hospitalized for evaluation.

In stable patients with suspected cardiac disease, outpatient exercise stress testing is indicated. Patients should have a baseline EKG to detect abnormalities such as a conduction defect or strain pattern that make interpreting a stress test difficult. Patients with baseline EKG abnormalities or a positive exercise stress test should undergo radionuclide testing, a stress echo, and/or coronary angiography.

An echocardiogram can detect wall motion abnormalities in areas damaged from ischemic myocardial disease, pericardial effusions, and valvular heart disease. If the cause of pericarditis is not evident, an antinuclear antibody, blood urea nitrogen, TSH, and tuberculosis skin test are indicated.

A chest x-ray can detect pneumonia, pneumothorax or other lung pathology. If pulmonary embolus is suspected, a ventilation-perfusion scan or a spiral CT scan is indicated. Patients with pulmonary embolus should also have a venous Doppler to rule out deep venous thrombosis.

Patients suspected of having musculoskeletal chest pain might not require any diagnostic testing. Evaluation for GI causes is discussed in part VII.

TREATMENT

Patients who present with myocardial infarction should be stabilized initially with oxygen, nitroglycerin, and morphine for pain control. Aspirin has been shown to reduce the mortality from acute myocardial infarction and as a result should be given as soon as possible. In patients who are allergic to aspirin, ticlopidine may be used. Other drugs used to treat an acute MI include beta-blockers, heparin, ACE inhibitors, and thrombolytics. Thrombolytics should be administered within 6 hours of onset of chest pain, although patients may benefit up to12 hours after the onset of pain. Contraindications for thrombolytics include active internal bleeding, history of cerebrovascular disease, recent surgery, intracranial neoplasm, arteriovenous malformation, aneurysm, bleeding diathesis, or severe uncontrolled hypertension.

Patients with stable angina may be treated in the outpatient setting and started on aspirin and sublingual nitroglycerin for angina episodes. Beta-blockers reduce the frequency of symptoms, increase anginal threshold, and reduce the risk of a subsequent MI in patients with a previous MI. Long-acting nitrates reduce anginal pain but do not increase longevity and require a daily nitrate-free period to avoid tolerance.

Aortic dissection is an emergency and requires hospitalization and surgical consultation. Pericarditis may improve with aspirin or other non-steroidal anti-inflammatory drugs (NSAIDs). Steroids should be considered in severe cases. Pulmonary embolus requires anticoagulation. Warfarin is started concomitantly with heparin and once the INR reaches the therapeutic level, heparin may be discontinued. A smaller pneumothorax (<30%) in a stable individual can be managed conservatively; a larger pneumothorax requires chest tube insertion. Treatment for patients with pneumonia or bronchitis is outlined in chapter 35. Costochondritis is treated with NSAIDs. Management for GERD and gastrointestinal causes for chest pain are outlined in chapter 28. Psychogenic disorders are discussed in part XV.

◆ KEY POINTS ◆

1. Chest pain can be due to pulmonary, gastrointestinal (GI), cardiac, musculoskeletal, or psychological causes.

2. The most common emergent causes of chest pain include myocardial infarction (MI), unstable angina, aortic dissection, pulmonary embolus, and pneumothorax.

3. Cardiac chest pain that lasts more than 30 minutes is most probably secondary to infarction.

4. The Beck's triad of jugular venous distention, muffled heart sounds, and decreased blood pressure indicates cardiac tamponade.

5. Signs of pneumothorax include hyperresonance to percussion, tracheal deviation, decreased breath sounds, and decreased tactile and vocal fremitus.

6. A patient who presents with myocardial infarction should be stabilized initially with oxygen, nitroglycerin, and morphine for pain control.

7. Contraindications for thrombolytics include active internal bleeding, history of cerebrovascular disease, recent surgery, intracranial neoplasm, arteriovenous malformation, aneurysm, bleeding diathesis, or severe uncontrolled hypertension.

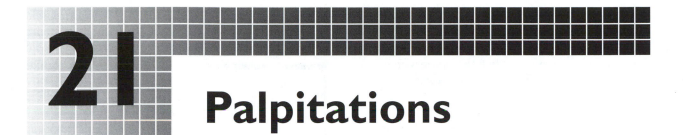

21 Palpitations

Palpitations are an abnormal awareness of the heartbeat. The patient may describe the sensation as a fluttering, skipping, pounding, or racing sensation. The causes for palpitations range from benign conditions requiring no therapy to life-threatening conditions requiring urgent monitoring, treatment and referral.

PATHOPHYSIOLOGY

Normally, individuals are unaware of the 60 to 100 heartbeats that occur each minute. Awareness of the heartbeat may occur when there are changes in the rate, rhythm, or contractility of the heart. Palpitations may occur as a result of cardiac or endocrine disease, an increase in sympathetic tone, or medications. Patients with underlying cardiac disease, such as valvular heart disease or a cardiomyopathy may have altered conduction within the cardiac chambers or an increased automaticity of foci within the heart leading to tachycardias such as atrial fibrillation or flutter. Disease within the conduction system may alter conduction of the cardiac impulses resulting in either a bradycardia or tachycardia. If impulses are blocked, then a bradycardia will result. If a reentrant circuit is present, then a tachycardia may result.

Hyperthyroidism results in increased metabolism and a hyperkinetic state. Tachycardia and palpitations are a frequent symptom associated with this disease. Pheochromocytoma is a rare adrenal disorder in which there are excess circulating catecholamines. The catecholamines can cause sympathetic overstimulation resulting in tachycardia and palpitations. Psychiatric conditions, such as anxiety, panic disorder, and depression are also associated with increased sympathetic tone. Other medical non-cardiac causes for palpitations include anemia and dehydration or hypovolemia.

Medications can cause disturbances in cardiac conduction. Common medications associated with palpitations include theophylline, digoxin, beta-agonists, over-the-counter stimulants such as pseudoephedrine, and antiarrhythmic medications. Alcohol, tobacco, and illicit drugs such as cocaine can also cause palpitations.

CLINICAL MANIFESTATIONS

History

The patient's description of symptoms and associated complaints such as lightheadedness, dizziness, or syncope is important. Patients with dizziness, near-syncope, or syncope may warrant hospitalization, monitoring, and aggressive evaluation. The onset and duration of symptoms may give clues to the cause. Paroxysmal episodes that begin abruptly and resolve abruptly are characteristic of paroxysmal atrial fibrillation or supraventricular tachycardia. Isolated extra or pounding beats are characteristic of PVCs or PACs. The duration of symptoms, as well as provocative or palliative factors, may help in determining the cause.

For example, sinus tachycardia and supraventricular tachycardias may be associated with exertion or emotional upset, whereas benign premature atrial or ventricular contractions will often disappear with exertion. The history should include inquiry about a history of heart disease, hypertension, thyroid disease or anemia. Medication use should be reviewed for possible toxicity or side effects. Diabetics may experience palpitations with hypoglycemic reactions. Patients taking stimulants by prescription or illicitly may experience palpitations as side effects. Alcohol use is associated with supraventricular tachycardia and atrial fibrillation. A review of systems should include assessment for other cardiac symptoms, pulmonary disease, abnormal bleeding, and symptoms suggestive of either thyroid or adrenal disease.

Physical Examination

Physical examination should include assessment of orthostatic pulse, blood pressure, and temperature. When taking the pulse, note should be made of the rate and any irregularity or extra beats. Pallor suggests anemia and exophthalmos or a goiter–hyperthyroidism. Special attention should be paid to the cardiopulmonary examination including not only the rhythm, but also the presence of rubs, murmurs, clicks, and gallops. A mental status exam, looking for signs of anxiety disorders, depression, or substance abuse—may provide clues to non-cardiac etiologies for palpitations.

DIFFERENTIAL DIAGNOSIS

Box 21–1 lists the differential diagnosis for palpitations and includes both cardiac and non-cardiac etiologies. A detailed history may suggest potential etiologies. For example, isolated extra heartbeats suggest PACs or PVCs as the cause. Sudden onset and cessation of episodes of palpitations suggests paroxysmal supraventricular tachycardia. A less abrupt onset and cessation of palpitations are more common with stimulant use or medication use. Sustained symptoms are associated with fever, dehydration, hyperthyroidism, or anemia.

DIAGNOSTIC APPROACH

Initial laboratory testing should include a hemoglobin, electrolytes, and thyroid stimulating hormone. Patients on medications such as digoxin should have levels

---

BOX 21–1

Causes for Palpitations

Cardiac
- —PVCs
- —PACs
- —Paroxysmal supraventricular tachycardia
- —Atrial fibrillation
- —Multifocal atrial tachycardia
- —Ventricular tachycardia
- —Mitral valve prolapse
- —Sick sinus syndrome (tachycardia-bradycardia syndrome)
- —Cardiomyopathy
- —Prolonged QT interval syndrome
- —Ischemic heart disease
- —Wolff-Parkinson-White syndrome

Non-cardiac
- —Exertion
- —Anxiety
- —Medications:
  - Theophylline
  - Beta-agonists
  - Pseudoephedrine
  - Antiarrhythmic drugs
  - Tricyclic antidepressants
  - Phenothiazines
  - Stimulants/cocaine
- —Alcohol
- —Tobacco
- —Caffeine
- —Hypoglycemia
- —Hyperthyroidism
- —Pheochromocytoma
- —Anemia
- —Electrolyte imbalance
- —Dehydration
- —Fever
- —Pregnancy
- —Panic disorder
- —Somatization
- —Hyperventilation

checked. Blood glucose should be checked in diabetic patients. In selected patients, screening for a pheochromocytoma by measuring urine and serum catecholamines may be warranted.

Cardiac evaluation begins with a 12-lead electrocardiogram which may detect an arrhythmia or abnormalities associated with arrhythmias. For example, a short PR interval and a delta wave occur with Wolff-Parkinson-White, which is associated with paroxysmal supraventricular tachycardias. Abnormalities in atrial or ventricular voltages and Q waves may signify presence of underlying cardiac disease.

Further cardiac evaluation often includes echocardiography to assess cardiac anatomy. Information can be gained about atrial and ventricular size, valvular abnormalities, ventricular systolic function and whether hypertrophic subaortic stenosis or wall motion abnormalities are present. A 24-hour Holter monitor records the cardiac rhythm for 24 hours and can detect an arrhythmia. During this period, the patient keeps a log of symptoms, and correlation with the monitor recording will show the heart's rhythm at the time of symptoms. For patients who do not have daily symptoms or for the patient who did not have symptoms while the monitor is being worn, an event monitor may be an effective tool. Event monitors can be carried for 30 days or more and are patient activated at the time of symptoms. The event recording can be transmitted by telephone to a monitoring station.

Stress testing should be considered for patients who have symptoms in association with exercise or who describe chest pain or pressure. Finally, invasive electrophysiologic study should be considered in syncopal or near-syncopal patients with heart disease, and those with suspected ventricular tachycardia or heart block. Electrophysiologic study may document the abnormality and direct therapy.

MANAGEMENT

Therapy will be directed by the underlying cause for the palpitations. Patients with anemia will need further evaluation for the cause of the anemia. Angioplasty or bypass surgery may be required for individuals with severe coronary artery disease. Treatment of underlying hyperthyroidism, anxiety, infection, and dehydration will resolve symptoms in patients affected with these diseases. For many patients, adjustment of medication or insulin dosages and avoiding stimulants such as caffeine may resolve symptoms. Treatment of supraventricular tachycardias may include use of medications (beta-blockers or calcium channel blockers) or catheter ablation of any identified bypass tracts. Patients with chronic or intermittent atrial fibrillation usually merit anticoagulation with coumadin to prevent thromboembolism. Younger, low-risk patients with atrial fibrillation (no hypertension, congestive heart failure [CHF], coronary artery disease, or history of transient ischemic attacks [TIAs] or a cerebrovascular accident [CVA]) may be treated with aspirin. Malignant ventricular arrhythmias may be treated with antiarrhythmics along with implantation of an automatic implantable cardiac defibrillator. Isolated PVCs or PACs do not require treatment, but may be treated for symptom relief with medications such as beta-blockers. If an antiarrhythmic drug is used, consultation with a cardiologist is often helpful since therapy can be complex and arrhythmia is a side effect of many of these drugs.

◆ KEY POINTS ◆

1. Palpitations are an abnormal awareness of the heartbeat, either in terms of rate or intensity of the perceived heartbeat.

2. Palpitations may occur due to the presence of cardiac or endocrine disease, increase in sympathetic tone, fever, dehydration, or medications.

3. Cardiac evaluation should include a 12-lead electrocardiogram, echocardiography, monitoring (Holter, event monitor) and in selected patients stress testing or electrophysiologic study.

4. Therapy is directed by the identified underlying cause.

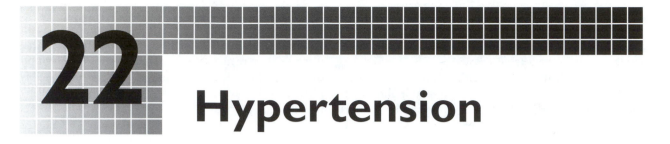

22 Hypertension

Hypertension is defined as a systolic blood pressure greater than or equal to 140 or diastolic pressure greater than or equal to 90. It affects 43 million Americans (24% of the adult population) and remains a major risk factor for the development of cardiovascular disease and cerebrovascular disease. Prevalence increases with age, such that by the age of 60, hypertension is present in approximately 71% of African-Americans, 61% of Mexican-Americans and 60% of non-Hispanic whites.

PATHOPHYSIOLOGY

Hypertension (HTN) can be either primary (essential), or secondary. Primary hypertension accounts for 90% to 95% of all cases of HTN. Primary hypertension is a complex process that results from a variety of physiologic and environmental factors that lead to an elevated blood pressure. Secondary hypertension causes about 5% to 10% of all adult hypertension and includes exogenous substances (e.g., stimulants, alcohol, NSAIDs), renal failure, sleep apnea, renovascular disease, primary aldosteronism, pheochromocytoma, and Cushings syndrome.

Insulin resistance is also associated with increased arterial blood pressure. Hyperinsulinemia can increase vascular tone by any of four mechanisms: (1) promoting Na+ retention, (2) promoting hypertrophy or hyperplasia of vascular smooth muscles through its mitogenic properties, (3) modifying ion transport leading to an increase in intracellular calcium and (4) sympathetic activation.

Poorly controlled hypertension leads to complications or damage in several target organs. Clinical manifestations include ischemic heart disease, stroke, peripheral vascular disease, renal insufficiency, retinopathy characterized by exudates or hemorrhages, and in severe hypertension, papilledema.

CLINICAL MANIFESTATIONS

History

Hypertension is referred to as the "silent killer" because it is generally asymptomatic until there is end organ damage. Hypertension is usually diagnosed during a routine office visit screening.

The history for hypertensive individuals should focus on symptoms of end organ damage, additional risk factors for cardiovascular disease and secondary causes of hypertension. It is essential to ask about cardiovascular symptoms, such as chest pain, shortness of breath, prior transient ischemic attacks or strokes and renal disease. Inquiring about a family history of heart disease, hypertension, hyperlipidemia, diabetes and renal disease is important. Additional behavioral risk factors such as tobacco and alcohol use, exercise and dietary habits should be elicited.

Features of the history that suggest a secondary cause include the following:

1. Early or late onset of HTN (younger than 20 and older than 50 years of age)

2. An associated history of tachychardia, sweating, and headache

3. A personal or family history of renal disease

4. Resistant hypertension in a compliant patient

5. History of amphetamine, cocaine, or alcohol abuse

6. Use of oral contraceptives, estrogens, cortico-steroids, NSAIDs

7. History of hirsutism or easy bruising

Physical Examination

The diagnosis of hypertension requires an elevated blood pressure (systolic blood pressures [SBP] ≥140 or diastolic blood pressures [DBP] ≥90 mm Hg) on at least *two consecutive visits* of at least *1* to 2 weeks apart. The exceptions are one SBP greater than or equal to 210, one DBP greater than or equal to 120, or the presence of significant end organ damage at the time of the first reading. Because several factors such as pain, fear, anxiety, physical activity, and exogenous substances or medication can influence blood pressure readings, a standard approach needs to be followed to ensure accurate blood pressure readings and avoid incorrectly labeling a patient as hypertensive (Box 22–1).

Additional elements of the physical examination include the *skin* exam looking for signs of Cushings syndrome or neurofibromatosis; *fundoscopy* looking for retinal hemorrhages, increased vascular tortuosity, "A-V nicking"; checking the *thyroid* for enlargement or nodularity; auscultating the *carotids* for bruits; listening to the *lungs* for signs of heart failure; palpating the *chest* for displacement of the PMI (suggestive of cardiomegaly); listening to the *heart* for murmurs and S3 or S4 heart sounds; examining the *abdomen* for bruits or masses; conducting a *neurologic* exam for focal deficits; and checking the *extremities* for pulses and the presence of edema.

BOX 22–1

Essentials of Blood Pressure Measurement

1. Seated at rest for 5 minutes

2. No caffeine or cigarettes in preceding 30 minutes

3. Bladder of blood pressure cuff encircles 80% of arm

4. Arm supported at heart level

5. Inflate cuff and determine systolic range by palpably checking for obliteration of radial pulse

6. Auscultate over brachial artery after inflating cuff 10–20 mmHg above palpable systolic pressure

7. Systolic pressure = onset of Korotkoff sounds

8. Diastolic = muffling or cessation of Korotkoff sounds

---

reading as well as "white coat" hypertension and "pseudohypertension."

Primary hypertension tends to run in families and the physical examination and laboratory screening do not identify a specific etiology for the elevated blood pressure. Although secondary hypertension accounts for only 5% of hypertensive individuals, it is important to identify these cases because they are potentially curable.

"White coat" hypertension and pseudohypertension are conditions where the patient does not truly have hypertension, but the blood pressure is elevated under the conditions or time it is being measured. For example, with white coat hypertension, the patient's blood pressure is elevated in the physician's office, but not at other times. In pseudohypertension, the patient is generally elderly, has calcified rigid blood vessels, and the intraarterial blood pressure is actually less than what can be measured with the blood pressure cuff.

DIFFERENTIAL DIAGNOSIS

The differential diagnosis generally involves distinguishing between primary hypertension and secondary hypertension. Additional considerations in evaluating elevated blood pressure readings are transient factors, such as stress or an acute illness causing the elevated

DIAGNOSTIC APPROACH

Once the diagnosis of hypertension has been made, four main questions must be addressed.

1. Is this HTN primary (essential) or secondary?

2. How many risk factors are present?

3. Is there evidence of target organ damage?

4. Are there any comorbid conditions that would affect the choice of therapy?

Laboratory and diagnostics are indicated to assess end organ damage, identify additional cardiovascular risk factors, to exclude secondary causes, and to assist in choice of medications. A *CBC* is recommended as a baseline for future evaluation in the event of medication-induced neutropenia or agranulocytosis. A *fasting serum glucose*, K+, serum *creatinine*, *urinalysis*, total *cholesterol* and *HDL* are recommended for newly diagnosed hypertensive patients. A high fasting serum glucose can indicate diabetes mellitus, unprovoked hypokalemia (<3.5 mEq/L) suggests hyperaldosteronism, an elevated creatinine may indicate renal insufficiency, and proteinuria or microalbuminuria may indicate renal end organ damage. Two other recommended tests are serum calcium (with albumin) and uric acid, since hypercalcemia or hyperuricemia may preclude the use of thiazide diuretics.

An *electrocardiogram* (ECG) is helpful in assessing for prior myocardial infarction (MI), heart block or left ventricular hypertrophy. A plain *chest x-ray* can detect cardiomegaly and rule out the remote possibility of coarctation of the aorta. In patients with suspected white coat hypertension, ambulatory blood pressure monitoring may help determine whether hypertension is an appropriate diagnosis.

MANAGEMENT

Once the diagnosis of hypertension has been established, treatment should be initiated. The 6th report of the Joint National Committee on Detection, Evaluation and Treatment of High Blood Pressure in 1997 classified HTN into three stages (Table 22–1).

The first step for non-diabetic patients with Stage 1 HTN is lifestyle modifications. About 60% of hypertensive patients are salt sensitive and may benefit from *sodium restriction* (<4 g/day) by avoiding added salt, and salty and processed food. Other lifestyle changes include *weight reduction*, regular aerobic *exercise* (30–60 minute sessions 3–4 times/week), *limiting alcohol* intake (<24 oz beer/day, <8 oz of wine/day, <2 oz of whisky/day), and *increasing dietary potassium*. Lifestyle modification alone effectively controls about 10% of patients.

If patients remain hypertensive after 3 to 6 months of lifestyle modifications, starting antihypertensive medication is appropriate. Patients with Stage 2 and 3

TABLE 22–1

Stages of Hypertension

Stage	Systolic Pressure Range	Diastolic Pressure Range
Optimal	<120	<80
Normal	120–129	80–84
High-normal	130–139	85–89
Stage 1	140–159	90–99
Stage 2	160–179	100–109
Stage 3	≥180	≥110

HTN and diabetic patients with systolic BP over 130 or diastolic BP over 85 warrant earlier initiation of pharmacologic therapy in addition to lifestyle recommendations. The therapeutic goal for non-diabetics is a blood pressure less than 140/90 mmHg, however, in diabetic individuals the goal is less than 130/85 mmHg. Isolated systolic hypertension (SBP ≥160 mmHg) is a common form of hypertension in the elderly. The Systolic Hypertension in the Elderly Program (SHEP) demonstrated that treating patients over 60 with isolated systolic hypertension (Stage 2) using low dose diuretics and beta-blockers significantly reduces the incidence of strokes and MIs in patients.

The four classes of medications that are most commonly used as first-line agents are diuretics, beta-blockers, calcium channel blockers, and angiotensin converting enzyme inhibitors.

Diuretics

Thiazides were the first major drugs introduced for the treatment of HTN and are still the most widely used. They inhibit Na+ reabsorption from the renal tubules and thus reduce total blood volume. In addition, they blunt the effect of endogenous vasoconstrictors on the vascular smooth muscles, causing a decrease in peripheral vascular resistance. Thiazides are useful in patients without renal impairment (glomerular filtration rate [GFR]>25 or creatinine levels <2 and <1.5 in the elderly). Although thiazides may cause adverse metabolic side effects, such as hypokalemia, hyperuricemia, carbohydrate intolerance, and hyperlipidemia, these side effects can be held to a minimum if the dose is kept below the equivalent of 25 mg/day of hydrochlorothiazide (*HCTZ*). Most patients can be successfully treated with 12.5 to 25 mg of

HCTZ. Side effects include sexual dysfunction, dyslipidemia, hyperglycemia, and elevations in uric acid levels.

For patients with renal impairment (Cr>2–2.5), loop *diuretics* (i.e., furosemide) are more effective. They tend to produce more diuresis and hypokalemia than thiazides. Concomitant use of NSAIDs interferes with the delivery of loop diuretics to their site of action. Loop diuretics tend to lower serum calcium, whereas thiazides tend to cause hypercalcemia.

Before diuretics are administered, the serum K+ level should be checked and monitored periodically after initiating diuretic therapy.

Beta-Blockers

Beta adrenergic receptor blockers work by decreasing heart rate and cardiac contractility. In addition, they modulate central and peripheral sympathetic nervous system output and decrease release of renin from the juxtaglomerular apparatus. Their renin-mediated mechanism of action may account for the decreased responsiveness in "low-renin" patients (elderly, African-Americans).

Within the beta-blocker class of medications, there are nonselective and selective beta-receptor blockers. Nonselective agents block both beta-1 and beta-2 receptors, whereas selective agents block only beta-1 receptors. Use of a selective agent is indicated in patients with a history of reactive airway disease where the selectivity may lessen the likelihood of medication-induced bronchospasm. In addition to selective and nonselective subcategories, there are beta-blockers with intrinsic sympathomimetic activity (ISA). Beta-blockers with ISA are thought to be less likely to elevate triglycerides and lower HDL cholesterol and cause less of a decrease in heart rate.

Side effects of beta-blockers include bradycardia, fatigue, insomnia, sexual dysfunction, and adverse effects on the lipid profile. Beta-blockers should be avoided or used cautiously in patients with asthma, chronic obstructive pulmonary disease, second or third degree heart block, peripheral vascular disease, and insulin dependent diabetes mellitus. Sudden withdrawal of these medications should be avoided as it can cause tachyarrhythmias and rebound hypertension due to upregulation of beta-receptors associated with chronic therapy.

Angiotensin Converting Enzyme Inhibitors

Angiotensin converting enzyme (ACE) inhibitors act through the renin-angiotensin system by inhibiting the enzyme that converts angiotensin I to angiotensin II. ACE inhibitors are particularly beneficial in patients with congestive heart failure and provide renal protection for those with diabetes. Patients epidemiologically associated with "low-renin" states, such as the elderly and African-American populations, may be less likely to respond to the antihypertensive effects of these medications. ACE inhibitors are generally well tolerated; the most common side effect is cough. Other less-common but serious reactions include angioedema and neutropenia. In those with renal artery stenosis ACE inhibitors may cause an acute reversible renal failure.

Calcium Channel Blockers

Calcium channel blockers include diltiazem, verapamil, and the dihydropyridines. Calcium channel blockers lower blood pressure through a peripheral vasodilatory action. Diltiazem and verapamil depress the AV node and myocardial contractility. The dihydropyridines have a more pure vasodilatory action and can cause a reflex tachycardia, but have less effect on cardiac contractility. The use of short-acting dihydropyridines to lower blood pressure may precipitate ischemic events in individuals with coronary artery disease because of reflex tachycardia. No such association has been associated with use of long-acting dihydropyridines. Other side effects of calcium channel blockers include dizziness, edema, constipation, headache, and flushing. Diltiazem and verapamil should be avoided or used cautiously in patients with second or third degree heart block, congestive heart failure and those already taking beta blockers.

◆ KEY POINTS ◆

1. Hypertension affects 43 million Americans and is a major risk factor for the development of cardiovascular disease and cerebrovascular disease.

2. Primary hypertension accounts for 90% to 95% of all cases of HTN.

3. The history, physical and laboratory evaluation of hypertensive individuals involves assessment for end organ damage, additional risk factors for cardiovascular disease, and secondary causes of hypertension.

4. The first step in therapy generally involves lifestyle modifications and if patients remain hypertensive after 3 to 6 months of lifestyle modifications, antihypertensive medications are started.

23 Congestive Heart Failure

Congestive heart failure (CHF) affects an estimated 4.9 million Americans and is the most frequent cause of hospitalization in the elderly. One percent of adults age 50 to 60 and 10% of adults in their 80s are affected by it. The overall 5-year mortality is 60% for men and 45% for women. The three major risk factors for heart failure are hypertension, coronary artery disease, and valvular heart disease.

PATHOPHYSIOLOGY

Congestive heart failure occurs if the heart is unable to adequately perfuse body tissues. Cardiac output depends on three factors: preload, contractility, and afterload. Preload (also referred to as the left-ventricular end diastolic pressure) is the pressure required to distend the ventricle at a given volume. The relationship of pressure and volume defines compliance. Contractility describes the functional state of the myocardial muscle. Normally as preload increases, the cardiac output and the amount of blood pumped by the heart muscle increases. Afterload is the resistance against which the heart contracts and is clinically reflected in the systolic blood pressure.

Heart failure begins with symptoms that occur only during periods of stress such as an illness or exercise but as the disease progresses symptoms may occur with rest. Heart failure may be due to either systolic or diastolic dysfunction. Systolic dysfunction is character-ized by decreased contractility of the left ventricle, resulting in a reduced ejection fraction. A decreased ejection fraction leads to a compensatory increase in preload to maintain cardiac output. Eventually there is a limit to which increases in preload can compensate and pulmonary congestion occurs, resulting in signs and symptoms such as orthopnea, paroxysmal nocturnal dyspnea, rales, jugular venous distention, and edema.

Decreases in cardiac output trigger a host of compensatory mechanisms, including activation of the renin-angiotensin-aldosterone system, increased levels of catecholamines, and the secretion of atrial natriuretic hormone. These compensatory mechanisms result in systemic vasoconstriction, fluid retention and increased afterload, which further inhibits cardiac output, thus creating a vicious feedback cycle. Late changes effected by these compensatory mechanisms include myocardial and vascular remodeling and fibrosis.

About 40% of patients have diastolic dysfunction. Diastolic dysfunction results from an inability of the ventricle to relax properly which leads to a higher filling pressure, pulmonary congestion and decreased cardiac return. Changes that occur with aging predispose elderly individuals to developing diastolic dysfunction. Other causes include ischemia, hypertension, ventricular hypertrophy, volume overload, and pericardial disease. It is also common for patients with systolic dysfunction to have some element of diastolic dysfunction.

CLINICAL MANIFESTATIONS

History

Symptoms of CHF include dyspnea, orthopnea, paroxysmal nocturnal dyspnea, nocturia, edema, weight gain, fatigue, chest pain, abdominal pain, anorexia, and mental status changes. When taking the patient's history it is useful to determine what activities make the patient short of breath, number of pillows the patient sleeps on, and other factors associated with their CHF (i.e., chest pain, increased salt intake). Previous and current medical conditions, risk factors for coronary artery disease (CAD), and all medications should be thoroughly reviewed.

Physical Examination

Checking general appearance and vital signs are important in order to determine if the patient is hypertensive or in respiratory distress. Examination of the neck may reveal jugular venous distention (JVD), a sign of elevated filling pressures. With examination of the chest, the point of maximal impulse (PMI) of the left ventricle is often displaced laterally and downward in individuals with cardiomegaly. Auscultation of the lungs may reveal bibasilar rales. When rales are present, measuring the lung field level at which they are heard is a useful way of following treatment. Auscultation of the heart may reveal third and fourth heart sounds, which are often present in patients who are fluid overloaded and/or who have a stiff ventricle. Murmurs may indicate valvular pathology as the cause of heart failure. Abdominal exam often reveals hepatomegaly, which is a sign of right-sided heart failure and indicates moderate to severe venous congestion. Lower extremity edema is a common finding and is often accompanied by stasis dermatitis. Quantifying the degree of edema is useful in determining effectiveness of treatment and chronicity of condition.

DIFFERENTIAL DIAGNOSIS

The differential diagnosis depends on the presenting symptom. For patients complaining of dyspnea, the major differential is pulmonary diseases such as chronic obstructive pulmonary disease, interstitial lung disease, pulmonary infections, and pulmonary embolus. Dyspnea may also be a sign of anemia.

For patients with fluid retention and edema, the differential diagnosis includes hypoalbuminemic states, cirrhosis, nephrotic syndrome, and chronic venous stasis. In the elderly, some common signs of heart failure may be misleading. For example many patients have edema from chronic venous insufficiency and may not have heart failure. In these patients, examination of the constellation of symptoms combined with diagnostic testing is needed to establish the presence or absence of heart failure.

DIAGNOSTIC EVALUATION

The goals of the diagnostic evaluation are to determine the underlying reason for heart failure and to search for causes of acute decompensation. Box 23–1 lists some causes of heart failure.

The chest x-ray remains an excellent and readily available test for identifying heart failure. Characteristic findings include cardiomegaly, redistribution of vascular markings, prominent interstitial markings, Kerley

---

BOX 23–1

Causes of Heart Failure

Myocardial Damage
- Infections
- Infarction
- Valvular heart disease
- Congenital heart disease
- Dilated cardiomyopathy
- Toxins (e.g., alcohol, Adriamycin)

Diastolic Dysfunction
- Ischemia
- Hypertensive cardiomyopathy
- Infiltrative heart disease (e.g., amyloid, sarcoid)
- Constrictive pericarditis

Extracardiac
- Anemia
- Renal failure
- Thyroid disease

B lines, and perihilar haziness. In more advanced cases pleural effusions may be identified. The chest x-ray may also identify pulmonary disease which may be causing or contributing to symptoms. An ECG is useful for detecting an arrhythmia or for providing evidence of ischemic disease, left ventricular hypertrophy, or left atrial enlargement.

Virtually all patients with heart failure should have an echocardiogram. The echocardiogram can determine if the mechanism of heart failure is primarily systolic or diastolic dysfunction. In patients with systolic dysfunction, the ejection fraction is reduced (<45%), whereas in diastolic dysfunction the ejection fraction is preserved or even high. Doppler ultrasound techniques help confirm diastolic dysfunction by identifying abnormal flow across the mitral valve. Echocardiograms can also detect left ventricular hypertrophy, valvular disease, pericardial disease, and wall motion abnormalities suggestive of ischemia.

Blood work should include a complete blood count, urine analysis, electrolytes, blood urea nitrogen, creatinine, albumin, and TSH. In patients with acute symptoms, cardiac markers are useful for detecting acute myocardial damage. Depending on the patient's initial clinical evaluation, other tests may be useful. For example, an exercise or pharmacological EKG stress test is helpful for detecting ichemic heart disease.

Common causes of cardiac decompensation are listed in Box 23–2 and should be considered in patients with previously stable heart failure. Coronary artery disease, atrial fibrillation, valvular disease, alcohol abuse, thyroid disease, and hypertension are examples of potentially treatable causes of heart failure.

MANAGEMENT

The goals of management are to reduce symptoms, prevent complications, and improve survival. All patients should follow a no-added sodium diet (<4 gm daily sodium), stop smoking, limit alcohol, monitor weights, and stay as active as possible. Box 23–3 outlines the goals of heart failure therapy. Diuretics are a mainstay of therapy for systolic dysfunction and acute pulmonary congestion in patients with diastolic dysfunction. Single larger doses of loop diuretics are more effective than smaller divided doses. Hypokalemia is a common side effect and requires treatment if less than 4.0 meg/l. Close monitoring of BUN and Cr as well as daily weights is important as an increase in either may indicate the need to adjust diuretic therapy.

ACE inhibitors slow the progression of heart failure, decrease the number of hospitalizations, and decrease mortality in patients with left ventricular systolic dysfunction (LVSD). Patients should start on a low dose of an ACE-inhibitor (e.g., 6.25 mg of captopril bid, 2.5–5 mg of lisinopril) and reduce concurrent diuretic therapy. Common side effects include hypotension, hyperkalemia, dehydration, and cough. Patients with pre-existing renal artery stenosis may experience renal impairment with an ACE. Any deterioration of renal

---

BOX 23–2

Causes of Cardiac Decompensation

Myocardial ischemia	Myocardial infarction
Arrhythmia	Anemia
Acute valvular disease	Superimposed medical illness
Pneumonia	Pulmonary embolus
Uncontrolled hypertension	Dietary indiscretion
Fever	Emotional stress
Excess exertion	

BOX 23–3

Treatment Principles of Heart Failure

- Identify and correct reversible causes
- Identify and correct causes for decompensation
- Determine if heart failure is primarily systolic or diastolic
- Use vasodilators in patients with systolic dysfunction
- Initiate low sodium diet to control fluid retention
- Cautious use of beta-blockers in systolic dysfunction
- Control heart rate in diastolic dysfunction
- Digoxin in patients with systolic dysfunction who remain symptomatic despite vasodilators/diuretics

function should result in either a dose reduction or discontinuation of the medication. If patients cannot tolerate an ACE inhibitor, an angiotensin receptor blocker (ARB) is an alternative. Another alternative to an ACE inhibitor is the combination of hydralazine and nitrates.

Randomized trials have shown a significant decrease in mortality and sudden death in patients with heart failure who are treated with beta-blockers. They should be added after ACE-inhibitors and diuretics in patients with stable heart failure. Beta-blockers are also helpful in heart failure secondary to ischemia, diastolic dysfunction and atrial arrhythmia. When adding beta-blockers to patients with heart failure, start with a low dose (e.g., 3.25 mg/d carvedilol or 12.5–25 mg/d of metoprolol) and titrate slowly upward to achieve a resting heart rate of 50 to 60 beats per minute. Patients should be monitored closely for fluid retention and clinical deterioration. Diuretic doses may need to be adjusted upward if fluid retention occurs.

Spironolactone, which blocks the effects of aldosterone, also significantly lowers the risk of hospitalization and sudden cardiac death from heart failure. Important side effects include renal and electrolyte abnormalities, especially hyperkalemia. The risk of hyperkalemia is especially high in patients on an ACE inhibitor and spironolactone.

Digoxin is useful in individuals with systolic dysfunction and moderate to severe failure whose symptoms are uncontrolled with an ACE inhibitor and diuretics. Digoxin is not useful in patients with diastolic dysfunction.

The goals for treating diastolic dysfunction are prevention of LVH and control of symptoms by reducing end diastolic pressure without reducing cardiac output. Rate control and maintaining sinus rhythm are essential. Slowing the heart rate allows more time for ventricular filling during diastole. Diuretics are indicated for volume overload and for correcting precipitating factors such as hypertension. If calcium channel blockers are used for diastolic failure, they should be in the nondihydropyridine class, such as verapamil and diltiazem. The dihydropyridine class causes a reflex tachycardia that decreases filling time.

◆ **KEY POINTS** ◆

1. One percent of adults age 50 to 60 and 10% of adults in their 80s are affected by CHF.

2. Systolic dysfunction is characterized by decreased contractility of the left ventricle, resulting in a reduced ejection fraction.

3. About 40% of patients with CHF have diastolic dysfunction. Diastolic dysfunction results from an inability of the ventricle to relax properly, which leads to a higher filling pressure, pulmonary congestion, and decreased cardiac return.

4. Characteristic chest x-ray findings in CHF include cardiomegaly, redistribution of vascular markings, prominent interstitial markings, Kerley B lines, and perihilar haziness.

5. The goals of management are reduction of symptoms, prevention of complications, and improvement of survival.

6. ACE inhibitors slow the progression of heart failure, decrease the number of hospitalizations, and decrease mortality in patients with LVSD and are recommended in patients with left ventricular systolic dysfunction (LVSD).

7. Randomized trials have shown a significant decrease in mortality and sudden death in patients with heart failure who are treated with beta-blockers.

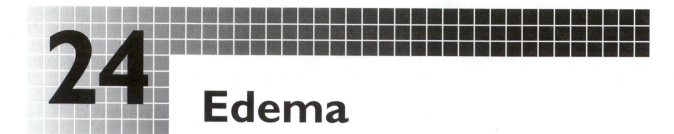

24

Edema

Edema is swelling that may be localized or generalized and is most common in dependent parts of the body, such as the legs. Leg edema is a common problem in primary care, occurring in about 15% of healthy subjects over 65. The importance of leg edema is its frequent association with illnesses such as congestive heart failure (CHF) or renal failure that can cause significant morbidity and mortality.

PATHOPHYSIOLOGY

Edema results from an imbalance of factors effecting the distribution of fluid between the intravascular and extravascular spaces. Edema forms when the production of interstitial fluid exceeds its removal through the venous or lymphatic system. Factors contributing to edema are:

1. Increased capillary hydrostatic pressure
2. Reduced intravascular oncotic pressure
3. Increased capillary permeability
4. Reduced lymphatic drainage from the interstitial space

As a result of the force of gravity, edema occurs most commonly in the lower extremities.

CLINICAL MANIFESTATIONS

History

Most patients with edema complain of leg swelling, but other symptoms include weight gain, tightness of shoes or clothing, puffiness in the eyes or face—especially in the morning—and an increase in abdominal girth. Patients with associated pulmonary edema may complain of exertional dyspnea, orthopnea, and paroxysmal nocturnal dyspnea. Reviewing medications is important since NSAIDs and vasodilators, such as nifedipine or prazosin, can cause fluid retention, and ACE inhibitors can cause localized facial edema. A history of diurnal variations of 4 to 5 pounds per day in healthy young women suggest idiopathic cyclic edema.

Physical Examination

A rapid increase in weight over a short period of time is one of the cardinal signs of edema. Generalized edema suggests renal disease, hypoalbuminemia hepatic disease, or CHF. The examination should focus on the cardiopulmonary, abdominal, and pelvic examinations. Neck vein distention along with peripheral edema and rales suggests congestive heart failure or pulmonary hypertension. Findings such as palmar erythema, spider telangiectasia, and ascites point to liver disease. The presence of a prostate or pelvic mass and inguinal adenopathy suggests the possibility of lymphatic obstruction. Obesity, previous episodes of phlebitis, and peripheral neuropathy all predispose individuals to chronic edema. Chronic venous insufficiency can cause leg edema and is associated with the physical exam findings of stasis dermatitis and venous varicosities.

The degree of edema should be noted, and whether it is unilateral or bilateral. The edema should be tested to see how easily it pits and whether the area is tender. Non-pitting leg edema may be a sign of hypothyroidism. Localized swelling that is not pitting is common in patients with lymphedema.

DIFFERENTIAL DIAGNOSIS

Generalized edema is usually a result of hypoalbuminemia or cardiac, renal, or hepatic disease. Although bilateral leg edema is associated with systemic diseases, in the primary care setting it is more commonly due to chronic venous insufficiency. Regional edema is usually due to increased capillary pressure from causes such as venous insufficiency or obstruction. Venous obstruction can be due to infection, trauma, thrombophlebitis, or immobility. It can also be a result of external obstruction due to fibrosis, radiation, surgery, neoplasm, or lymph nodes. Box 24–1 lists the causes of leg edema.

DIAGNOSTIC APPROACH

Routine laboratory tests for patients with generalized edema include a chemistry panel, a complete blood count (CBC), urinalysis (UA), and chest x-ray. The chemistry panel measures renal function, albumin levels, and assesses electrolytes. A UA provides important information about the presence of renal disease and can detect nephrotic range proteinuria. The chest x-ray can detect pulmonary congestion, effusions, assess heart size, and provide clues to the presence of pericardial disease. A thyroid stimulating hormone (TSH) can rule out hypothyroidism in cases of suspected myxedema. Further cardiac testing such as an EKG and echocardiogram is indicated for patients with CHF.

For patients with unilateral leg edema, an ultrasound can test for a deep vein thrombosis (DVT). Failure of the vein to compress and impaired venous flow correlate with the presence of a DVT. A CT scan of the

---

BOX 24–1

Causes of Leg Edema

Bilateral or Generalized Edema

CHF

Pulmonary hypertension from lung disease

Cirrhosis

Hypoalbuminemia

Renal disease
  Chronic renal failure
  Glomerulonephritis
  Nephrotic syndrome

Medications

Myxedema (hypothyroidism)

Idiopathic edema

Allergic reaction

Unilateral Leg Edema

Acute
  Cellulitis
  Deep vein thrombosis
  Hematoma or soft tissue tear
  Baker's cyst

Chronic
  Venous insufficiency
  Lymphedema
  Extrinsic compression
  Neoplasm
  Lymphoma

---

abdomen and pelvis is indicated in cases of suspected obstruction from a mass.

MANAGEMENT

Treating the underlying cause is important. For example, lymphedema may resolve with treatment of an underlying malignancy. Therapy for generalized edema should be tailored to the underlying cause. For example, nephrotic syndrome may respond to corticosteroids. Diuretics and ACE inhibitors can help edema associated with CHF. Edema due to a medication usually responds to withdrawal of the medication.

Non-pharmacological measures, such as leg elevation, compression stockings, and salt restriction are important. Patients with leg edema should routinely avoid prolonged sitting with their knees bent and may benefit from sleeping with a pillow underneath their legs. Support stockings or custom-made pressure gradient hose can reduce dependent edema. Stockings above the knee may work better, but are often poorly tolerated. Compressive stockings are contraindicated in patients with arterial insufficiency. Initial salt restriction consists of eliminating added salt and avoiding high sodium foods.

Diuretics should be used cautiously as an adjunct to non-pharmacological therapy. Lymphedema and edema due to chronic venous insufficiency do not typically respond to diuretics. Patients receiving diuretics should be monitored to avoid over-diuresis. Monitoring includes following weights, checking orthostatic blood pressure, and measuring electrolytes and renal function periodically to detect hypokalemia or prerenal azotemia.

◆ KEY POINTS ◆

1. Leg edema is a common problem in primary care occurring in about 15% of healthy subjects over 65. The importance of leg edema is its frequent association with illnesses such as CHF or renal failure that can cause significant morbidity and mortality.

2. Generalized edema is usually a result of hypoalbuminemia or cardiac, renal, or hepatic disease.

3. Non-pharmacological measures for treating edema such as leg elevation, compression stockings, and salt restriction are important.

4. Diuretics should be used cautiously as an adjunct to non-pharmacological therapy. Lymphedema and edema due to chronic venous insufficiency do not typically respond to diuretics.

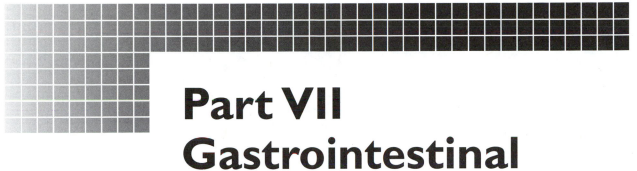

Part VII
Gastrointestinal Diseases

25 Nausea and Vomiting

Nausea is the sensation of having to vomit and often precedes or accompanies vomiting. Vomiting, which can be either voluntary or involuntary, is the forceful expulsion of gastric contents through the mouth. In most instances in the primary care setting, the symptoms are caused by self-limited illness, such as viral gastroenteritis. However, vomiting can be a presenting symptom for a more serious illness.

PATHOPHYSIOLOGY

Vomiting is under the control of two central nervous system (CNS) centers, the vomiting center in the medullary reticular formation and the chemoreceptor trigger zone in the fourth ventricle. Vagal nerve irritation and impulses from the sympathetic nerves in the throat, head, abdomen, and gastrointestinal tract can send impulses to the vomiting centers. Vestibular disturbances, drugs, and metabolic abnormalities can activate the chemoreceptor trigger zone and cause vomiting. Efferent impulses from the CNS then travel to the effector muscles, causing a stereotypical vomiting response that varies little regardless of cause.

CLINICAL MANIFESTATIONS

History

A thorough history is critical to effectively sorting out the many causes of nausea and vomiting. Characteriz-

ing the duration, timing, frequency, and type of vomiting is important. Acute symptoms lasting less than one week suggest an infection, intoxication, drug effect, metabolic abnormality, or visceral disease. Early-morning nausea and vomiting is common with pregnancy, but is also typical of vomiting associated with uremia and adrenal insufficiency. Symptoms precipitated by eating are common with gastrointestinal disorders, such as acute gastritis, peptic ulcer disease, gastric outlet obstruction, or psychogenic factors. Vomiting several hours after eating can occur with diabetic gastroparesis, or gastric malignancy. Projectile vomiting may indicate pyloric stenosis in children or occasionally CNS disease causing increased intracranial pressure. Characterizing the type of vomitus can be helpful. The presence of bile indicates an open pylorus, while feculent vomitus is seen in patients with a lower gastrointestinal obstruction or gastrocolic fistula. Bloody or coffee-ground emesis indicates bleeding from the esophagus, stomach, or duodenum. Less commonly, bloody vomitus is seen in patients with blood swallowed from bleeding in the mouth or nose.

Nausea and vomiting accompanied by fever, watery diarrhea, and abdominal cramps is typical for viral gastroenteritis. Food poisoning usually begins within 6 hours of eating the offending substance and resolves within 24 to 48 hours. Abdominal pain may indicate a surgical problem, such as appendicitis or cholecystitis. Cramps may be caused by gastroenteritis or an early obstruction. Visceral pain syndrome, seen with myocardial infarction, renal colic, and pancreatitis, can commonly cause nausea. Vestibular vertigo suggests an acute vestibular cause such as labyrinthitis. Recurring vertigo, tinnitus, and vomiting are consistent with Meniere's disease. Headache and other neurological symptoms suggest a CNS cause.

Medications are a common cause of vomiting. Common examples include macrolide antibiotics, metronidazole, opiates, NSAIDs, estrogen, digitalis, theophylline, and chemotherapeutic agents. The medical and surgical history often suggests possible causes. Diabetic ketoacidosis should always be considered in diabetic individuals with nausea and vomiting. A history of coronary artery disease or renal insufficiency raises the possibility that nausea and vomiting is caused by one of these conditions. Previous abdominal surgeries increase the risk of obstruction.

Physical Examination

The physical examination includes an overall assessment of appearance, vital signs, and volume status. The abdominal exam can provide clues to the underlying etiology that is essential in patients with abdominal pain. Localized tenderness may indicate a specific cause. For example, a large tender liver suggests hepatitis. Tenderness with guarding, or rebound tenderness, occurs with peritoneal irritation. High-pitched bowel sounds are consistent with an early obstruction, whereas decreased or absent bowel sounds are consistent with peritonitis, ileus, or obstruction.

With vestibular disorders, head movement will reproduce the patient's symptoms of vertigo, nausea, and vomiting in association with the physical finding of nystagmus. A neurological examination can detect signs such as papilledema indicating increased intracranial pressure, ataxia indicating a cerebellar disorder, or a stiff neck suggesting meningitis.

DIFFERENTIAL DIAGNOSIS

In addition to GI diseases, the list of diseases that can cause nausea and vomiting encompasses a wide range of conditions. The most common causes of acute nausea and vomiting in the family practice setting are infection, gastroenteritis, and metabolic and medication side effects.

Chronic nausea and vomiting are commonly related to structural lesions in the upper gastrointestinal tract such as peptic ulcer disease, gastroparesis, and gastric

outlet obstruction. Other causes include metabolic abnormalities such as uremia or chronic hepatitis. Psychological causes are common in younger individuals, especially women. Persistent early-morning vomiting without another explanation such as pregnancy, raises the possibility of increased intracranial pressure and an underlying neurological disease.

DIAGNOSTIC APPROACH

The history and physical may suggest a cause for nausea and vomiting, such as pregnancy, dietary indiscretion, labyrinthitis, gastroenteritis, food poisoning, or medications. In these instances, testing may be indicated only to confirm the diagnosis (e.g., pregnancy testing) or in situations of more protracted vomiting, to check for electrolyte abnormalities. Significant volume depletion elevates the BUN and can cause hemoconcentration with a rise in hematocrit. Drug levels, such as a digoxin level, are useful in suspected drug toxicity. Liver function tests are useful when hepatitis is suspected. Visceral pain syndromes causing nausea, such as a myocardial infarction or renal colic, usually have associated symptoms that indicate the need to investigate these possibilities. However, in diabetic individuals and the elderly it is not uncommon for a myocardial infarction to present primarily with nausea and vomiting. The threshold for obtaining an EKG in these individuals should be low.

Patients with nausea and vomiting may need imaging tests along with blood tests. Plain films can help rule out an acute obstruction. An ultrasound can detect gallstones and changes compatible with pancreatitis.

Chronic nausea and vomiting are most commonly related to structural lesions affecting the upper gastrointestinal tract. Endoscopy and barium studies are helpful in identifying outlet obstruction and motility disorders. Evidence of extrinsic compression on a barium study needs either an ultrasound or CT scan for further evaluation.

Persistent early-morning nausea in the absence of a pregnancy or metabolic disease raises the possibility of increased intracranial pressure, and a head CT or MRI should be considered. Recurring vomiting of unknown cause may be due to a psychological problem. These include vomiting around meal times, inappropriate attention to body image, abnormal appetite, and a conflict-filled social environment.

MANAGEMENT

Management should be directed at the underlying cause. For most individuals with self-limited illnesses, simple dietary measures are sufficient. Nausea and vomiting resulting from medication usually resolves by discontinuing the medication. If the drug is essential, decreasing the dosage of the medication or changing to an alternative medication may help nausea. Phenothiazines such as prochlorperazine (Compazine) and promethazine (Phenergan) are among the most commonly used agents and are centrally acting agents used for controlling symptoms from drugs, metabolic diseases, or gastroenteritis. Their most common side effects include sedation, but they can also cause extrapyramidal symptoms, especially in children. Trimethobenzamide (Tigan) is a non-phenothiazine centrally acting agent. In patients with vestibular symptoms, the antihistamine, meclizine (Antivert) is helpful. Other antihistamines such as dimenhydrinate (Dramamine) or diphenolate are also effective. Antihistamines can cause drowsiness and patients should be cautioned about driving or operating machinery when taking these drugs.

Patients with motility disorders may benefit from a prokinetic agent such as metoclopramide (Reglan). Side effects include anxiety, extrapyramidal reactions, and rarely, tardive dyskinesia. Scopolamine, an anticholinergic, is used primarily for motion sickness prophylaxis. It comes as both a pill and a patch. Psychogenic vomiting is best managed with a psychiatric consultation.

◆ KEY POINTS ◆

1. In most instances, patients seen in the primary care setting with nausea and vomiting have a self-limiting illness.

2. Nausea and vomiting accompanied by fever, watery diarrhea, and abdominal cramps are typical for viral gastroenteritis.

3. Common medications causing nausea include the macrolide antibiotics, metronidazole, opiates, NSAIDs, estrogen, digitalis, theophylline, and chemotherapeutic agents.

4. Phenothiazines are commonly used, centrally acting agents that help control nausea. Side effects include sedation and extrapyramidal symptoms, especially in children.

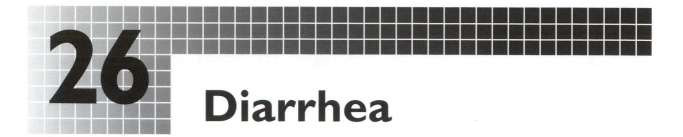

26 Diarrhea

Diarrhea is defined as an increase in stool weight to more than 200 grams per day. Clinically, diarrhea is defined as the passage of more than three abnormally loose stools per 24 hours. Acute diarrhea lasts less than three weeks, while chronic diarrhea is a persistent or recurring condition that lasts more than three weeks.

PATHOPHYSIOLOGY

Fluid balance in the gastrointestinal system represents a dynamic flux between absorption and secretion. Conditions that either increase fluid secretion or decrease absorption lead to diarrhea. Inflammation, hormones, or enterotoxins may trigger increased fluid secretion. A functional or anatomical decrease in the absorptive capacity of the bowel may cause diarrhea. Osmotically active solutes that retain fluid in the intestinal lumen may also increase stool volume. Altered bowel motility can impair absorption, either by decreasing the contact time of intestinal contents with the bowel mucosa or by preventing the effective mixing of intestinal contents. Although the basic mechanisms of diarrhea are straightforward, more than one mechanism may contribute to diarrhea in an individual patient. For example, in a patient with Crohn's disease, an abnormal ileum may

cause decreased fluid absorption and increased secretion due to diffuse inflammation.

CLINICAL MANIFESTATIONS

History

Acute diarrhea has two common clinical presentations: either a watery non-inflammatory diarrhea, or an inflammatory diarrhea with the presence of either blood or white blood cells in the stool. Symptoms may be mild with no change in activity, moderate with some limitation in activity, or severe where patients are confined to bed.

It is important to ask patients with acute diarrhea about exposure to patients with similar symptoms, recent travel, and whether they are taking antibiotics or other medications. A diet history is important since excessive caffeine or alcohol intake, and sorbitol-containing foods can all cause transient diarrhea. Overindulgence of milk or milk products in a lactose intolerant individual can cause bloating, cramps, and diarrhea. Antibiotic use within two weeks suggests that diarrhea may be caused by either an alteration in bowel flora or a *Clostridium difficile* infection. Severe abdominal pain in an elderly individual accompanied by acute diarrhea suggests the possibility of ischemic colitis.

Watery stools accompanied by a low-grade fever, headache, nausea or vomiting, and achiness is consistent with a viral gastroenteritis. Traveler's diarrhea, due to toxogenic *Escherichia coli*, presents similarly to viral gastroenteritis. Bacterial infections, such as shigella, salmonella, and Campylobacter, present with a prodrome of fever, headache, anorexia, fatigue, and stools that may initially be watery before becoming bloody. Salmonella is usually a self-limited infection and is acquired by ingesting contaminated poultry or eggs. Campylobacter infection is more common than either shigella or salmonella and is usually acquired from ingesting contaminated poultry. *Escherichia coli* 0157:H7 accounts for up to a third of cases of bloody diarrhea. Its presentation ranges from mild, crampy, non-bloody diarrhea to life-threatening hemorrhagic colitis, complicated by hemolytic uremic syndrome or thrombocytopenic purpura.

Diarrhea from food poisoning usually occurs several hours after eating contaminated food. A common food source and an absence of other associated symptoms are characteristic findings. *Staphylococcal aureus* commonly contaminates custard-filled pastries while *Clostridium perfringens* is especially common in foods warmed on a steam table.

Chronic diarrhea can be either persistent or recurrent. Irritable bowel syndrome (IBS) typically affects young or middle-aged adults with a 2:1 female-to-male predominance. It can present as diarrhea alternating with constipation or chronic recurring diarrhea. Other symptoms include abdominal pain that is relieved by defecation, fecal urgency, bloating, the need to strain to pass stool, and occasionally having a small amount of mucus in the stool. This condition may wax or wane over the years. Any rectal bleeding that occurs in patients with IBS is usually due to anal trauma from passing a hard stool. In the active phase, inflammatory bowel disease (IBD) is associated with abdominal pain, bloody stools, and fever. Extraintestinal manifestations include arthritis, liver disease, uveitis, and skin lesions.

Giardiasis, amoebiasis, and *C. difficile* can present with acute, intermittent, or chronic symptoms. Giardia is the leading cause of parasitic diarrhea. The organism is endemic to areas such as the Rocky Mountains and Russia. It is also common in areas such as third world countries where the water supply may be contaminated. Foul greasy bulky stools characterize malabsorption syndromes causing diarrhea. Associated symptoms such as weight loss or neuropathy may be a function of malabsorption.

Physical Examination

Generally the physical exam is more helpful for assessing the severity of the disease than in determining a specific cause. Vital signs should be checked and the patient assessed for signs of significant dehydration. The abdomen should be carefully examined and a rectal examination performed, checking for occult blood.

DIFFERENTIAL DIAGNOSIS

Box 26–1 lists causes of diarrhea. Viral gastroenteritis is the most common cause of acute diarrhea. Rotavirus is

---

BOX 26–1

Causes of Chronic Diarrhea

Increased secretion
  Clostridium toxin
  Cholera toxin
  Non-invasive microbial gastroenteritis (e.g., viral gastroenteritis, campylobacter)
  Carcinoid syndrome
  Vasoactive intestinal peptide secreting tumors
  Villous adenoma

Increased osmotic load
  Sorbitol ingestion (dietetic candy)
  Bile salt malabsorption
  Pancreatic insufficiency
  Lactose intolerance
  Malabsorption
  Post-gastrectomy syndrome
  Magnesium containing laxatives

Inflammation
  Ulcerative colitis
  Crohn's disease
  Radiation induced colitis
  Invasive microbial gastroenteritis (e.g., shigella)

Altered motility
  Thyrotoxicosis
  Irritable bowel syndrome
  Autonomic neuropathy (e.g., diabetic associated enteropathy)

the most common virus in children, while the Norwalk virus is the most common in adults. Food poisoning from staphylococcal toxins, clostridium toxins and ingestion of campylobacter, salmonella, shigella and enteropathogenic *E. coli* are common bacterial entities. Giardia and amoebiasis are less frequent causes of diarrhea in the United States. Traveler's diarrhea is usually due to *E. coli* but can be due to other bacterial diseases. Dietary indiscretion, alcohol, caffeine, and drug side effects are common non-infectious causes (Box 26–2). In the primary care setting, the most common causes for persistent diarrhea are IBS, IBD, lactose intolerance, and chronic or relapsing gastrointestinal infections, such as giardiasis, amoebiasis, and *C. difficile*.

DIAGNOSTIC APPROACH

Most cases of acute diarrhea are self-limiting and diagnostic tests are usually not indicated. Signs of more severe disease, such as significant dehydration, more than six stools per 24 hours, bloody stools, high temperatures, severe abdominal pain, and failure to improve after 48 to 72 hours suggest a need for a more detailed evaluation. The threshold for evaluating immunocompromised or elderly individuals should be lower.

Examining a stool specimen for leukocytes and occult blood are useful first tests in patients with acute diarrhea. A stool specimen with less than three to four white blood cells per HPF usually indicates a non-inflammatory, self-limiting process. If there is either blood in the stool or an inflammatory process is suspected, a stool culture should be sent along with an assay for *C. difficile* toxin in those patients with recent antibiotic exposure. Patients at risk for giardia or other parasitic infections should have stools evaluated for ova and parasites.

The diagnostic evaluation for chronic diarrhea should be individualized. The history should help focus the approach. Box 26–3 lists signs suggestive of a serious underlying disorder. For patients whose history and physical exam suggest a benign illness, only a limited evaluation is needed. For example, a patient with suspected lactose intolerance who responds to a lactose-free diet needs no further testing. About 5% of cases of chronic diarrhea are due to medications and no further evaluation is needed in individuals who respond to either stopping or decreasing a medication known to cause diarrhea. For patients with chronic diarrhea whose cause is not readily apparent, an initial evaluation may consist of a CBC, ESR, and checking stools for occult blood, leukocytes, and ova and parasites and an assay for *C. difficile* toxin for patients with recent antibiotic exposure. For patients with associated left lower quadrant pain or bloody diarrhea, a sigmoidoscopy is indicated and can detect mucosal ulcerations, friability and masses.

Suspected IBD may be confirmed by biopsy. A biopsy can also detect less common diseases, such as amyloi-

BOX 26–2
Common Medications Associated with Diarrhea

- Alpha-glycoside inhibitors (e.g., acarbose)
- Antacids
- Anti-depressants (SSRIs)
- Antibiotics
- Colchicine
- Lactulose
- Laxatives
- Loop diuretics
- Protein pump inhibitors
- Quinidine
- Theophylline
- Thyroxine

BOX 26–3
Symptoms Suggestive of a Serious Underlying Etiology for Diarrhea

- New onset in patients greater than age 40
- Nocturnal symptoms
- Aggressive course
- Weight loss
- Rectal fissures
- Anemia
- Elevated sed-rate
- Greasy stools that are difficult to flush

dosis and collagenous colitis. In individuals with suspected IBS, a limited evaluation, including sigmoidoscopy, may be sufficient to exclude more serious disorders. Often cases of chronic diarrhea with unclear etiology or suspected IBD may need referral to a gastroenterologist for evaluation.

MANAGEMENT

Most patients with acute diarrhea can be managed with an alteration in diet and fluid therapy. Oral rehydration is sufficient unless the patient is severely dehydrated. Commercial rehydration solutions, such as Pedialyte or Rice-Lyte, designed to replace fluids and electrolytes, are most commonly used for infants or children. Sports drinks, fruit drinks, and flat soft drinks supplemented with crackers, soup, or bland foods, are usually adequate for treating older children and adults.

Boiled starches, such as rice, noodles, or potatoes and avoiding milk products or caffeine-containing foods are usually recommended for patients with acute diarrhea. For children, a BRAT diet (bananas, rice, applesauce, and toast) is traditionally used despite limited evidence demonstrating its efficacy. Preparations containing kaolin and pectate are available over-the-counter but are of uncertain value. Bismuth subsalicylate (Pepto-Bismol) is also used for diarrhea and may have an anti-secretory effect. The anti-motility drugs, such as loperamide, are considered the drugs of choice for non-specific treatment. They should not be used in febrile patients with inflammatory or infectious diarrhea.

Specific management depends on the cause of the diarrhea. The decision to use antibiotics in patients with bacterial diarrhea depends on the organism, health of the individual, and systemic symptoms. All cases of shigella should be treated with a fluoroquinolone or trimethoprim sulfamethoxazole (TMP/SMZ). Salmonella infections causing mild to moderate symptoms should generally not be treated since antibiotics may prolong the carrier state. Patients with salmonella who have severe symptoms or those at risk for bacteremia (easily infected individuals or elderly patients) should be treated with a fluoroquinolone.

Erythromycin or a fluoroquinolone shortens the duration of a campylobacter infection if symptoms are still present when the culture results become available. Invasive *E. coli* with bloody diarrhea should be treated with a fluoroquinolone or TMP/SMZ. Traveler's diarrhea due to toxigenic *E. coli* responds to a short course of a fluoroquinolone or TMP/SMZ. *C. difficile* infections should be treated with metronidazole (an alternative is oral vancomycin). Giardia is treated with metronidazole.

For lactose intolerant patients, a 1 to 2 week trial of a lactose-free diet is usually sufficiently long to decrease symptoms. Lactase-containing capsules taken orally before consuming dairy products are also an effective treatment. Antimotility agents such as loperamide may provide relief for IBS patients with significant diarrhea. Antispasmodics, such as dicyclomine, can benefit patients with crampy abdominal pain. A high fiber diet may be helpful for IBS patients with alternating diarrhea and constipation.

Management goals for IBD are to control active disease, monitor emission, detect complications, and refer for surgery when appropriate. Commonly used medications are sulfasalazine and corticosteroids. Patients are generally managed conjointly with a gastroenterologist.

◆ KEY POINTS ◆

1. Most cases of diarrhea are due to infectious agents, particularly viruses.

2. A bacterial infection, inflammatory bowel disease, ischemic colitis, or malignancy can all cause bloody diarrhea.

3. The most common viral pathogens causing diarrhea are the Norwalk virus, Rotavirus, and enterovirus.

4. Fluoroquinolones are active against salmonella, shigella, and *E. coli*.

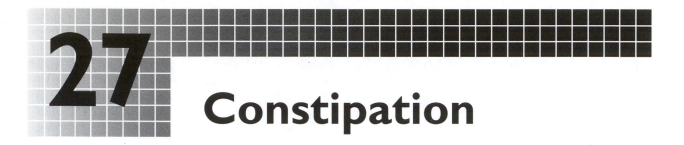

Constipation

Constipation most often occurs in patients at the extreme ages of life. Most individuals eating an average diet will pass at least three stools per week, making it useful to clinically define constipation as the passage of less than three stools per week.

PATHOPHYSIOLOGY

Passing stool depends on stool volume, colonic motility, and patency of the colon lumen. Defecation requires a complex interaction between the central nervous system and the muscles that increase intra-abdominal pressure, relax the sphincter, and open the canal. Alteration of any one of these components can cause constipation. Anorectal disorders such as anal fissures or thrombosed hemorrhoids that cause pain can also lead to constipation by causing avoidance of defecation. Mechanical obstruction as seen in cancer, strictures, or external compression is another cause of constipation.

Patients with diminished fluid and fiber intake have decreased stool volume and can experience constipation. Colonic motility can be inhibited by a variety of medical conditions including hypothyroidism, hypercalcemia, hypokalemia, scleroderma, diabetes, and neurological disorders such as multiple sclerosis, Parkinson's disease, and paraplegia. Medications such as calcium channel blockers (e.g., verapamil), narcotics, and anticholinergics commonly cause a delay in colonic motility. Irritable bowel syndrome is characterized by abnormal colonic motility with delayed colonic transit followed by periods of more frequent and loose stools. A sedentary lifestyle or imposed bed rest (e.g., post-operative patients) results in significant slowing of fecal matter through the colon. Congenital disorders such as Hirschsprung's disease may also lead to delayed emptying of the colon.

CLINICAL MANIFESTATIONS

History

Since many patients have misconceptions regarding normal stool patterns, the frequency of bowel movements and consistency of stool must be accurately determined. Inquiring about symptoms such as pain with defecation, abdominal distention, gas, nausea, emesis, abdominal discomfort, and the presence of blood in the stool is important. A dietary history should include questions about the type and quantities of liquid, fruits, vegetables, and fiber as well as any recent change in diet.

Past medical history, previous surgeries, exercise frequency, and family history should be elicited. Reviewing medications, including over-the-counter medications, may identify the underlying cause. The review of systems should include questions about weight loss, fatigue, depression, and anxiety.

Physical Examination

Physical exam begins with a general assessment of nutritional status, weight, and vital signs. The thyroid should be examined for abnormalities and the skin assessed for pallor and signs of scleroderma. The abdominal exam should note the frequency and pitch of bowel sounds, the presence of any distention or masses and focal tenderness. Rectal exam is useful for determining the stool consistency, detecting occult blood, and for ruling out rectal abnormalities such as fissure, ulcers, masses, or hemorrhoids and detecting impaction. A neurological exam may detect signs of dementia, Parkinson's disease, or neuropathy.

DIFFERENTIAL DIAGNOSIS

Box 27–1 lists the differential diagnosis for constipation. Causes can be related to colonic disease, structural abnormalities, anorectal disease, extracolonic disease, medications, diet, and psychological factors. In the primary care setting, dietary factors (particularly inadequate fiber), medications, irritable bowel syndrome, and poor fluid intake are common causes of constipation.

DIAGNOSTIC EVALUATION

The history and physical examination determines the need for further testing. In younger persons with a reasonable explanation for constipation, management can be instituted without further evaluation. Further testing is indicated in cases refractory to treatment, in older adults with new onset constipation, if the etiology is uncertain, or if the clinical evaluation suggests an underlying disorder that merits further evaluation. Laboratory evaluation should include a complete blood count, serum electrolytes, thyroid stimulating hormone (TSH), and calcium level. Anoscopy is helpful if there is concern about anal pathology such as internal hemorrhoids and fissures.

Abdominal x-rays are of limited value unless obstruction or fecal impaction is suspected. Further evaluation using flexible sigmoidoscopy, coupled with a barium enema or colonoscopy, may be necessary to detect strictures, masses, polyps, or diverticular disease. A full colonoscopy is indicated in patients with anemia, weight loss, heme-positive stools, or other situations in which a malignancy is suspected. During colonoscopy, biopsies of mucosa can be performed to rule out amyloidosis, Hirschsprung's disease, and cancer. The absence of neurons on rectal biopsy demonstrates the presence of Hirschsprung's disease.

BOX 27–1

Causes of Constipation

—Insufficient dietary fiber
—Inactivity
—Medications:
  —Opiates
  —Calcium channel blockers
  —Anticholinergics
  —Tricyclic antidepressants
  —Diuretics
  —Antacids
  —Clonidine
  —Levodopa
  —Laxative abuse
—Metabolic abnormalities:
  —Hypokalemia
  —Hypercalcemia
  —Hypothyroidism
—Scleroderma
—Amyloidosis
—Pregnancy
—Neurological disorders
  —Parkinson's disease
  —Paraplegia
—Prior pelvic surgery
—Diabetes mellitus
—Irritable bowel syndrome
—Colonic mass
—Hirschsprung's disease
—Peri-anal pathology:
  —Fissure
  —Hemorrhoids
  —Rectocoele
  —Rectal prolapse
  —Diverticular disease

MANAGEMENT

Disorders causing constipation such as hypothyroidism, bowel obstruction, or anal fissure should be treated accordingly. Some patients may only require education and reassurance that their bowel pattern is normal.

Increasing fluid and fiber is the cornerstone for treating cases of functional constipation. Patients should drink at least eight 8-ounce glasses of water and consume large amounts of bran, fresh fruit, vegetables, beans, and whole grains. If possible, medications suspected to be causing or contributing to constipation should be discontinued or changed.

Patients may also benefit from "bowel retraining." Specifically, patients should devote 10 to 15 minutes each day of quiet and unhurried time on the commode. This should take place at the same time each day and occur after a meal to utilize the gastric-colic reflex. Bowel retraining often requires 2 to 3 weeks to become effective and should become a part of the patient's daily routine.

If the above modalities fail to alleviate the patient's symptoms and bowel obstruction has been ruled out, medications may be required. There are numerous medications available to treat constipation and some have significant side effects. However, with adequate knowledge of mechanism of action and risks most medications for constipation can be administered safely.

Bulk-forming Agents

Bulk-forming agents are high in fiber and increase stool volume by absorbing water. Examples include psyllium (Metamucil), methylcellulose (Citrucel), and polycarbophil (Fibercon). Common side effects include bloating and flatulence and if not taken with enough water may paradoxically worsen constipation.

Osmotic Laxatives

Osmotic laxatives are non-absorbable solutes that draw fluid into the intestinal lumen by creating an osmotic gradient. Examples include lactulose, magnesium salts (Milk of Magnesia), and sorbitol. Side effects include bloating, excess gas, and abdominal cramping. Magnesium salts are contraindicated in renal failure patients.

Stimulant Agents

Stimulant agents work by altering mucosal permeability and by stimulating intestinal smooth muscle activity.

Examples include phenolphthalein (Ex-Lax) and bisacodyl (Dulcolax). Chronic abuse of these may lead to melanosis coli and constipation secondary to enteric nervous system damage.

Stool Softeners

Docusate sodium (Colace) is a commonly prescribed stool softener that is often used for patients complaining of hard stools that are difficult to pass. It decreases surface tension and allows water and fat to mix in the stool. To work optimally, stool softeners need to be taken with plenty of fluid.

Enemas and Suppositories

Warm tap water enemas and suppositories work by distention and stimulation of the rectum, which then leads to evacuation. This is especially useful in bedridden patients and those with stool impaction. In patients with severe idiopathic constipation, surgeries such as hemicolectomy with ileorectal anastomosis may be a last resort.

◆ KEY POINTS ◆

1. Constipation is defined clinically as less than three stools per week.

2. Poor fluid intake and a lack of fiber are common causes of constipation in the primary care setting.

3. Indications for laboratory testing include refractory cases, new onset constipation in an older individual, heme-positive stools, and situations in which the etiology is unclear or the clinical evaluation suggests underlying pathology.

4. The types of laxatives include bulk-forming agents, osmotic laxative, stimulant laxative, stool softeners, suppositories, and enemas.

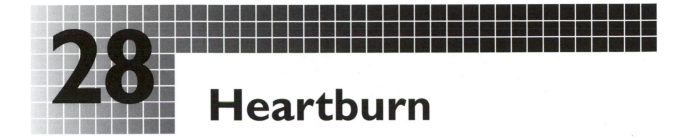

28 Heartburn

Heartburn from gastroesophageal reflux disease (GERD) is experienced on a daily basis by 7% of the population, on a weekly basis by 15%, and at least monthly by up to 40%. Peptic ulcer disease is present in 1.5% of the population and has a lifetime incidence of about 10%. Duodenal ulcers occur more commonly than gastric ulcers and at a younger age. Peptic ulcer disease affects males slightly more than females. Non-ulcer dyspepsia occurs in up to 25% to 30% of the population at some point.

PATHOPHYSIOLOGY

Gastroesophageal reflux occurs when gastric contents reflux or enter the esophagus. Decreased lower esophageal sphincter pressure or increased intra-abdominal pressure play a significant role in this process. The low pH of the gastric contents can cause inflammatory changes leading to esophagitis. Long-term acid exposure can cause the normal squamous cells (lining the distal esophagus) to undergo adenomatous metaplastic transformation (Barrett's esophagus). Patients with Barrett's esophagus are at a higher risk (30- to 40-fold) for developing esophageal cancer. Continued inflammatory reaction can also lead to scarring within the esophagus and development of a stricture with resultant dysphagia.

Peptic ulcer disease and gastritis have similar causes and risk factors. Typically, the gastric and duodenal mucosa are resistant to any damage from acid secretion. Peptic ulcers and gastritis occur when the defense mechanisms are compromised or, rarely, when acid secretion is sufficient to overwhelm the defenses.

Helicobacter pylori infection is the most significant risk factor for peptic ulcer disease. In 10% to 20% of infected individuals, gastric or duodenal ulcers develop. Exactly why peptic ulcers occur and why the ulcers are more prevalent in the duodenum is unclear. Infection with *H. pylori* is also associated with an increased risk of gastric adenocarcinoma and gastric lymphoma.

NSAIDs contribute to gastritis and ulcer formation by blocking cyclooxygenase-1 production of prostaglandins that maintain mucosal blood flow, mucous secretion, and bicarbonate. Without these protective factors, acid-induced inflammation and ulcers may result. Stress-induced gastritis and ulcers are thought to occur due to impaired mucosal defense resulting from vasoconstriction and resultant tissue hypoxia.

Non-ulcer dyspepsia is a poorly understood disease with symptoms like those of GERD and peptic ulcer disease. The pathophysiology is thought to be related to altered gastrointestinal motility, gastrointestinal contractile patterns, and transit of food.

CLINICAL MANIFESTATIONS

History

Initial evaluation of individuals with heartburn includes the patient's detailed description of the episodes along with assessment of risk for the different diseases with heartburn as a presenting symptom.

GERD is characterized by burning pain in the epigastric, sternal, and throat regions accompanied by a sour taste in the mouth and is aggravated by lying down or bending over. Burning, aching, or gnawing pain in the epigastric region or upper quadrants of the abdomen is typical of peptic ulcer disease. Pain brought on by exertion and relieved by rest, and chest tightness, rather than burning, is more typical of cardiac disease. Colicky upper abdominal pain is indicative of cholecystitis, nephrolithiasis, and irritable bowel syndrome or non-ulcer dyspepsia as possible etiologies.

Esophageal reflux may be alleviated by antacids or food, but frequently recurs within 1 to 2 hours. Commonly, the pain of peptic ulcer disease is more intense in the middle of the night, typically mid-epigastric, and relieved by eating. Eating usually aggravates cholecystitis and sometimes gastric ulcers. The pain of nephrolithiasis is independent of ingestion of food. The pain of non-ulcer dyspepsia is more variable, but often related to eating.

GERD can cause respiratory symptoms of cough, wheezing, sore throat, and laryngitis. Heartburn associated with shortness of breath and chest pain should raise concerns about a cardiac etiology for the patient's symptoms.

Eliciting a past history of previously diagnosed gastrointestinal diseases can aid in directing the evaluation. Connective tissue and neuromuscular disease can bring about esophageal symptoms from associated motility disorders. Medications, such as theophylline and calcium channel blockers, can precipitate or exacerbate symptoms associated with GERD. Nonsteroidal anti-inflammatory drugs (NSAIDs) are associated with gastric and duodenal ulcers, as well as heartburn. Any medications the patient is using to alleviate symptoms should also be elicited, particularly with availability of over-the-counter (OTC) H2 blockers.

In addition to its association with cardiac disease, smoking can worsen gastroesophageal reflux and is a risk factor for peptic ulcer disease. Dietary factors associated with lowering the pressure of the esophageal sphincter include consumption of coffee, chocolate, mints, fatty foods, and alcohol. There are no specific dietary correlates for peptic ulcer disease. However, alcohol can cause gastric irritation with resultant gastritis.

Physical Examination

The physical examination generally will not be able to distinguish between gastritis, peptic ulcer disease, non-ulcer dyspepsia, and GERD. All of these typically have minimal physical findings other than epigastric tenderness. A hemoccult test may show evidence of blood loss and makes the presence of peptic ulcer disease and erosive gastritis or esophagitis more likely diagnoses than simple gastroesophageal reflux.

Cardiac findings such as S3, S4, pulmonary rales, or irregular rhythm signify underlying cardiac disease. Abdominal tenderness with pancreatitis is typically periumbilical, while the tenderness with cholecystitis occurs in the right upper quadrant and is associated with a positive Murphy's sign. Nephrolithiasis typically presents no physical findings other than possible costovertebral angle tenderness. Palpation of a mass suggests the presence of a neoplasm.

DIFFERENTIAL DIAGNOSIS

Table 28–1 presents a comprehensive differential diagnosis for patients with heartburn complaints. The most common causes for heartburn symptoms are GERD, peptic ulcer disease, gastritis, and non-ulcer dyspepsia.

Non-ulcer dyspepsia is a poorly understood disease with symptoms overlapping GERD, peptic ulcer disease, and gastritis. Patients may have symptoms consistent with GERD, peptic ulcer disease, gastritis, or may present with dysmotility symptoms such as abdominal bloating or cramping. This is generally considered a diagnosis of exclusion. In patients younger than age 45, if the initial laboratory evaluation (complete blood count, hemoccult testing of the stools, *H. pylori* serology) is normal, empiric therapy can be initiated based upon the patient's predominant symptoms. Patients presenting after age 45 require more aggressive evaluation since organic disease becomes more prevalent as patients get older.

DIAGNOSTIC APPROACH

No single test is accepted as the standard for diagnosing GERD. However, several tests may prove useful in evaluating patients with heartburn. Early diagnostic evaluation is indicated when complications such as

TABLE 28–1

Differential Diagnosis of Heartburn

Condition	Typical Symptoms
Gastroesophageal reflux disease (GERD)	Regurgitation, dysphagia
Peptic ulcer disease	Gnawing epigastric pain, nausea, vomiting, bloating
Gastritis	Same as peptic ulcer disease
Non-ulcer dyspepsia	Upper abdominal/epigastric pain, bloating, belching, flatulence, nausea
Coronary artery disease/Angina	Chest pressure, nausea, diaphoresis, palpitations
Cholelithiasis	Colicky right upper quadrant pain, with meals, radiation to scapular region
Pancreatitis	Severe constant mid-abdominal pain
Infectious esophagitis	Dysphagia, associated immunocompromised condition
Medication or chemical esophagitis	Dysphagia, associated ingestion
Scleroderma/Polymyositis with secondary gastroesophageal reflux	Associated signs of connective tissue disease, potential risk of stricture/dysphagia

weight loss, vomiting, or bleeding are present, or when a patient fails to respond to therapy.

Esophagogastroduodenoscopy (EGD) is the diagnostic tool most frequently used in evaluating the symptoms of heartburn or dysphagia and in assessing the upper gastrointestinal tract in patients with gastrointestinal blood loss. EGD will detect esophagitis, erosions, ulceration, malignancies, webs, diverticula, and strictures, and it can be therapeutically useful in treating ulcer disease and strictures.

Barium studies, such as the barium swallow or upper gastrointestinal series, can reveal anatomical abnormalities, esophageal spasm, and may detect reflux. However, barium studies have a lower sensitivity than EGD for detecting ulceration, erosions, and tumors, and do not allow tissue diagnosis.

Ambulatory esophageal pH monitoring can be useful for patients with suspected GERD who have normal endoscopy and have either atypical symptoms or are refractory to therapy. A thin pH probe is placed through the patient's nose into the esophagus 5 centimeters above the lower esophageal sphincter. The percentage of time the esophageal pH is below 4, in conjunction with the patient's symptoms, provides diagnostic information. The reported sensitivity and specificity for this test are both 95%.

Esophageal manometry involves monitoring of lower esophageal sphincter pressures and esophageal peristalsis. Its primary role is to evaluate patients for motility disorders.

H. pylori testing can be useful in assessing patients with heartburn. Currently, there are four different tests: the rapid urease test, histologic staining, serologic tests, and urea breath tests.

The rapid urease test analyzes tissue samples obtained during endoscopy for the presence of urease, a marker of *H. pylori* infection. This test has a sensitivity of approximately 90% and a specificity of 98%. The test itself is inexpensive and quickly performed, but obtaining samples is expensive because of the costs associated with endoscopy.

If the rapid urease test is negative in a patient with ulcers or gastritis, then a separate sample can be sent for histologic staining for *H. pylori*. Histologic staining is very sensitive and specific for *H. pylori*, however, results are less readily available and testing is more expensive than the urease test.

Serologic tests have the advantage of being noninvasive, inexpensive, and highly sensitive and specific (>90%). The disadvantages are that serology will remain indefinitely positive, and a positive test indicates only prior infection, not necessarily current activity; and patients in their 20s are rarely positive, whereas more than 50% of those in their 60s are positive. Serologic testing is most useful in younger populations and for diagnosing *H. pylori* in radiographically diagnosed duodenal ulcers.

Urea breath tests involve having the patient ingest urea labeled with radioactive carbon. If *H. pylori* is present, urease hydrolyzes the urea and the patient exhales labeled carbon dioxide. The test is both sensitive and specific but can be expensive and may not be readily available.

MANAGEMENT

Table 28–2 outlines common heartburn treatments. Typical GERD symptoms of heartburn and regurgitation can be treated empirically with lifestyle modifications and acid suppressive therapy using H2 blockers or proton pump inhibitors. Lifestyle modifications include elevating the head of the patient's bed, weight loss if obese, avoiding foods that lower LES tone, and for smokers stopping tobacco use. Patients with symptoms persisting beyond 6 weeks merit referral for diagnostic evaluation such as endoscopy.

The rate of recurrence with GERD is high because the underlying pathophysiologic process is unchanged when therapy is discontinued. Moderate to severe esophagitis and atypical symptoms, particularly respiratory symptoms, may require long-term treatment. Nonetheless, attempts to step down therapy should be attempted after 8 weeks of symptom control.

TABLE 28–2

Treatments for Common Causes of Heartburn

Disease	Treatments	Example
GERD	Behavioral changes	— Avoid fatty foods, spicy foods, chocolate, mints, citrus
		— Avoid alcohol, caffeine
		— Avoid large meals and reclining after meals
	Medications	
	— H2 blockers	Cimetidine, ranitidine, famotidine, nizatidine
	— Proton pump inhibitors	Omeprazole, lansoprazole, pantoprazole, rabeprazole
PUD/Gastritis		
— *H. pylori*-positive	Medications	
	Antibiotics *and*	Clarithromycin, amoxicillin, metronidazole
	Proton pump inhibitors	Omeprazole, lansoprazole, pantoprazole, rabeprazole
— *H. pylori*-negative	Medications	
	— H2 blockers	Cimetidine, ranitidine, famotidine, nizatidine
	— Proton pump inhibitors	Omeprazole, lansoprazole, pantoprazole, rabeprazole
Non-ulcer dyspepsia	Behavioral changes	Avoid offending foods Reassurance
Dysmotility symptoms	Medications	Metoclopramide
Ulcer-like or reflux	Medications	
	— H2 blockers	Cimetidine, ranitidine, famotidine, nizatidine
	— Proton pump inhibitors	Omeprazole, lansoprazole, pantoprazole, rabeprazole

Some patients may require only intermittent therapy along with continued lifestyle modifications. Severe esophagitis, Barrett's esophagus, and stricture are markers of severe reflux and require long-term treatment, even in the absence of symptoms, in order to reduce the risk of esophageal carcinoma, bleeding, or stricture.

Therapy for peptic ulcer disease and gastritis depends on whether *H. pylori* is present. If *H. pylori* is present, then therapy directed against this organism is indicated. Regimens include triple therapy with combinations of omeprazole (a proton pump inhibitor), clarithromycin, and amoxicillin or metronidazole for 7 to 14 days. Triple therapy regimens have cure rates of approximately 90%. After completing the antibiotic regimen, proton pump inhibitors are generally continued for 4 to 8 weeks for duodenal ulcers and for 6 to 12 weeks for gastritis or gastric ulcers.

Patients with NSAID-related ulcers are generally treated with acid suppression therapy and discontinuance of the NSAID. If NSAIDs must be used, options include switching the patient to a nonacetylated salicylate such as salsalate (Disalcid), or a Cox-2 inhibitor, using an enterically coated preparation and prescribing the lowest effective dose. If NSAIDs must be used in patients with a history of ulcer, misoprostol (Cytotec) or a proton pump inhibitor can help prevent recurrence.

Therapy for non-ulcer dyspepsia involves avoiding foods or medications that aggravate symptoms, reassurance regarding the absence of serious disease, and medications directed at the predominant symptoms. In patients with ulcer-like or reflux symptoms, acid-suppressing agents are helpful while dysmotility related symptoms, such as nausea, bloating, or early satiety respond better to motility agents. If treatment is initially successful, 4 weeks of continuous therapy is followed by a trial off medication. Some patients need only intermittent therapy, whereas others may require continuous treatment. In such cases, periodic attempts to wean off medication should be attempted to see if symptoms recur.

◆ KEY POINTS ◆

1. Heartburn is a common symptom, affecting 40% or more of the population every month.

2. Gastroesophageal reflux disease, peptic ulcer disease, gastritis, and non-ulcer dyspepsia are the major causes for heartburn symptoms.

3. Atypical symptoms of dysphagia, early satiety, weight loss, or blood loss should trigger a gastrointestinal work-up.

4. Esophagogastroduodenoscopy is the most useful diagnostic tool for evaluating heartburn.

5. *Helicobacter pylori* is a leading causative factor for peptic ulcer disease and gastritis.

6. H2 blockers, proton pump inhibitors, and behavioral changes are the cornerstones of therapy for *H. pylori*-negative disease. Antibiotic therapy, along with proton pump inhibitors, is used to treat *H. pylori*-positive patients with peptic ulcer disease or gastritis.

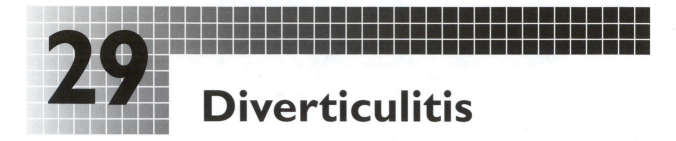

29 Diverticulitis

Diverticuli are herniations in the colonic mucosa that are present in many patients over the age of 40. Twenty percent of individuals over the age of 40 and up to 70% of people over age 70 have diverticuli. Most patients with diverticuli are asymptomatic, however, up to 15% will develop complications such as diverticulitis, gastrointestinal obstruction, or bleeding. Diverticulitis is an inflammation of the diverticuli that most commonly affects the sigmoid colon. Risk factors for the development of diverticulitis include older age, low fiber diet, a previous history of diverticulitis, and the presence of a large number of diverticuli in the colon.

PATHOPHYSIOLOGY

Diverticuli are outpouchings, or herniations, of the colonic mucosa through the muscularis layer. These occur most commonly in areas of mucosal weakness, usually where an artery penetrates the muscularis to reach the submucosa and the mucosa. The sigmoid colon is more commonly involved because the luminal size is smaller and the pressures generated are greater than in other areas of the colon. Normally, diverticuli are asymptomatic, however they may become obstructed with fecal material, which can cause inflammation and microabscess formation within and around the diverticulum. This inflammatory process is called diverticulitis. The inflammation may progress to involve a larger segment of colon and cause a narrowing or stric-

ture. Larger abscesses may form and encroach on neighboring structures leading to development of fistulae. Diverticular bleeding is usually not associated with pain and occurs when fecal matter traumatizes one of the perforating arteries at the site of a diverticulum.

CLINICAL MANIFESTATIONS

History

The clinical manifestations of diverticular disease vary from asymptomatic disease to abdominal pain or bleeding. Only 10% to 25% of diverticulosis sufferers will develop symptoms. Patients with diverticulitis usually present with complaints of colicky left lower quadrant abdominal pain that may be aggravated by eating and relieved with bowel movement. On occasion, the abdominal pain may occur in other locations, such as the right lower quadrant. These patients also experience fever, chills, nausea, vomiting, decreased appetite, and are often constipated. Patients may present with massive gastrointestinal bleeding, but without other symptoms or pain. Colon cancer should be suspected in elderly patients with weight loss, abdominal pain, and changes in bowel habits.

Physical Examination

Physical exam may reveal peritoneal signs such as rigidity, rebound tenderness, and guarding. The abdomen may be distended and tympanic. Often a mass or fullness is palpated in the left lower quadrant. The physical exam should include a rectal exam to rule out any bleeding. In cases of severe bleeding, patients may have signs of hypovolemia and anemia.

DIFFERENTIAL DIAGNOSIS

Box 29–1 lists some causes for lower quadrant abdominal pain. The differential diagnosis for rectal bleeding will include polyps, colon cancer, angiodysplasia, as well as diverticular disease. Patients with left lower quadrant abdominal pain may have infectious, inflammatory or ischemic colitis, irritable bowel syndrome, or colon cancer. In right-sided abdominal pain, appendicitis needs to be considered. Nephrolithiasis may cause abdominal pain but is usually not associated with tenderness or fever. In females, gynecologic complaints such as an ovarian mass, ruptured ovarian cyst, torsion, and endometriosis are part of the differential diagnosis.

DIAGNOSTIC APPROACH

Diverticulitis is initially a clinical diagnosis that is then supported by laboratory and diagnostic testing. An elevated white blood count along with a left shift suggests an inflammatory process. Hemoglobin testing is useful for evaluating gastrointestinal bleeding and urinalysis is useful in evaluating urinary tract disorders such as stones or infection. Plain abdominal films do not show any specific findings with diverticulitis, but may show an

---

BOX 29–1
Causes for Lower Abdominal Pain

Diverticulitis
Inflammatory bowel disease
Irritable bowel syndrome
Carcinoma of the colon
Ischemic colitis
Nephrolithiasis
Appendicitis
Ileus
Urinary tract infections
Gynecological disorders

---

ileus pattern. Computed tomography (CT) of the abdomen is the imaging test of choice for patients with suspected diverticulitis and will provide diagnostic evidence of diverticulitis in more than 90% of cases. A CT scan can also be helpful in detecting other causes for a patient's abdominal pain. Barium enema can reveal diverticulitis, but is often not advisable during an acute episode for fear of causing perforation and spillage of barium into the abdomen. In patients with diverticulitis, follow-up testing should include a colonoscopy 6 weeks after resolution of symptoms in order to detect an underlying malignancy.

TREATMENT

Patients with diverticulosis should be encouraged to eat high-fiber diets and to avoid nuts and fruits with small seeds. Fiber supplements such as psyllium are helpful. In addition to dietary maneuvers, anticholinergic drugs or antispasmodic drugs may be helpful for the relief of crampy abdominal pain. Stool softeners may be helpful.

Patients with diverticulitis may be treated as outpatients or inpatients depending upon the severity of illness and the reliability of the patient in adhering to therapy and follow-up. Patients with mild symptoms, stable vital signs, and who are not vomiting may be placed on a clear liquid diet and oral antibiotics with follow-up in 2 to 3 days. If the patient is improving, the diet may be advanced and the antibiotic continued for 7 to 10 days. The patient should undergo colonoscopy in 6 weeks to evaluate the possibility of colon carcinoma. Patients with more severe pain, vomiting, or unstable vital signs will require hospitalization. The patient initially takes nothing by mouth and is provided with intravenous fluids and antibiotics. As the pain subsides, a diet is introduced and the patient is placed on oral antibiotics. Again, follow-up colonoscopy is recommended. Both inpatients and outpatients with diverticulitis are monitored for complications that may require surgical intervention. These include abscess formation, stricture formation with obstruction, fistulae, and peritonitis. Recurrent episodes may prompt surgical intervention.

Antibiotic selection for patients with diverticulitis should provide coverage for gram negative and anaerobic bacteria. Common oral outpatient choices are trimethoprim-sulfamethoxazole, amoxicillin-clavulanate, doxycycline, or ciprofloxacin plus metronidazole. Common inpatient antibiotic choices are ampicillin-sulbactam or cefoxitin.

Diverticular bleeding is managed with supportive care and evaluation of the source of the bleeding. The bleeding will generally stop without intervention, but may recur in up to 25% of cases.

◆ KEY POINTS ◆

1. Diverticular disease is a common disease in the elderly.

2. Risk factors for diverticulitis include age over 40 years, low fiber diet, history of diverticulitis, and the number of diverticuli in the colon.

3. The clinical manifestations of diverticular disease vary from total asymptomatic disease to severe pain, bleeding, or diverticulitis.

4. Patients with diverticulitis will often have left lower quadrant pain along with fever and chills.

5. Elderly patients with weight loss, abdominal pain, and changes in bowel habits should be suspected of having colon cancer.

6. In acute cases of diverticulitis, CT scan is the test of choice.

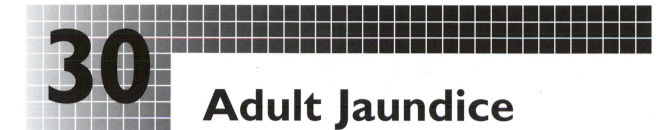

30 Adult Jaundice

Jaundice (icterus) is defined as yellowing of the sclera, skin, and other tissues due to hyperbilirubinemia. The increased level of bilirubin can be due to unconjugated or conjugated bilirubin. Total serum bilirubin in a healthy person is normally 0.2–1.2 mg/dl. This consists of both conjugated and unconjugated bilirubin. Jaundice becomes clinically evident when the bilirubin level reaches 2.0–2.5 mg/dl. Increased levels of bilirubin can be due to overproduction, impaired uptake by the liver or due to impaired excretion. In adults, jaundice is most often due to liver disease or obstruction of the common bile duct. Hepatitis accounts for up to 75% of the cases of jaundice in young adults. Hereditary disorders such as Gilbert's syndrome and Crigler-Najjar syndrome are less common causes of jaundice. Gilbert's syndrome is a life-long disease and is often diagnosed early in life. It affects 3% to 5% of the population. Crigler-Najjar syndrome is a rare disorder that is diagnosed early in life.

PATHOPHYSIOLOGY

Bilirubin is the major breakdown product of hemoglobin. Bilirubin, which is water insoluble, binds to albumin and is transported to the liver for conjugation with glucuronic acid to form bilirubin diglucuronide (conjugated bilirubin or direct bilirubin). The unconjugated bilirubin cannot pass the glomerular membrane and as a result does not appear in the urine. However, the conjugated bilirubin (bilirubin diglucuronide) is water-soluble and can be present in the urine, giving it a tea color. This color is typical of hepatocellular or cholestatic jaundice and results in a positive urine dipstick test for bilirubin. Once direct bilirubin is formed, it is excreted into the biliary system and thus enters the small intestine. In the intestine, the bacterial flora deconjugates the bilirubin to stercobilinogens, which gives the brown color to the stools.

An elevated bilirubin can either be unconjugated or conjugated. The causes of unconjugated hyperbilirubinemia are secondary to overproduction, hemolysis, or defects in bilirubin conjugation. Overproduction of bilirubin can be due to diseases such as thallasemia, sideroblastic anemia, and B12 deficiency, all of which result in ineffective erythropoiesis. Gilbert's syndrome and Crigler-Najjar syndrome cause unconjugated hyperbilirubinemia by a defect in the liver's ability to conjugate bilirubin. Decreased hepatic uptake of bilirubin, secondary to sepsis or right heart failure, can also elevate unconjugated bilirubin.

Conjugated hyperbilirubinemia can be due to impaired excretion of bilirubin from the liver. This can happen at the cellular level due to hepatocellular disease, in the ductule due to medication exposure (e.g., phenothiazines), or in the septal ducts due to primary biliary cirrhosis. In addition, obstruction of the common bile duct by gallstones or pancreatic cancer can cause conjugated hyperbilirubinemia.

CLINICAL MANIFESTATIONS

History

A complete history helps formulate the differential diagnosis. The presence of right upper quadrant pain suggests a hepatobiliary cause. Nausea and vomiting accompanied by flu-like symptoms that precede jaundice may indicate hepatitis. Other questions in the history of the present illness should include the presence of pruritus, urine discoloration, increased abdominal girth (ascites), fever, and weight loss. Patient should be asked about IV drug use, alcoholism, contact with hepatitis patients, recent blood transfusions, recent travel, and prior history of immunizations. A family history of episodic jaundice in the setting of intercurrent illness is consistent with Gilbert's disease. Current and past medicines and any herbal medicines should be noted. Drugs that may cause jaundice include acetaminophen, isoniazid, nitrofurantoin, methotrexate, sulfonamides, and phenytoin.

Physical Examination

Patients with unconjugated hyperbilirubinemia may present with weakness, abdominal pain, or back pain. Since unconjugated bilirubin is water insoluble, the urine and the stool color in these patients are normal. However on physical exam, splenomegaly may be present indicating hemolysis as a possible cause of jaundice.

Patients with hereditary cholestatic syndromes or intrahepatic cholestasis may present with pruritus, light colored stool, and malaise, or they may be totally asymptomatic. Patients with hepatocellular disease such as hepatitis will present with malaise, anorexia, low-grade fever, and right upper quadrant pain. Also the urine may appear tea colored because of the excretion of conjugated bilirubin. Patients who present with right upper quadrant pain without any fever or anorexia may have gallstones obstructing the common bile duct, resulting in jaundice. In patients who present with Charcot's triad (high fever, right upper quadrant pain, and jaundice) cholangitis needs to be ruled out. Jaundice and weight loss are findings associated with carcinoma of the head of the pancreas.

Jaundice can be noted in the sclera, skin, and mucous membranes. The eyes should be closely examined for Kayser-Fleischer rings, which indicate Wilson's disease. In the abdominal exam, any tenderness should be noted. Liver span should be measured by percussion. A palpable gallbladder (Courvoisier's sign) indicates gallstones as a cause of jaundice. Viral hepatitis usually causes a mildly tender liver with slight to moderate enlargement. A fluid wave and shifting dullness indicates ascites. Findings such as a small liver, ascites, splenomegaly, spider angiomas, gynecomastia, palmar erythema, and other stigmata of cirrhosis suggest advanced hepatocellular disease. Severe liver disease may cause fetor hepaticus and on the neurologic exam, patients may have asterixis and other neurologic deficits.

DIFFERENTIAL DIAGNOSIS

Box 30–1 lists the causes of jaundice grouped by pathophysiology and whether the hyperbilirubinemia is conjugated. Obstruction, intrahepatic cholestasis, and hepatocellular disease cause the majority of cases of jaundice. In young patients, hepatitis is the most common cause of jaundice. In older individuals, obstruction from stones or tumors is more common.

DIAGNOSTIC APPROACH

The diagnostic approach begins with the history and physical exam, which should provide clues as to the etiology of the patient's jaundice. Testing usually begins with a complete blood count, urinalysis, and a liver panel test, including transaminases, total bilirubin, alkaline phosphatase, and albumin. An anemia or sudden drop in the hemoglobin level suggests a hemolytic process as the cause of jaundice. If the conjugated bilirubin level is elevated and the urine dipstick is positive for bilirubin, this most likely indicates obstruction, cholestasis, or hepatocellular injury. If the urine dipstick is negative, then the jaundice is most likely due to a hemolytic process or a hereditary hyperbilirubinemia, most commonly Gilbert's syndrome. A reticulocyte count, lactate dehydrogenase, peripheral smear, and haptoglobin can detect hemolysis. Gilbert's syndrome is characterized by a mild recurrent elevation of bilirubin precipitated by fasting or mild illness. Patients with Gilbert's syndrome generally have no systemic symptoms and no other liver test abnormalities.

In patients with elevated conjugated bilirubin, the pattern of the liver enzyme elevations provides clues to the cause of the jaundice. Transaminases elevated out of proportion (>5x normal) to the alkaline phosphatase suggest liver dysfunction. Conversely, an obstructive enzyme pattern is characterized by an elevated alkaline phosphatase (>3x normal) out of proportion to the rise

BOX 30–1

Differential Diagnosis for Adult Jaundice

Unconjugated hyperbilirubinemia
  Increased production
    Hemolytic anemias secondary to
    ineffective erythropoiesis
      Thalassemia
      Sideroblastic anemia
      Pernicious anemia
  Impaired uptake
  Gilbert's syndrome
  Crigler-Najjar syndrome

Conjugated hyperbilirubinemia
  Hereditary cholestatic syndromes
  Faulty excretion of bilirubin
    Dubin-Johnson syndrome
    Rotor's syndrome
  Hepatocellular dysfunction
    Biliary epithelial damage
      Hepatitis
      Cirrhosis
    Intrahepatic cholestasis
      Drugs
      Biliary cirrhosis
      Sepsis
  Biliary obstruction
    Choledocholithiasis
    Biliary atresia
    Carcinoma of biliary duct
    Sclerosing cholangitis
    Pancreatic cancer

in transaminases (<4–5× normal). Gamma glutamyl transpeptidase usually parallels the rise in alkaline phosphatase. This test is useful for confirming that an elevated alkaline phosphatase is caused by liver disease since an increase in alkaline phosphatase can also occur in bone disease.

If liver disease is suspected as the cause of jaundice, then the following tests should be performed as indicated by the history and physical exam:

1. Hepatitis profile to look for hepatitis as a cause

2. Antimitochondrial antibody to screen for primary biliary cirrhosis

3. Serum iron, transferrin saturation, and ferritin to screen for hemochromatosis

4. Serum ceruloplasmin and urine copper levels to screen for Wilson's disease

Imaging tests are useful for patients with obstructive disease. Ultrasound is a noninvasive test for detecting dilated bile ducts indicative of obstruction. The sensitivity and specificity of this test is in the 90% to 95% range. Although an ultrasound can detect obstruction, it is less helpful in determining the site and cause of the obstruction. A CT scan is more likely to identify the site or cause of obstruction but is more expensive than ultrasound.

If an obstruction is identified and additional anatomic detail is needed, endoscopic retrograde cholangiopancreatography (ERCP) can provide visualization. This test is also useful if obstructive jaundice is suspected despite negative imaging procedures. An ERCP may be therapeutically helpful, since an obstructing stone might be removed during the procedure, a sphincterotomy performed, or a stent placed. Complications of ERCP include infection and pancreatitis.

MANAGEMENT

The treatment of jaundice should focus on the underlying disease process. Any drug that may cause jaundice should be discontinued. If there is complete resolution of laboratory abnormalities within 2 weeks of withdrawing the offending agent, no further workup or treatment is needed. Symptomatic pruritus can be treated with cholestyramine and antihistamines such as diphenhydramine. Pernicious anemia, which may cause a hemolytic anemia, can be treated with vitamin B12 replacement.

Patients with obstructive jaundice may need to be treated surgically. For patients with gallstones, either open or laparoscopic cholecystectomy is indicated.

In some cases of obstructive jaundice, an ERCP can be both diagnostic and therapeutic. Common bile duct stones may be removed via the endoscope or a stent placed to relieve the biliary obstruction and to reduce inflammation and prepare a patient for surgery. Most patients with neoplasm require surgery. This surgery can either be palliative or for definitive treatment. Patients with obstructive jaundice and a fever and chills need to be hospitalized for possible cholangitis. These patients require intravenous antibiotics.

Hepatitis can be treated on an outpatient basis. However, patients with severe nausea and vomiting who become dehydrated need to be hospitalized.

◆ KEY POINTS ◆

1. Jaundice becomes clinically evident when the bilirubin level is greater than 2.0–2.5 mg/dl.

2. An elevated bilirubin can be due to overproduction, impaired uptake by the liver, or impaired excretion.

3. Hepatitis can account for as much as 75% of the causes of jaundice in younger adults.

4. Biliary obstruction from gallstones or malignancy is more common in older patients.

5. Drugs causing jaundice: acetaminophen, isoniazid, nitofurantoin, methotrexate, sulfonamides, and phenytoin.

6. Charcot's triad (high fever, right upper quadrant pain, and jaundice) indicates cholangitis.

7. Weight loss and painless jaundice are signs of pancreatic cancer.

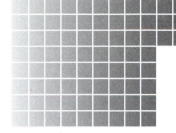

Part VIII
Genitourinary
Disease

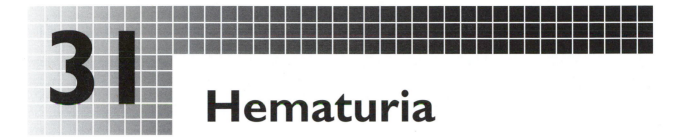

31 Hematuria

Hematuria can be either microscopic or grossly visible. Microscopic hematuria is defined as more than three red blood cells per high-power field (phpf). Although hematuria may be asymptomatic, it is important to evaluate the cause since up to 10% of cases have a serious underlying etiology.

PATHOPHYSIOLOGY

Normally, the amount of RBCs excreted in the urine per day is 2000 cells/ml, equivalent to about 1 RBC phpf. Hematuria may be caused by systemic illnesses, intrarenal or glomerular disease and extrarenal or structural disease such as a neoplasm that erodes into blood vessels. Prostatic disease can enlarge and dilate mucosal vessels and cause bleeding if these vessels leak or rupture. Kidney or bladder stones can inflame the mucosa and blood vessels as they move through the urinary tract.

CLINICAL MANIFESTATIONS

History

Pyelonephritis, renal infarction, and a kidney mass can all present with flank pain. Flank pain radiating into the groin suggests a kidney stone. Urgency, frequency, and dysuria occur with inflammation of the lower urinary tract from conditions such as cystitis. Fever is common with pyelonephritis but is sometimes associated with advanced renal cell carcinoma. Hematuria is present in 90% of renal cell carcinoma cases, and painless hematuria may be a presenting sign of a urinary tract malignancy. It is the most common presenting symptom of bladder cancer in individuals over age 50 and is a common cause of hematuria in this age group.

In women, the menstrual history is important since menstrual bleeding may be mistaken for hematuria. A history of trauma increases the likelihood of a renal, ureteral, or urethral injury. Inquiring about recent infectious illnesses is also important. A recent streptococcal infection may be a clue for poststreptococcal glomerulonephritis, while exposure to tuberculosis (TB) increases the risk for a TB infection. A recent upper respiratory infection may cause hematuria in a patient with IgA nephropathy (Berger's disease). A previous history of kidney stones, nephritis, cystitis, or bladder cancer suggests a recurrence as a possible cause of hematuria. Valvular heart disease in association with recent dental work or a history of intravenous drug use increases the risk for subacute bacterial endocarditis. Hemoptysis combined with hematuria is a symptom of Goodpasture's syndrome.

Reviewing the patient's medications is important. Interstitial nephritis can result from a number of medications such as NSAIDs, cephalosporins, and ciprofloxacin. It may cause hematuria accompanied by fever and a skin rash. Chemotherapeutic agents, particularly cyclophosphamide, can cause hemorrhagic cystitis. Medications that discolor the urine such as pyridium and rifampin may be mistaken for hematuria.

Family history is valuable for recognizing risk factors for certain diseases. For example, sickle cell disease or trait is much more prevalent in African-American patients with a family history of the illness. Patients with benign familial hematuria have normal renal function and often have family members similarly affected. Polycystic kidney disease can either be adult onset (autosomal dominant) or found in childhood. Alport's syndrome (autosomal recessive) is associated with deafness.

Physical Examination

Costovertebral angle tenderness is common with pyelonephritis and tumors that stretch the kidney capsule. Kidney stones may cause severe pain, with patients finding it difficult to sit still. An abdominal mass may be present with polycystic kidney disease or renal cell carcinoma. Suprapubic tenderness occurs with cystitis, while a urethral discharge suggests urethritis. In men, a rectal examination may reveal an enlarged smooth prostate gland consistent with BPH or a nodular hard prostate found in prostate cancer. A tender boggy prostate is a sign of prostatitis.

Findings such as a malar rash, fatigue, and joint pain suggest systemic lupus erythematosis (SLE). In children and young adults, palpable purpura, arthritis, and abdominal pain are signs of Henoch-Schonlein purpura. Hypertension and peripheral edema are common findings with glomerulonephritis. Patients with atrial fibrillation are at risk for developing emboli and renal infarction. A pelvic examination in a female may reveal a pelvic source for the bleeding.

DIFFERENTIAL DIAGNOSIS

Lesions involving the kidney, ureters, bladder, prostate, and urethra can all present with hematuria. Gross hematuria is usually associated with infection, stones, and neoplasm. In children, benign familial hematuria, glomerular disease, hypercalciuria, infection, and perineal irritation or trauma are the most common etiolo-gies. In young adults, the most likely causes are infection, stones, trauma, and a urinary tract tumor. In older age groups, bladder cancer and prostate disease increase in prevalence. The underlying prevalence of a serious disease such as a neoplasm or polycystic kidney disease varies but may be as high as 10%.

SLE may present with hematuria. Blood disorders such as sickle cell, coagulopathies, and leukemia are possible but infrequent causes of hematuria. As noted earlier, drugs may cause hematuria. Although anticoagulants can cause bleeding, those individuals on anticoagulants who have hematuria should still be evaluated because underlying lesions are frequently found. Table 31–1 lists the differential diagnosis for hematuria.

DIAGNOSTIC APPROACH

The quantity of bleeding, the clinical setting, and other associated findings on the U/A determine the extent of the evaluation. The presence or absence of dysmorphic red blood cells, such as RBC casts, is pivotal since RBC casts suggest bleeding from a glomerular source. The finding of heavy proteinuria also suggests that the bleeding is glomerular in origin.

Pyuria, defined as greater than 4 to 5 WBCs phpf, points to infection as the cause for hematuria. Even in asymptomatic individuals, the initial test for hematuria is a urine culture. An entirely normal repeat study after treating an infection in a healthy individual less than 35 to 40 usually requires no further evaluation other than a follow-up U/A in 1 to 2 months. Similarly, a repeat U/A to confirm the presence of hematuria in an individual suspected of having a benign cause such as menstrual bleeding or vigorous exercise is helpful before starting an extensive workup. If interstitial nephritis is suspected, eosinophiluria may be present.

Persistent hematuria or hematuria in individuals over 40 merits further investigation. In the absence of significant proteinuria (>2+ proteinuria), dysmorphic RBCs or infection, hematuria usually indicates a structural abnormality of the urinary tract.

After obtaining routine chemistries, such as a CBC, platelet count, BUN, and creatinine, an intravenous pyelogram (IVP) is usually the initial test. This imaging procedure can detect stones, masses, cysts, and hydronephrosis. An ultrasound is an alternative for indi-

TABLE 31–1

Differential Diagnosis of Hematuria

Hematologic	coagulopathy, sickle hemoglobinopathies (e.g., Sickle cell)
Renal/glomerular	glomerulonephritis
	benign familial hematuria
	multisystem disease (systemic lupus erythematosus, Henoch-Schonlein purpura, hemolytic uremic syndrome, polyarteritis nodosa, Wegener's granulomatosis, Goodpasture's syndrome)
Renal/nonglomerular	renal vein or artery embolus, tuberculosis, pyelonephritis, polycystic kidney disease, medullary sponge kidney, acute interstitial nephritis, tumor, vascular malformation, trauma, papillary necrosis, exercise
Postrenal	stones, tumor of ureter/bladder/urethra, cystitis, tuberculosis, prostatitis, urethritis, Foley catheter placement, exercise, benign prostatic hypertrophy

viduals allergic to contrast media, at risk for contrast nephropathy, or with renal insufficiency. Suspicious lesions on IVP or US usually require further evaluation by CT or MRI and possibly biopsy. Rarely, renal arteriography is needed to evaluate for traumatic injury, a suspicious renal mass, and A-V malformation.

If imaging reveals normal upper tracts, cystoscopy is indicated in patients over 40 and can detect bladder neoplasm, bladder stones, BPH, and cystitis. Since bladder cancer is rare in those under 40, the value of cystoscopy is less certain in younger individuals. Urine cytology is a safe test that can detect some bladder cancers and may be an alternative in younger individuals. If performed on three consecutive first-voided morning urine specimens, it has a sensitivity of about 30%. Cystoscopy should still be considered in persistent hematuria in younger individuals and in those with risk factors for bladder cancer such as smoking or exposure to aniline dyes.

For patients with evidence of glomerular bleeding such as RBC cast or heavy proteinuria (>3 or 4+), a more extensive laboratory workup is indicated. Tests include an ESR, ANA, cryoglobulins, antistreptococcal enzyme tests (anti-ASO, anti-DNAse B), and an antineutrophil cytoplasmic antibody (ANCA) to screen for Wegener's granulomatosis and vasculitis. Also plasma complement levels should be tested, since low levels are associated with SLE and poststreptococcal glomerulonephritis. Other useful tests include checking for eosinophiluria in patients with suspected interstitial nephritis and TB cultures in cases of persistent sterile pyuria. A hemoglobin electrophoresis can detect sickle cell disease and other hemoglobinopathies. Serum IgA levels may be helpful in patients suspected of having Berger's disease or Henoch-Schonlein purpura. Serum antiglomerular basement membrane antibodies can be positive in Goodpasture's syndrome and serum and urine immunoelectrophoresis can help diagnose multiple myeloma.

MANAGEMENT

Management depends on the underlying cause. The presence of a defined lesion or the need to undergo cystoscopy merits referral to a urologist. Poststreptococcal glomerulonephritis therapy is generally limited to treating the associated hypertension. Rapid or progressive deterioration of renal function merits consultation. Most other patients with suspected glomerulonephritis should be referred for consideration of renal biopsy.

Despite an extensive evaluation, no cause of hematuria can be found in 10% to 15% of patients. These individuals require long-term follow-up with monitoring of the urine sediment and renal function at 6-month intervals.

◆ KEY POINTS ◆

1. Asymptomatic microscopic hematuria is defined as more than three red blood cells per high-power.

2. Under age 20, glomerulonephritis and urinary tract infection (UTI) are most common. In the age group between 20 and 40, one should consider UTI, stone, trauma and neoplasm of the urinary tract. In the age group 40 to 60, the most common cause of hematuria is bladder carcinoma, followed by kidney stone, UTI, kidney carcinoma and benign prostate hypertrophy.

3. Familial causes of hematuria are benign familial hematuria, sickle cell disease or trait, polycystic kidney disease, Alport's syndrome and familial hypercalciuria.

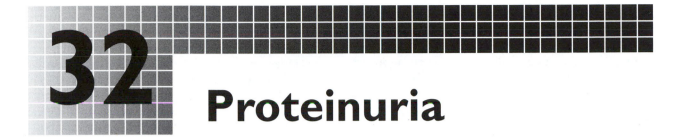

32 Proteinuria

Proteinuria is defined in adults as protein excretion greater than 150 mg per 24 hours. In children proteinuria varies with the age and size of the child. Nephrotic range proteinuria is defined as the daily excretion of more than 3.5 grams of protein over 24 hours. The causes for proteinuria range from benign conditions such as orthostatic proteinuria to life-threatening conditions such as glomerular nephritis and rapidly progressive renal failure. Proteinuria is often first identified as an incidental finding on urinalysis during a routine office visit.

PATHOPHYSIOLOGY

The glomerulus allows the easy passage of water while providing a barrier to protein excretion. Each day the normal glomerular filtrate contains between 500 and 1500 mg of low molecular weight proteins. Most of this protein is resorbed and metabolized by the renal tubular cells. Normally excretion is less than 150 mg per day. Since urine testing may turn positive at 100 mg/ml, normal individuals may test trace positive for proteinuria on an office dipstick.

Significant proteinuria can occur from glomerular damage and increased permeability, renal tubular diseases that affect resorption, and overflow proteinuria. Glomerular disease can be either primary or secondary. Primary glomerular diseases include minimal change disease, focal glomerular sclerosis, membranous glomerular nephropathy and IgA nephropathy. Secondary causes include infections such as post-streptococcal glomerular nephritis and systemic diseases such as lupus or a drug-related effect on the glomerulus. Overflow proteinuria occurs when there is production of abnormal proteins, such as Bence-Jones proteins as seen in multiple myeloma, that easily pass through the glomerulus. The type of protein found in the urine differs depending on the cause. Glomerular disease usually results in excess albumin excretion while tubular disease is associated with an array of low molecular proteins. Plasma proteins are found in multiple myeloma or monoclonal gammopathy.

CLINICAL MANIFESTATIONS

History

Proteinuria can either be transient or persistent. Transient, or functional proteinuria, can occur with exercise, febrile illness, seizures, abdominal surgery, congestive heart failure, and epinephrine administration. Persistent proteinuria is defined as the presence of proteinuria on at least two separate occasions. Orthostatic or postural proteinuria accounts for 60% of patients with asymptomatic proteinuria. Typically patients are less than 30 years old, have protein secretion less than 2 gm/day, and the proteinuria occurs when the patient is in the upright position, but normalizes in the supine position.

Nephrotic range proteinuria (>3.5 gm/24 hours) is usually the consequence of glomerular damage.

Proteinuria can either be primary or occur in the setting of renal or systemic diseases. Glomerular nephritis patients usually present with hematuria, red blood cell casts, and mild to moderate hypertension. These patients typically have proteinuria and edema, but not as severe as those patients seen with nephrotic syndrome. Nephrotic syndrome consists of massive proteinuria, hypoalbuminemia, hyperlipidemia, lipiduria, and edema.

The focus of the history is to determine possible causes for proteinuria and to assess the severity of the condition. Edema suggests nephrotic range proteinuria, and hypertension the possibility of significant renal disease. The history may reveal the presence of systemic illnesses that are associated with proteinuria such as long-standing diabetes mellitus, systemic lupus erythematosis, congestive heart failure, multiple myeloma, and amyloidosis. A detailed review of medications is important since medications such as penicillin and cephalosporins may cause proteinuria. Other medications causing proteinuria include ACE inhibitors, cyclosporins, NSAIDs, heavy metals, aminoglycosides, and sulfonamides. Heroin abuse is also a cause. Chronic renal disease suggests possible polycystic disease. Dysuria and frequency along with a fever indicate a possible urinary tract infection.

Physical Examination

Skin changes such as malar rashes, vasculitis, and purpura can be signs of a connective tissue disease. Diabetic retinopathy is strongly associated with proteinuria and the fundi should be carefully examined. The presence of lymphadenopathy, heart failure, abdominal masses, hepatosplenomegaly, peripheral edema, and blood pressure measurements are important parts of the physical exam. Fever may be present in infectious causes.

DIFFERENTIAL DIAGNOSIS

The differential diagnosis for proteinuria is extensive. Benign transient proteinuria is a common problem that resolves spontaneously and is most often seen in children or young adults. Exercise, congestive heart failure, fever, urinary tract infection, and orthostatic proteinuria are common causes of transient proteinuria in patients without significant renal disease.

Although individuals may have isolated proteinuria without other urinary symptoms or disease, persistent isolated proteinuria suggests underlying glomerular or tubular disease. Primary renal diseases include acute renal failure, acute tubular necrosis, acute glomerular nephritis, and polycystic disease. Systemic illnesses listed in Box 32–1 may all cause proteinuria. Diabetes, in particular, is an important cause of proteinuria. About one-third of Type 1 and one-fourth of individuals with Type 2 diabetes have persistent proteinuria. Drugs and toxins that cause proteinuria include antibiotics, analgesics, anticonvulsants, ACE inhibitors, and heavy metals. Infectious causes include bacterial (SBE, syphilis, post-streptococcal glomerular nephritis), viral (CMV, EBV, HIV, and hepatitis B), and parasitic disease (malaria and toxoplasmosis). In patients with nephrotic range proteinuria, about 50% to 75% of cases are due to intrinsic renal disease. The remainder is due to systemic illnesses such as diabetes, lupus, amyloidosis, and other diseases that cause glomerular injury.

DIAGNOSTIC APPROACH

A urine dipstick is a simple, readily available screening tool for proteinuria. A 1+ protein level usually represents approximately 300 mg/dl of protein excreted per

---

BOX 32–1

Systemic Illnesses Causing Proteinuria

Amyloidosis
Carcinoma
Cryoglobulinemia
Diabetes mellitus
Drugs/Toxins
Goodpasture's syndrome
Henoch-Schonlein purpura
HIV associated nephropathy
Leukemia
Lymphoma
Multiple myeloma
Polyarteritis nodosa
Preeclampsia
Sarcoidosis
SLE
Transplant nephropathy

24 hours. A 4+ usually indicates over 1 g/dl per day. A urine dipstick reacts to albumin and can fail to detect abnormal proteins such as Bence-Jones proteins. A sulfosalicylic acid test measures the total concentration of proteins, including Bence-Jones proteins. False positive dipstick results can be seen with dehydration, gross hematuria, or highly alkaline urine.

If the patient has two or more positive dipstick tests, a 24-hour urine protein collection is indicated along with a urine creatinine clearance determination. If orthostatic proteinuria is suspected, an orthostatic test should be performed. The patient is instructed to urinate and discard the urine the night before a collection. A 16-hour daytime collection should stop before bedtime, followed by an overnight specimen collection. Patients with true orthostatic proteinuria have elevated proteinuria during the day that returns to normal at night.

A total 24-hour protein excretion exceeding 1 gram suggests significant renal impairment. A qualitative urine protein electrophoresis to rule out a monoclonal component is indicated. Further evaluation includes a complete urinalysis, a chemistry panel (including a BUN, creatinine, albumin and total protein), lipid profile, ESR, ASO titer, and a C3-C4 complement level. The presence of red cell casts in the urine indicates glomerular disease. White blood cell casts may be seen in pyelonephritis and interstitial nephritis. Oval fat bodies, if present, are due to lipiduria seen in nephrotic syndrome. A chemistry panel will identify electrolyte imbalances and assess renal function. The complete blood cell count identifies a normocytic normochromic anemia seen when chronic renal insufficiency or multiple myeloma is present. Serum complement levels are low in acute glomerulonephritis and lupus nephritis and an ESR screens for connective tissue diseases and other inflammatory states. ASO titers indicate if there has been a recent strep throat. An ANA, hepatitis panel, RPR, HIV testing, and serum protein electrophoresis should be ordered selectively based on the history, physical, or previous lab results. An ultrasound is helpful in determining kidney size, ruling out polycystic kidney disease or masses, and in detecting an obstructive nephropathy.

MANAGEMENT

Treatments for proteinuria depend on the underlying cause. Those with renal insufficiency, nephrotic range proteinuria, hematuria or red blood cell casts, or with an uncertain underlying cause should be referred to a nephrologist. A nephrologist may perform a renal biopsy to rule out treatable forms of glomerulonephritis, such as membranous glomerulonephropathy, which may respond to steroids or immunosuppressive therapy. ACE inhibitors benefit patients with diabetes and proteinuria. Asymptomatic patients with low range proteinuria may be observed with periodic blood pressure monitoring and an annual assessment of renal function. Referral to a nephrologist should be considered if renal insufficiency or hypertension develops.

◆ KEY POINTS ◆

1. Proteinuria is defined in adults as protein excretion greater than 150 mg per 24 hours. Nephrotic range proteinuria is defined as the daily excretion of more than 3.5 grams of protein over 24 hours.

2. Glomerular nephritis patients usually present with hematuria, red blood cell casts, and mild to moderate hypertension. Nephrotic syndrome consists of massive proteinuria, hypoalbuminemia, hyperlipidemia, lipiduria, and edema.

3. Diabetes is an important cause of proteinuria. About one-third of Type 1 and one-fourth of individuals with Type 2 diabetes have persistent proteinuria.

4. A total 24-hour protein excretion exceeding 1 gram suggests significant renal impairment.

5. Patients with renal insufficiency, nephrotic range proteinuria, hematuria or red blood cell casts, or with proteinuria of uncertain etiology should be referred to a nephrologist.

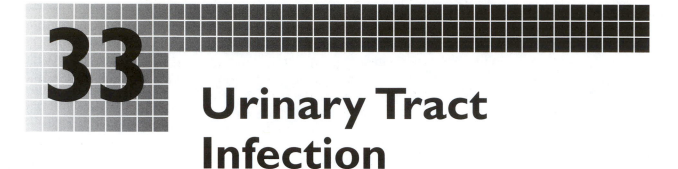

33 Urinary Tract Infection

Urinary tract infections (UTIs) affect women more often than men. Bacteriuria is present in 1% of infants of both sexes, 1% to 2% of school-age girls and 3% to 4% of women of childbearing age while males have a prevalence of bacteriuria of 0.3% after infancy. With increasing age the occurrence of bacteriuria increases for both sexes to about 15% of the geriatric population.

PATHOPHYSIOLOGY

Normal urine is sterile as a result of the antibacterial properties of the bladder mucosa and of the urine itself and because of the removal of bacteria through voiding. In most UTIs, bacteria gain access to the bladder via the urethra. Women are prone to UTIs because bacteria can access the bladder through their shorter urethra. Further ascent of bacteria from the bladder is the pathway for most renal parenchymal infections.

UTIs can be divided into lower tract infection (urethritis, cystitis, and prostatitis) and upper tract infection (acute pyelonephritis and intrarenal and perinephric abscesses), which may occur together or independently. Infections of the urethra and bladder are usually superficial infections, while prostatitis, pyelonephritis, and renal suppuration signify tissue invasion.

Gram-negative bacilli are the most common cause of infection. *Escherichia coli* is the most common pathogen and accounts for 70% to 80% of cases of UTI. Other gram-negative rods, such as Proteus, Klebsiella, Enterobacter, Serratia and Pseudomonas account for a smaller proportion of infections and are associated with urologic manipulation, calculi, obstruction, and catheter-associated infections. Proteus species, by virtue of urease production, and Klebsiella species, through the production of extracellular slime and polysaccharides, predispose individuals to form stones.

Although gram-positive cocci are less common, *Staphylococcus saprophyticus* accounts for 10% to 15% of acute symptomatic UTIs in young females. Enterococci and *Staphylococcus aureus* cause infections in patients with renal stones or previous instrumentation. Isolation of *S. aureus* from the urine should arouse suspicion of bacteremic infection of the kidney.

Sexual intercourse increases the likelihood of cystitis. In addition, the use of a diaphragm and/or a spermicide has been associated with increases in vaginal colonization with *E. coli* and in the risk of urinary infection. Any impediment to the free flow of urine, such as tumor, stricture, stone, neurologic disease or prostatic hypertrophy is associated with an increased frequency of UTI. Urinary infections are detected in 2% to 8% of pregnant women, and 20% to 30% of pregnant women with asymptomatic bacteriuria subsequently develop pyelonephritis. This predisposition to upper tract infection during pregnancy results from decreased ureteral tone and peristalsis, and temporary incompetence of the vesicoureteral valves.

Vesicoureteral reflux is associated with UTIs in children and can lead to renal scarring and chronic renal disease. Vesicoureteral reflux occurs during voiding or with elevation of pressure in the bladder. Reflux of urine from the bladder predisposes individuals to upper tract infections. Vesicoureteral reflux is common among children with anatomic abnormalities of the urinary tract.

CLINICAL MANIFESTATIONS

History

Patients with dysuria, frequency, urgency, and suprapubic pain usually have cystitis. The urine often becomes grossly cloudy and malodorous, and is bloody in about 30% of cases. Symptoms of acute pyelonephritis include fever (>101°F), shaking chills, nausea, vomiting, diarrhea, and flank pain. Symptoms of cystitis may or may not precede an upper tract infection. Patients should be asked about previous urinary tract infections, renal disease, kidney stones, and recent surgical procedures or antibiotic use. Other medical problems, such as diabetes, should be noted. The patient should be asked about sexual activity and contraceptive use.

Older children experience UTI symptoms similar to those found in adults. In infants and younger children, irritability, fever, nausea, vomiting, bed-wetting, and diarrhea may be presenting symptoms of a UTI. Elderly patients may also present with nonspecific symptoms such as change in mental status, malaise, incontinence, and poor appetite.

Physical Examination

Physical examination should include temperature, an abdominal examination and checking for costovertebral angle tenderness. For individuals who are unable to distinguish between the "internal" dysuria associated with urethritis and cystitis and the "external" dysuria that may occur with vaginitis, a genital examination can be helpful.

DIFFERENTIAL DIAGNOSIS

The differential diagnosis of dysuria includes UTI, vaginitis, and urethritis. Approximately 30% of patients with acute dysuria, frequency, and pyuria have mid-stream urine cultures with either no growth or insignificant bacterial growth. Clinically, these patients cannot be readily distinguished from those with cystitis. In this situation, sexually transmitted pathogens, such as *C. trachomatis*, *N. gonorrhoeae*, or herpes simplex virus and a low-count *E. coli* or staphylococcal infection may account for the symptoms. Chlamydial or gonococcal infection should be suspected when there is a gradual onset of illness, no hematuria, no suprapubic pain, and more than 7 days of symptoms. A new sex partner or exposure to chlamydial or gonococcal urethritis should heighten suspicion for a sexually transmitted infection. Infection with *C. trachomatis*, *N. gonorrhoeae*, Trichomonas, Candida, and herpes simplex virus should be considered in patients with vaginal discharge, mucopurulent cervicitis, genital lesions and urethritis symptoms but negative cultures.

Non-infectious causes such as urethral or bladder irritation from conditions such as trauma, exposure to chemical irritants (e.g., coffee, spicy foods, citrus) may also cause dysuria. A negative culture and a normal U/A characterize interstitial cystitis, which is most common in young women. Cystoscopy may reveal inflammation and mucosal hemorrhage. Bladder tumors, instrumentation, and trauma may also cause cystitis symptoms.

Dysuria is less common in men. In younger sexually active men, urethritis is the usual etiology. Older men usually have a UTI or irritative symptoms secondary to BPH. Other considerations in men include prostatitis or epididymitis.

Patients with upper tract infection usually experience back pain. Non-infectious causes of flank pain include renal stones, renal infarction, and papillary necrosis.

DIAGNOSTIC APPROACH

Many experts recommend treating healthy young women with characteristic symptoms of acute uncomplicated cystitis and pyuria without an initial urine culture. The absence of pyuria suggests an alternative diagnosis. The leukocyte esterase "dipstick" method is less sensitive than microscopy in identifying pyuria but is a useful alternative when microscopy is not available. Pyuria in the absence of bacteriuria (sterile pyuria) may indicate infection with organisms, such as *C. trachomatis*, *U. urealyticum*, Mycobacterium tuberculosis or fungi, or non-infectious urologic conditions such as calculi, anatomic abnormality, nephrocalcinosis, or polycystic disease. White blood cell casts suggest upper tract involvement.

A urine culture is indicated if the diagnosis is uncertain, in patients with suspected upper tract infections, and in those with complicating factors such as pregnancy or diabetes.

Growth of more than 10^5 organisms per milliliter from a properly collected midstream clean-catch urine sample indicates infection. In urine specimens obtained by suprapubic aspiration or catheterization, colony counts of 10^2 to 10^4 per milliliter generally indicate infection. In some circumstances (antibiotic treatment, high urea concentration, high osmolarity, low pH), relatively low bacterial colony counts may still indicate infection. Dilute urine or recent voiding also reduces bacterial counts in urine.

MANAGEMENT

Table 33–1 outlines treatment for urinary tract infections in adults. The following principles underlie the treatment of UTIs:

1. A urine analysis, gram stain, or culture is indicated to confirm infection before starting treatment. If a culture is obtained, antimicrobial sensitivity testing should be used to direct or modify therapy.

2. Factors predisposing to infection, such as obstruction and calculi, should be identified and corrected if possible.

3. In general, uncomplicated infections and lower tract infections respond to shorter courses of therapy, while upper tract infections require longer treatment. Early recurrences usually mean relapse. Recurrences more than 2 weeks after completing therapy nearly always represent reinfection with a new strain.

4. Community-acquired infections, especially initial infections, are usually due to antibiotic-sensitive strains.

5. In patients with repeated infections, instrumentation, or recent hospitalization, the presence of antibiotic-resistant strains should be suspected.

Cystitis usually responds to shorter courses of antibiotics. Single doses of trimethoprim-sulfamethoxazole (four single-strength tablets), trimethoprim alone (400 mg), and most fluoroquinolones (norfloxacin, ciprofloxacin, ofloxacin) have been used successfully to treat acute uncomplicated episodes of cystitis, but the higher relapse rate makes longer courses (3 to 7 days) more desirable. With upper tract infections, the majority of cases respond to 10 to 14 days of therapy. Longer periods of treatment (2 to 6 weeks) aimed at eradicating a persistent focus of infection may be necessary in some cases.

Males with UTI often have urologic abnormalities or prostatic involvement and should receive a 7- to 14-day antibiotic course. In women, acute uncomplicated pyelonephritis without accompanying clinical evidence of calculi or urologic disease is due to *E. coli* in most cases. A 14-day course of trimethoprim-sulfamethoxazole, a fluoroquinolone, an aminoglycoside, or a third-generation cephalosporin is usually adequate. Ampicillin or amoxicillin should not be used as initial therapy because 20% to 30% of strains of *E. coli* are now resistant to these drugs. Trimethoprim-sulfamethoxazole (TMP-SMX) should not be used as initial therapy in areas where more than 20% of *E. coli* strains are resistant to TMP-SMX.

Acute cystitis in pregnancy can be treated with amoxicillin, nitrofurantoin, or a cephalosporin. All pregnant women should be screened and if positive, treated for asymptomatic bacteriuria. Acute pyelonephritis in pregnancy usually requires hospitalization and parenteral antibiotic therapy, generally with a cephalosporin or an extended-spectrum penicillin. After treatment, a culture to document clearing of the infection is indicated, and cultures should be repeated monthly thereafter until delivery. Continuous low-dose prophylaxis with nitrofurantoin is indicated for pregnant women with recurrent infections.

In a child or infant who is toxic, dehydrated, or unable to tolerate oral intake, initial antimicrobial therapy should be given parenterally, and hospitalization should be considered. Reevaluation and repeat urine testing is indicated in children who do not improve after 2 days of antibiotic therapy.

Intravenous pyelography and cystoscopy is indicated in women with relapsing infection, a history of childhood infections, stones or painless hematuria, or recurrent pyelonephritis. Most males with a single urinary tract infection require investigation. Men or women presenting with acute infection and signs or symptoms suggestive of an obstruction or stones should undergo

TABLE 33–1

Urinary Tract Infections in Adults

Category	Diagnostic Criteria	Principal Pathogens	First-line Therapy	Comments
Acute uncomplicated cystitis	Urinalysis for pyuria and hematuria (culture not required)	• Escherichia coli • Staphylococcus saprophyticus • Proteus mirabilis • Klebsiella pneumoniae	• TMP-SMX DS (Bactrim, Septra) • Trimethoprim (Primsol) • Ciprofloxacin (Cipro) • Ofloxacin (Floxin) • Norfloxacin (Noroxin)	• Quinolones may be used in areas of TMP-SMX resistance or in patients who cannot tolerate TMP-SMX
Recurrent* cystitis in young women	Symptoms and a urine culture with a bacterial count of more than 100 CFU per mL of urine	• Same as for acute uncomplicated cystitis	• If the patient has more than three cystitis episodes per year, treat prophylactically with postcoital, or continuous daily therapy (see text)	• Repeat therapy for 7–10 days based on culture results and then use prophylactic therapy*
Acute cystitis in young men	Urine culture with a bacterial count of 1,000 to 10,000 CFU per mL of urine	• Same as for acute uncomplicated cystitis	• Same as for acute uncomplicated cystitis	• Treat for 7–10 days
Acute uncomplicated pyelonephritis	Urine culture with a bacterial count of 100,000 CFU per mL of urine	• Same as for acute uncomplicated cystitis	• If gram-negative organism, oral fluoroquinolone • If gram-positive organism, amoxicillin • If parenteral administration is required, ceftriaxone (Rocephin) or a fluoroquinolone • If Enterococcus species, add oral or IV amoxicillin	• Switch from IV to oral administration when the patient is able to take medication by mouth; complete a 14-day course

TABLE 33–1

(Continued)

Category	Diagnostic Criteria	Principal Pathogens	First-line Therapy	Comments
Complicated urinary tract infection	Urine culture with a bacterial count of more than 10,000 CFU per mL of urine	• E. coli • K. pneumoniae • P. mirabilis • Enterococcus species • Pseudomonas aeruginosa	• If gram-negative organism, oral fluoroquinolone • If Enterococcus species, ampicillin or amoxicillin with or without gentamicin (Garamycin)	• Treat for 10–14 days
Asymptomatic bacteriuria in pregnancy	Urine culture with a bacterial count of more than 10,000 CFU per mL of urine	• Same as for acute uncomplicated cystitis	• Amoxicillin • Nitrofurantoin (Macrodantin) • Cephalexin (Keflex)	• Avoid tetracyclines and fluoroquinolones • Treat for 3–7 days
Catheter-associated urinary tract infection	Symptoms and a urine culture with a bacterial count of more than 100 CFU per mL of urine	• Depends on duration of catheterization	• If gram-negative organism, a fluoroquinolone • If gram-positive organism, ampicillin or amoxicillin plus gentamicin	• Remove catheter if possible, and treat for 7–10 days • For patients with long-term catheters and symptoms, treat for 5–7 days

TMP-SMX = trimethoprim-sulfamethoxazole; CFU = colony-forming unit; IV = intravenous.
*—Patient is given a prescription for an antibiotic to take if symptoms develop.
(Adapted from Stamm WE, Hooton TM. Management of urinary tract infections in adults. N Engl J Med 1993;329:1328–1334.)

ultrasound or CT scan. Girls with recurrent UTI, boys with a single UTI, and children with pyelonephritis should undergo evaluation including renal ultrasound and voiding cystourethrogram (VCUG). The VCUG is generally performed after completing a course of antibiotics and sterilizing the urine since infection itself may cause reflux.

Patients with frequent symptomatic infections may benefit from long-term administration of low-dose antibiotics to prevent recurrences. Daily or thrice-weekly administration of a single dose of trimethoprim/sulfamethoxazole (80/400 mg), trimethoprim (100 mg), or nitrofurantoin (50 mg) is effective. Prophylactic antibiotics and voiding after sexual intercourse reduce recurrences in women whose infections are temporally related to intercourse. Other patients for whom prophylaxis appears to have some merit include men with chronic prostatitis; patients undergoing prostatectomy, both during the operation and in the postoperative period; and pregnant women with asymptomatic bacteriuria. Asymptomatic bacteriuria in older women is common and does not require therapy.

◆ KEY POINTS ◆

1. Urinary tract infections (UTIs) affect women more often than men.

2. Gram-negative bacilli are the most common cause of infection. *Escherichia coli* is the most common pathogen and accounts for 70% to 80% of cases of UTI.

3. The differential diagnosis of dysuria includes UTI, vaginitis, and urethritis.

4. Pyuria is present in almost all urinary infections and the absence of pyuria suggests an alternative diagnosis.

5. In general, uncomplicated infections and lower tract infections respond to shorter courses of therapy, while upper tract infections require longer treatment.

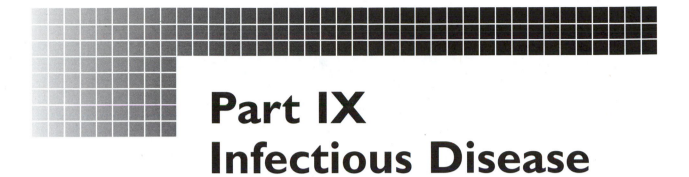

Part IX
Infectious Disease

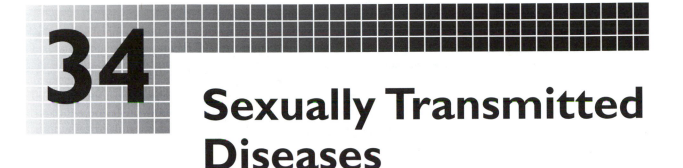

34

Sexually Transmitted Diseases

Sexually transmitted diseases (STDs) are among the most common infections. More than 8 to 12 million STDs are diagnosed annually in the United States. Although HIV is considered an STD, it is discussed in chapter 36.

PATHOPHYSIOLOGY

Sexually transmitted organisms enter through the mucosa or skin to cause disease. On mucosal surfaces, the organisms attach to the surface and cause an inflammatory reaction that can allow the organism to penetrate. Organisms that produce skin ulcers usually gain access by small abrasions in the upper layers of the epidermis. These abrasions occur related to micro-trauma associated with sexual intercourse, accounting for the fact that the most common locations for STD lesions are the penis, vagina, labia, and rectal surfaces.

Younger women are at a greater risk for STDs than older women because they have a more exposed transformation zone (squamous-columnar junction). Exposed columnar cells have a higher affinity for *C. trachomatis* and *N. gonorrhoeae* than squamous cells, and are also more vulnerable to infection by HPV. In addition, progesterone deficiency, commonly seen in younger women, results in a thinner protective mucus layer on the cervix, which facilitates pathogens migrating to the upper genital tract.

CLINICAL MANIFESTATIONS

History

Most individuals with STDs seek care because of genitourinary symptoms or because they notice a genital lesion. The most commonly encountered symptoms in men are related to urethritis and epididymitis. In women, urethral symptoms and vaginal discharge are the most common presenting complaints. Both men and women can develop genital lesions such as ulcers and genital warts.

Some patients are asymptomatic but seek care because of exposure to a partner with a STD or because of a high-risk sexual contact. A sexual history inquiring about numbers of partners, sexual practices, history of sexually transmitted diseases, and any high-risk sexual contacts identifies individuals at risk.

Physical Examination

Careful examination of the genitalia is critically important for evaluating a patient with a suspected STD. The examination should focus on detecting skin lesions, rashes, lymphadenopathy, ulcers, and mucosal lesions. Specific clinical syndromes are listed below and summarized in Table 34–1.

Urethritis

In men the most common symptom of a gonorrhea infection is a urethral discharge. Typically the discharge

TABLE 34–1

Clinical Characteristics of STDs

Disease	Characteristics
Urethritis	urethral discharge, dysuria, periurethral irritation
Hepatitis B	flu-like prodrome, nausea, vomiting, arthralgias, rash, jaundice
Hepatitis A	nausea, vomiting, diarrhea, jaundice
Human papilloma virus	genital warts, abnormal Pap smear
Herpes simplex	painful genital vesicles and ulcers, dysuria, fever (primary infection), recurrences
Chancroid	painful ulcer and inguinal lymphadenopathy
Syphilis	primary: nontender, painless ulcers; secondary: rash, flu-like illness; tertiary: aortic insufficiency, aortic aneurysm, peripheral neuropathy, meningitis, psychiatric disease
Cervicitis	vaginal discharge, dysuria
Bacterial vaginosis	malodorous vaginal discharge, pruritus
Epididymitis	testicular pain and swelling, urethral discharge

from gonococcal urethritis is more purulent than from a nongonococcal urethritis (NGU). NGU is usually caused by a chlamydial infection, but may be from Ureaplasma or Mycoplasma infections.

Hepatitis B

Sexual transmission accounts for 30% to 60% of hepatitis B cases. Common signs and symptoms of hepatitis B infections include jaundice, nausea, vomiting, arthralgias, fever, and abdominal pain.

Hepatitis A

Hepatitis A infection is usually transmitted fecal-orally. However, the most frequent source for hepatitis A infection is household or sexual contact with a person with hepatitis A.

Genital Warts

The human papilloma virus (HPV) causes anogenital warts (condylomata acuminata). The lesions are typically cauliflower-like, but can be smooth and either flesh colored or pigmented. The lesions are usually asymptomatic and discovered by the patient or physician upon examination.

Genital Ulcers

Herpes simplex virus (HSV) and chancroid cause painful ulcers, whereas syphilis ulcers are painless. HSV is the most common cause of genital ulceration. Primary genital herpes usually presents 2 days to 2 weeks after exposure with widespread vesicles and ulcers on genitalia. Symptoms such as dysuria and fever are common and can be mistaken for a urinary tract infection. The initial infection is usually more severe than recurrences, presumably because of the body's immune response. Reactivation triggers include sunlight, skin trauma, cold or heat, stress, concurrent infection, and menstruation.

Chancroid is caused by *Haemophilus ducreyi* and is associated with inguinal lymphadenopathy and painful genital ulcers. Chancroid ulcers are deep and tender, with irregular borders and a purulent base.

Syphilitic chancres are caused by the spirochete *Treponema pallidum* and are painless, nontender, indurated ulcers with a clean base. The chancre develops about 3 weeks after exposure. Even without treatment, the primary lesion usually resolves within 4 to 6 weeks. The secondary stage of syphilis typically presents with a generalized maculopapular rash, often involving the palms and soles. Other symptoms include general malaise, fever, rhinorrhea, sore throat, myalgias, headaches, and generalized lymphadenopathy. Secondary syphilis may evolve into a latent asymptomatic stage with no symptoms but with positive serology testing. One-third of these patients eventually develop tertiary syphilis, which can cause significant morbidity and a shortened lifespan due to the associated cardiovascular and neurological complications.

Cervicitis and PID

Either chlamydia or gonorrhea most commonly causes cervicitis. Many women with cervicitis are asymptomatic, while others may experience a vaginal discharge, dysuria, or spotting. Pharyngeal and anorectal gonorrhea infections can develop in patients who engage in oral or rectal sex. Pelvic inflammatory disease (PID), often marked by the development of abdominal pain and fever, can occur if the upper tracts are involved. Physical examination may reveal pain with cervical motion, adnexal tenderness, and rebound tenderness. Table 34–2 lists the diagnostic criteria for PID. Although PID is most commonly caused by *N. gonorrhoeae (GC)* and *Chlamydia trachomatis*, other pathogens including anaerobes, gram-negative facultative bacteria (e.g., *Bacteroides fragilis*) and *streptococci* may play a role. Perihepatitis, also known as Fitzhugh-Curtis syndrome, is a rare complication of PID. Long-term complications include tubal scarring which can cause infertility, chronic pain, and an increased risk of ectopic pregnancy.

Approximately 1% to 2% of patients with gonorrhea infections develop bacteremia. These individuals can develop septic arthritis and petechial or pustular skin lesions found primarily on the dorsal aspect of the distal extremities, ankle, or wrist joints.

BV

Although BV is associated with multiple sexual partners, it is still controversial whether BV is transmitted sexually. BV is discussed in chapter 39.

Vaginitis (chapter 39)

Trichomonas is usually asymptomatic in men and is passed to women. Candida may be harbored under the foreskin in men and passed on to women.

Epididymitis

Epididymitis is most common in young sexually active men and is usually caused by gonorrhea or chlamydia. On examination, the epididymis, which is located on the posterior aspect of the testis, is tender and swollen.

DIFFERENTIAL DIAGNOSIS

Lesions that can mimic condyloma acuminata (HPV infection) are seborrheic keratosis, nevi, molluscum contagiosum, pearly penile papules, and condyloma latum (syphilitic lesions). Urethral symptoms such as dysuria can be present in urinary tract infections, prostatitis, and vaginitis. The differential diagnosis for PID includes appendicitis, ectopic pregnancy, ovarian torsion, ruptured ovarian cyst, endometriosis, irritable bowel syndrome, and somatization disorder.

DIAGNOSTIC EVALUATION

Evaluation of STDs begins with a clinical assessment. In male patients with urethritis, a gram stain of the discharge looking for neutrophils and the presence of

---

TABLE 34–2

Criteria for the Diagnosis of PID

Minimal criteria	lower abdominal pain, adnexal tenderness, cervical motion tenderness
Additional criteria	oral temp >101°F (38.3°C), abnormal cervical or vaginal discharge, elevated ESR, C-reactive protein, documented *N. gonorrhoeae* or *C. trachomatis* infection
Definitive criteria	histopathologic evidence of endometritis on endometrial biopsy; transvaginal U/S or other imaging modes showing thickened fluid-filled tubes with or without free pelvic fluid or tubo-ovarian complex; laparoscopic abnormalities c/w PID

organisms is helpful. A urethral swab can also be sent for culture, DNA analysis, and either culture or immunofluorescence testing for chlamydia. Finding intracellular gram-negative diplococci on the gram stain is diagnostic for gonorrhea. In women with urethral symptoms, it is important to rule out a urinary tract infection or vaginitis. Vaginal discharge can also be a sign of cervicitis or PID and swabs of the discharge should be sent for culture, DNA analysis, or immuno-fluorescent testing. Gram stains are less valuable in women. A wet mount, KOH, pH determination, and whiff test are useful in characterizing a vaginal discharge.

Painful genital ulcers suggest HSV or chancroid. Painless ulcers suggest syphilis. The presence of multi-nucleated giant cells on a smear or a positive viral culture can diagnose HSV, while *H. ducreyi* can be isolated by cultures. Spirochetes seen on a darkfield examination from a scraping of an ulcer or direct immunofluorescent microscopy can confirm the diagnosis of syphilis.

The common serological screening tests for syphilis—a RPR or VDRL—turn positive as early as 4 to 7 days after a chancre appears. The VDRL or RPR titer can be used to determine disease activity following treatment. False positive tests for syphilis may occur in conditions such as antiphospholipid syndrome, advancing age, narcotic use, chronic liver disease, HIV, tuberculosis, and acute herpetic infection. Generally higher titers (>1 : 8) are more likely to represent true disease. A fluorescent treponemal antibody absorption (FTA-Abs) test should be used to confirm a positive RPR or VDRL result. The FTA-Abs will remain positive indefinitely and therefore cannot be used to determine disease activity.

HPV is commonly diagnosed by its appearance, but if necessary the diagnosis can be confirmed by tissue biopsy. Pap smears can detect cervical changes associated with HPV infection.

TREATMENT

Primary prevention, by encouraging condom use and avoiding high-risk sexual activity, is an important part of STD management. Vaccination for hepatitis B remains the most effective measure to prevent this disease. Hepatitis B immune globulin can be used in conjunction with the vaccine series in unimmunized individuals who have been exposed to the virus.

The treatment for genital warts depends on the number, size, morphology, and anatomic sites of the warts. Treatments include patient-applied therapies such as podofilox and imiquimod, and provider-applied therapies such as cryotherapy, trichloroacetic acid, bichloroacetic acid, or surgical removal. Podofilox is not recommended for perianal, vaginal, or urethral warts and should not be used during pregnancy. Imiquimod directly eradicates HPV but has not been studied in pregnant women. Cryotherapy with liquid nitrogen eradicates warts by thermally induced cytolysis. Generally, two to three sessions are required for treating the warts.

Acyclovir and two newer agents, valacyclovir (valtrex) and famciclovir (famvir) are used to treat HSV. Treatment shortens the course of the infection and reduces the length of time that the virus is shed. Suppressive therapy is indicated for patients who have frequent recurrences.

Uncomplicated chlamydial infections can be treated with doxycycline, erythromycin, or ofloxacin for 7 days. A single 2 GM oral dose of azithromycin is also effective. Uncomplicated gonorrhea can be treated with intramuscular ceftriaxone, or single oral doses of cefixime, ciprofloxacin, or ofloxacin. Treatment for gonorrhea should generally be followed by a regimen effective against chlamydia. Erythromycin, ceftriaxone, or azithromycin are each active against chancroid.

Two regimens of oral antibiotics are recommended for mild PID. Either (A) ofloxacin plus metronidazole for 14 days; or (B) an 1M dose of ceftriaxone (better coverage against *N. gonorrhoeae*) or cefoxitin (better coverage against anaerobes) with concurrent probenecid plus oral doxycycline. The indications for hospitalizing patients with PID include pregnancy, failed outpatient therapy, the inability to follow or tolerate an outpatient oral regimen, severe illness, high fever, a tubo-ovarian abscess, immunodeficiency, or in cases when the diagnosis is uncertain.

Recommended regimens for women with bacterial vaginosis include oral metronidazole and topical metronidazole or clindamycin. Penicillin is the treatment of choice for syphilis. For individuals with penicillin allergy, doxycycline or tetracycline can be used.

◆ KEY POINTS ◆

1. Both hepatitis B and A are considered STDs because sexual transmission accounts for the majority of reported incidences.

2. HSV and chancroid cause painful ulcers, whereas syphilis ulcers are painless.

3. Either chlamydia or gonorrhea most commonly causes cervicitis. Pelvic inflammatory disease (PID), often marked by the development of abdominal pain and fever, can occur if the upper tracts are involved.

4. The differential diagnosis for PID includes appendicitis, ectopic pregnancy, ovarian torsion, ruptured ovarian cyst, endometriosis, irritable bowel syndrome and somatization disorder.

5. The treatment for genital warts depends on the number, size, morphology, and anatomic sites of the warts. Treatments include patient-applied therapies such as podofilox and imiquimod, and provider-applied therapies such as cryotherapy, trichloroacetic acid, bichloroacetic acid, or surgical removal.

6. Uncomplicated chlamydial infections can be treated with doxycycline, erythromycin, or ofloxacin for 7 days. A single 2 gm oral dose of azithromycin is also effective. Uncomplicated gonorrhea can be treated with intramuscular ceftriaxone, or single oral doses of cefixime, ciprofloxacin, or ofloxacin.

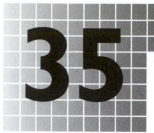

35 Respiratory Infections

Respiratory tract infections are the leading cause of illness among children and adults. Clinically, it is useful to distinguish between upper and lower respiratory tract infections. Upper respiratory tract infections (URIs) consist of infections affecting the respiratory structures above the larynx. Lower respiratory tract infections encompass the larynx, trachea, and pulmonary structures.

Upper respiratory tract infections include the common cold, sinusitis, and pharyngitis. Adults average two to four colds per year. Although most individuals with URIs do not seek medical care, it is still among the most common reasons for physician visits. Rhinoviruses account for 30% to 50% of the cases of the common cold; coronaviruses for another 10% to 20%. The remaining cases are either from an unidentifiable virus or from a host of viruses including influenza, parainfluenza, respiratory syncytial virus, and adenovirus. Laryngitis is viral in origin in 90% of cases, most commonly due to influenza, rhinovirus, adenovirus, and parainfluenza virus. The etiological agent of pharyngitis and otitis media are described in other chapters.

Lower respiratory tract infections include bronchitis and pneumonia. Bronchitis is an inflammation of the lining of the bronchial tube. Viral infections cause approximately 95% of bronchitis cases in healthy adults. Non-viral causes include chemical irritation, mycoplasma, and chlamydia.

Pneumonia is defined as inflammation of the lung parenchyma. Each year in the U.S. there are over 3 million cases of community acquired pneumonia (CAP), resulting in 500,000 hospitalizations. Pneumonia is the sixth leading cause of death.

PATHOPHYSIOLOGY

Most URIs are caused by viruses, which replicate in the nasopharynx, and cause inflammation with edema, erythema, and nasal discharge. Transmission occurs primarily by hand contact with the infected agent.

Sinusitis is a bacterial infection that occurs when inflammation and swelling of the mucosal membranes block the ostia draining the sinuses thus allowing pooling of mucus and bacterial proliferation. Sinusitis may also occur if anatomical abnormalities, such as polyps, obstruct the ostia. Occasionally, sinusitis results from a dental abscess. Bronchitis is characterized by edematous mucosal membranes, increased bronchial secretions, and diminished mucociliary function. Acute exacerbations of chronic bronchitis are frequently precipitated by a viral infection, but bacteria colonized in the airway appear to play a role in the infection.

Pneumonia is an inflammation of the terminal airways, alveoli, and lung interstitium usually from infection. The primary mechanism by which pneumonia occurs is aspiration of oropharyngeal secretions colonized by respiratory pathogens. Aspiration of gastric contents or hematogenous spread is less common. Factors that predispose an individual to pneumonia are abnormal host defenses (e.g., malnutrition, immuno-compromised) altered consciousness (which can lead to aspiration), ineffective cough (such as seen in patients with neuromuscular diseases or following surgery), or abnormal mucociliary transport (which is seen in smokers, COPD patients, and following a viral bronchitis).

CLINICAL MANIFESTATIONS

History

The clinical symptoms of a cold are well known and typically begin with a scratchy sore throat followed by sneezing, nasal congestion, and rhinorrhea. General malaise, fever, hoarseness, cough, low-grade fever and headache are also frequent symptoms. The acute syndrome usually resolves in about one week; however, a cough may persist for several weeks.

Persistent purulent nasal discharge, facial pain exacerbated by leaning forward, and a maxillary toothache are symptoms of sinusitis. Many patients with acute sinusitis may experience "double sickening" with improvement in their cold symptoms followed by a relapse with increased pain and nasal discharge.

Acute bronchitis usually presents with a productive cough and is often accompanied by URI symptoms. Low-grade fever and fatigue are common.

Pneumonia may present with symptoms very similar to bronchitis. However, patients with pneumonia are more likely to have a high fever, experience dyspnea and chills, have chest pain, and develop complications such as hypoxia or cardiopulmonary failure. Common organisms for community acquired pneumonia (CAP) in previously healthy adults are Streptococcus pneumonia, Hemophilus influenzae, Mycoplasma pneumoniae, or Chlamydia pneumoniae.

In patients with suspected pneumonia it is important to obtain a history of underlying diseases such as diabetes mellitus, COPD, asthma, alcohol abuse, and HIV. It is important to inquire about recent travel, seizures, and environmental or occupational exposures. HIV positivity increases the likelihood of an opportunistic infection, such as *Pneumocystis carinii*, cytomegalovirus, fungus, or mycobacterial tuberculosis.

Physical Examination

The history and physical examination are often sufficient to make the diagnosis. Important examination ele-ments include measuring vital signs; an ear, nose, and throat exam; palpation of the neck and sinuses; and a thorough cardiopulmonary exam.

Patients with URIs usually have a swollen, red nasal mucosa. Fever accompanied by purulent nasal discharge, facial tenderness, and a loss of maxillary transillumination suggests sinusitis. Although most patients with bronchitis will have clear lungs, some may have rhonchi, hoarse rales, or wheezing. Patients with pneumonia are more likely to have abnormal vital signs such as fever, tachypnea, tachycardia, and tend to look more ill. The vital signs and general appearance are also important in assessing the degree of illness. Marked abnormalities of the vital signs and poor general appearance suggest the need for hospitalization. Although the lungs may be clear in patients with pneumonia, usually there are abnormalities such as localized rales, bronchial breath sounds, wheezing, or signs of consolidation such as dullness to percussion.

DIFFERENTIAL DIAGNOSIS

The diagnosis of a cold is usually self-evident. Occasionally, allergic or vasomotor rhinitis can be confused with a URI. Influenza should be differentiated from the common cold since specific treatment may be effective. The differential diagnosis of acute sinus pain includes dental disease, nasal foreign body, and migraine or cluster headaches. Table 35–1 lists some clinical

TABLE 35–1

Distinguishing Features of Lower Respiratory Tract Infections

Bronchitis	Pneumonia
Antecedent URI	Acute onset of cough, fever, & tachypnea
Cough	
No or low-grade fever	Chest pain
Clear lungs or coarse rhonchi	Leukocytosis
Normal chest x-ray	Pulmonary infiltrate on chest x-ray

features that help distinguish between pneumonia and bronchitis.

Although most patients with fever, cough, and an infiltrate on chest x-ray have an infection, non-infectious causes need to be considered. These include cardiac disease, pulmonary embolus, atelectasis, or malignancy. Generally, the presentation of non-infectious causes tends to be more insidious and the patient is afebrile.

DIAGNOSTIC APPROACH

Most patients with URIs are diagnosed clinically. Blood tests or imaging is not required for patients with acute sinusitis, unless the patient appears toxic or has a complication of sinusitis, such as orbital cellulitis or cavernous thrombosis. CT is the imaging procedure of choice, and is also indicated in patients with chronic sinusitis, in recurrent sinusitis, in individuals showing poor response to therapy, if a tumor is suspected, and when surgery is contemplated.

If pneumonia is suspected by history and physical, a chest x-ray is indicated. A chest x-ray can distinguish between bronchitis and pneumonia, assess the extent of disease, detect pleural effusions, and help distinguish between infectious and non-infectious causes. Lab tests for suspected pneumonia include a CBC, electrolytes, BUN, creatinine, pulse oximetry, sputum for gram stain and culture, and liver function tests. Patients admitted to the hospital should have blood cultures, and based on the clinical evaluation, HIV testing and serology testing (e.g., legionella testing) may be indicated.

MANAGEMENT

Fluids, rest, and either NSAIDs or acetaminophen to relieve pain and fever help URI symptoms. Sympathomimetics such as pseudoephedrine can reduce nasal congestion. Topical decongestants (e.g., phenylephrine) have fewer side effects than oral decongestants but their use needs to be limited to 3 to 4 days to avoid tolerance and rebound congestion. Ipratropium bromide nasal spray is an anticholinergic agent that reduces rhinorrhea, but is of limited benefit in reducing congestion. Vitamin C and zinc may shorten the duration of symptoms. Treating sinusitis should be directed at improving drainage and eradicating pathogens. Decongestants,

hydration, analgesics, warm facial packs, humidification, and sleeping with the head of the bed elevated are types of adjunctive care. Mucolytics such as guaifenesin may be of benefit. Most patients with a URI have some element of sinusitis that is self-limited and will resolve with symptomatic care. If symptoms persist for more than a week, antibiotics are usually started and administered for 10 to 14 days. Amoxicillin or trimethoprim sulfamethoxazole are suitable for initial therapy. For patients allergic to these medications, cephalosporins, macrolides, or quinolones may be substituted. Most individuals respond within 5 days of initiating treatment.

For patients who fail to respond, a broader spectrum antibiotic is indicated. For individuals whose symptoms persist despite therapy, a CT scan and ENT referral is appropriate. In toxic-appearing patients or those with suspected complications such as osteomyelitis, orbital cellulitis, or intracranial disease, urgent hospitalization and consultation are indicated.

Treatment for bronchitis includes symptomatic care with fluids, decongestants, smoking cessation, and cough suppressants. Although controversial, some authorities advocate using antibiotics for severe or persistent cases of bronchitis.

In patients with pneumonia, an important consideration is the locus of care. Box 35–1 lists some indications for hospitalization. For those patients suitable for outpatient therapy, antibiotics are started and close

BOX 35–1
Indications for Hospitalization
Systolic blood pressure less than 90
Pulse rate greater than 140
O_2 sat less than 90% or PO_2 less than 60 mmHg
Presence of abscess or pleural effusion
Marked metabolic abnormality

Concomitant disease such as
    CHF
    Renal failure
    Malignancy
    Diabetes mellitus
    COPD

Age greater than 65
Unreliable social situation

monitoring is begun. If possible, therapy is guided by the sputum gram stain results. However, gram stains are often impractical or unobtainable in the outpatient setting, and most family physicians start empiric antibiotic therapy. For healthy adults less than 60 years old, erythromycin or a newer extended spectrum macrolide such as azithromycin is a suitable choice. Doxycycline is an acceptable, less expensive alternative. For patients over 60, a fluoroquinolone with good activity against pneumococcus (e.g., levofloxacin), a newer macrolide, or a second-generation cephalosporin are good choices for empiric therapy.

◆ **KEY POINTS** ◆

1. Adults average two to four colds per year. Rhinoviruses account for 30% to 50% of the cases of the common cold; coronaviruses for another 10% to 20%.

2. Common organisms for community acquired pneumonia (CAP) in previously healthy adults are Streptococcus pneumoniae, Hemophilus influenzae, Mycoplasma pneumoniae, or Chlamydia pneumoniae.

3. A chest x-ray can distinguish between bronchitis and pneumoniae, assess the extent of disease, detect pleural effusions, and help distinguish between infectious and non-infectious causes.

4. Blood tests or imaging is not required for patients with acute sinusitis, unless the patient appears toxic or has a complication of sinusitis, such as orbital cellulitis or cavernous thrombosis.

5. Erythromycin or a newer extended spectrum macrolide such azithromycin or doxycycline are suitable choices for healthy adults less than 60 years old with pneumonia. For patients over 60, a fluoroquinolone with good activity against pneumococcus (e.g., levofloxacin), a newer macrolide, or a second-generation cephalosporin is suitable for empiric pneumonia therapy.

36

Human Immunodeficiency Virus

Human Immunodeficiency Virus (HIV) is a disease that a family doctor will often encounter in practice. A 1997 study found that approximately 1% of primary care patients were HIV positive. HIV infection is often a disease of families, involving spouse and children, giving the family doctor an important role in the diagnosis, treatment, and prevention of the Acquired Immunodeficiency Syndrome (AIDS).

PATHOPHYSIOLOGY

HIV-1 is a retrovirus that infects lymphocytes and cells bearing the CD4 marker. CD4 lymphocytes are T-cells involved in cell-mediated immunity. The depletion of CD4 lymphocytes also impairs B-cell activation against foreign antigens and limits antibody production. This contributes to the immunocompromised state termed AIDS.

HIV is transmitted from person to person through blood and body fluids. HIV transmission is linked to sexual contact and intravenous drug use. HIV may also be transmitted to health care workers from needle-stick injuries or from mother to infant during labor (65%) or through breastfeeding (10%–20%). The transmission rate with sexual activity from a male to a female is 0.5 to 1.5 per 1000 episodes, whereas the transmission rate from female to male is 0.3 to 0.9 per 1000 episodes. There is a 1.5 times greater risk of transmission during menstruation. Health care workers suffering an infected

needle stick have a risk of seroconversion of approximately 3.2 in 1000 with hollow bore needles and a lower rate with a suture needle stick. Blood splashed on intact skin poses a very low risk of transmission.

CLINICAL MANIFESTATIONS

History

Manifestations of acute HIV infection are fever, fatigue, rash, headache, lymphadenopathy, pharyngitis, myalgia, GI upset (i.e., diarrhea, vomiting), night sweats, aseptic meningitis, and oral or genital ulcers. Symptoms of acute HIV infection usually develop within days to weeks after exposure and usually last less than 14 days. During the acute infection, HIV disseminates widely and spreads into lymphoid tissue. Seroconversion or the development of antibodies to the virus takes place 3 to 4 weeks after the exposure. A prolonged asymptomatic period of clinical latency (up to 12 years) may ensue with measurable HIV-1 RNA and antibody levels as the only evidence of infection. Ultimately AIDS develops, characterized by a constellation of symptoms: collapse of immune system, high-level viremia, opportunistic infections, and death (Figure 36–1).

A complete history should include risks for transmission, pre-existing comorbid conditions, social history, and previous antiretroviral treatments. A patient's spouse or partner(s) and children should be evaluated for HIV infection. Patients should be ques-

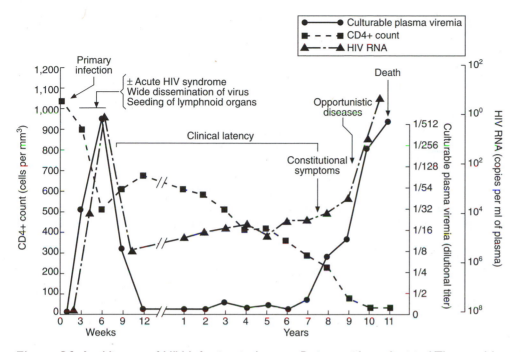

Figure 36–1 History of HIV Infection in Average Patient without Antiviral Therapy. Natural History of human immunodeficiency virus (HIV) infection in the average patient without antiretroviral therapy, from the time of HIV transmission to death at 10 to 11 years. The initial burst of viremia with very high HIV-1 RNA levels (circle icon) is followed by a prolonged period during which viral replication continues with lower but measurable HIV-1 RNA levels (triangle icon). With the decline of the CD4 lymphocyte count (square icon) and the collapse of the immune system, high-level viremia, symptoms and opportunistic infections develop, and death ultimately occurs. Reprinted with permission from Fauci AS, Pantaleo G, Stanley S, Weissman D. Immunopathic Mechanisms of HIV Infection. Ann Intern Med 1996; 124: 654–63.

tioned about symptoms associated with opportunistic infections such as dyspnea, dysphagia, and skin lesions. Past and current history of genital symptoms or lesions should be obtained. Even though many HIV patients live longer because of new combinations of antiretroviral regimens, many patients still view HIV infection as untreatable. Patients may become depressed and even suicidal. Learning about patients' previous psychiatric illnesses and family support can help them to cope with the disease and adhere to treatments. Inquiring about prior medications used by the patient, duration of use, response, intolerance, and toxicities may help clinicians to choose appropriate medications and antiviral therapy.

Physical Examination

Physical examination should focus on weight change, the presence of fever, skin lesions, signs of opportunis-

tic infections, presence of STDs, neurological function, and emotional state. A weight loss of more than 10% requires aggressive evaluation and treatment. *Pneumocystis carinii* pneumonia is the most common cause of fever and patients may have a normal lung examination despite active infection. Sinusitis is also common in early-stage disease and the presence of sinus tenderness should be noted. Other opportunistic infections that may be apparent on physical examination include oral thrush (candidiasis), cytomegalovirus retinitis (with a ketchup-and-cottage-cheese fundus), toxoplasmosis (an intracranial lesion manifested as deficits in extraocular movements), and cryptococcal meningitis (headache, fever, mental status change). Common skin lesions are Kaposi sarcoma, an exacerbation of psoriasis, seborrheic dermatitis, drug-related eruptions, dry skin, molluscum contagiosum, and herpes zoster. HIV infection increases the risk for pelvic inflammatory disease and cervical carcinoma in women, making a gynecologic exam including Pap smear and STD evaluation (such as syphilis) necessary. Mild confusion and memory loss may be found relatively early in HIV disease and may indicate AIDS dementia complex. Myopathies, sensory and motor neuropathies, and central lesions (CNS lymphoma) may also be found in HIV disease.

DIFFERENTIAL DIAGNOSIS

Box 36–1 lists the differential diagnosis. Early HIV infection can be confused with acute viral infections or other immunocompromised states. Primary care physicians should be alert to the possibility of HIV in patients presenting with fever, fatigue, and STD.

Diagnostic Approach

HIV is officially defined as the presence of HIV antibodies confirmed by a positive Enzyme-Linked Immunosorbent Assay (ELISA) and a positive Western blot test. A positive ELISA test should always be followed by a Western blot test. A positive Western blot test reacts with two out of three (p24, gp41, and gp120/180) different antigens. False-negative ELISA or indeterminate Western blot tests may occur in the first 3 to 4 weeks after HIV exposure (acute seroconversion state). On the other hand, plasma viral load (PVL) can detect HIV infection as early as 11 days. Laboratory evaluation is performed to determine the stage of HIV disease preferably using the CD4 count and PVL. Other suggested screenings for related cancers, STDs, and HIV-related infections are listed in Box 36–2.

MANAGEMENT

The U.S. Department of Health and Human Services (HHS) updated guidelines for antiretroviral therapy in adults and adolescents with HIV infection in 2001. The current recommendation is to offer antiretroviral therapy in asymptomatic HIV patients who have fewer than 350 CD4 cells/mm^3 or PVL more than 30,000-copies/ml by bDNA or 50,000-copies/ml by PCR. For those asymptomatic patients whose CD4 cells are more than 350/mm^3 and PVL is less than 30,000 copies, it is recommended to defer the treatments. The treatments should be instituted aggressively in advanced HIV disease and antiretroviral therapy may need to be changed to overcome resistance. Effectiveness of treatments is measured against baseline CD4 and PVL with follow-up labs drawn 4 to 6 weeks from the start of

---

BOX 36–1

Differential Diagnosis for Acute HIV Infection

Infectious diseases:
Infectious mononucleosis, Influenza, Primary cytomegalovirus infection, Streptococcal pharyngitis, Viral hepatitis, Secondary syphilis, Primary herpes simplex virus infection, Toxoplasmosis, Malaria

Immunocompromised state:
Primary immunodeficiency disease in both B/T cells (i.e., Immunoglobulin A deficiency, most commonly found in adults >21 years old), lymphoma

Others:
Drug reactions

BOX 36–2

Initial Laboratory Evaluation of an HIV-Positive Patient

(1) CD4 cell counts, PVL*, CBC for HIV-related anemia or thrombocytopenia

(2) Pap smear, GC/Chlamydial cultures, VDRL

(3) Hepatitis B and C panel, Tuberculin skin test, Toxoplasma titer, Cytomegalovirus titer

(4) Metabolic profile: BUN, creatinine, electrolytes, liver function tests, total protein, serum albumin

* PVL can be done via branched DNA (bDNA) assay, polymerase chain reaction (PCR), or the nucleic acid sequence-based amplification (NASBA). Sensitivity of all three assays is between 200 and 500 HIV RNA copies/ml. The new ultrasensitive assay can detect as low as 20 to 50 copies/ml.

TABLE 36–1

Primary Prophylaxis Against Opportunistic Infections

Infection	Indications	Primary tx	Secondary
PCP[a]	CD 4 cells <200/mm^3	Bactrim	Dapsone
Toxoplasmosis	CD 4 cells <100/mm^3	Bactrim	Dapsone
MAC[b]	CD 4 cells <50/mm^3	Clarithromycin	Rifabutin
TB	PPD >5 mm	INH w/pyridoxine	Rifampin
VZV	exposure	VZIG	Acyclovir

[a] In neonates, PCP prophylaxis treatment (Bactrim or dapsone) begins when zidovudine therapy is stopped or the child reaches age six weeks, and continued until the child is found to be HIV-free or for at least one year.
[b] MAC (*Mycobacterium avium* complex), VZV (*Varicella zoster virus*).

therapy. Desired results would be a 1- to 2-log reduction in PVL (i.e., 50,000 copies to 500 copies) and a rise in CD4 counts. The viral load should become undetectable after 16 to 20 weeks of therapy. Treatment regimens for HIV infection should include a combination of antiretroviral medications continued indefinitely. Three different categories of antiviral agents are available, the nucleoside reverse transcriptase inhibitors (NRTIs), protease inhibitors (PI), and nonnucleoside reverse transcriptase inhibitors (nNRTIs). Two NRTIs (e.g., zidovudine + didanosine or zidovudine + lamivudine) plus a protease inhibitor (e.g., indinavir) or a non-NRTI (e.g., efavirenz) are recommended for initial therapy. Resistance to antiretroviral therapy can develop and changing medications and resistance testing may be necessary in cases of therapeutic failure. Guidelines for providing prophylaxis against opportunistic infections are presented in Table 36–1. Dosages for adolescents and children will need to be adjusted based upon weight and Tanner stages. A full discussion of medication dosing and side effects is beyond the scope of this chapter.

Studies in obstetric HIV patients have shown that elective cesarean section appears to decrease the vertical transmission rate by 50% and by 87% with concurrent zidovudine therapy. Since maternal immunoglobulins against HIV cross the placenta, all neonates born to an HIV-positive mother will have a positive ELISA test/Western blot test for HIV in the first 6 months. Current recommendations for children born to HIV-positive mothers state that infants should receive zidovudine for at least the first 4 to 6 weeks of life. Repeat testing at 1 month, 2 to 3 months and 4 months of age is indicated until two tests are concordant.

The Public Health Service (PHS) has recommended prophylactic antiviral treatment for occupational exposure to HIV infections. Since there are 3 to 4 weeks before seroconversion occurs, early chemoprophylaxis may destroy the virus and prevent long-term infection. The optimal window to initiate prophylaxis is 24 to 72 hours after exposure.

◆ **KEY POINTS** ◆

1. Symptoms of acute HIV infection usually develop within days to weeks after exposure and usually last less than 14 days. The development of antibodies (seroconversion) takes place at 3 to 4 weeks after the exposure.

2. HIV is officially defined as presence of HIV antibodies confirmed by a positive Enzyme-Linked Immunosorbent Assay (ELISA) and a positive Western blot test.

3. Treatment regimens for HIV infection should include a combination of antiretroviral medications continued indefinitely.

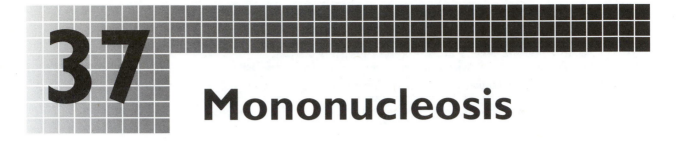

37 Mononucleosis

Fever, sore throat, malaise, lymphadenopathy, atypical lymphocytosis, and splenomegaly mark the classic syndrome of infectious mononucleosis (IM). IM is caused by heterophile-positive Epstein-Barr virus (EBV), a herpes virus.

In countries with higher standards of hygiene, like the United States, infection with EBV is often delayed until adulthood. In lower socioeconomic groups and in areas of the world with lower standards of hygiene, EBV tends to infect children at an early age, and symptomatic IM is less common.

PATHOPHYSIOLOGY

EBV is spread by contact with oral secretions, usually from asymptomatic persons shedding the virus. The virus is frequently transmitted from adults to infants and among young adults by transfer of saliva during kissing. Transmission by less intimate contact is rare. EBV has also been transmitted by blood transfusion and by bone marrow transplantation.

The virus infects the epithelium of the oropharynx and the salivary gland and then spreads through the bloodstream and disseminates throughout the body. The proliferation of EBV-infected B cells along with reactive T cells during IM results in lymphadenopathy and lymphatic tissue enlargement.

CLINICAL MANIFESTATIONS

History

Most EBV infections in infants and young children either are asymptomatic or present as mild pharyngitis with or without tonsillitis. In contrast, up to 75% of these infections in adolescents present with the classic syndrome of fever, fatigue, and lymphadenopathy. Occasionally patients may present with a hepatitis picture.

The incubation period for IM in young adults is about 4 to 6 weeks. A prodrome of fatigue, malaise, and headache may last for 1 to 2 weeks before the onset of fever, sore throat, and lymphadenopathy. The classic fever, sore throat, and lymphadenopathy are most prominent during the first 2 weeks of the illness. Splenomegaly is more prominent during the second and third week. Most patients have the above signs and symptoms for 2 to 4 weeks, but malaise and difficulty concentrating can persist for months.

Pharyngitis is the most common symptom and is present in over 80% of symptomatic patients. A morbilliform or papular rash, usually on the arms or trunk, develops in about 5% of cases. Most patients treated with ampicillin develop a macular rash, which is not an allergic reaction and does not predict future adverse reactions to penicillins. In elderly patients, pharyngitis, lymphadenopathy, splenomegaly, and atypical lymphocytes are less common and patients may present with nonspecific symptoms such as fever and fatigue.

Most cases of IM are self-limited. Deaths are very rare and most often are due to central nervous system (CNS) complications, splenic rupture, upper airway obstruction, or bacterial superinfection.

If CNS complications develop, they typically occur during the first 2 weeks of EBV infection. In some patients—especially children—meningitis, cranial nerve palsies, and encephalitis may be the only clinical manifestation of IM. Most cases resolve without neurologic sequelae.

Hematological complications include autoimmune hemolytic anemia, which may occur with hemoglobinuria and jaundice. Spontaneous splenic rupture is extremely rare, but may occur with relatively minor trauma.

EBV is associated with several human tumors, including nasopharyngeal carcinoma, Burkitt's lymphoma, Hodgkin's disease, and B-cell lymphoma in patients with immunodeficiencies (i.e., AIDS and organ/bone marrow transplant recipients on immunosuppressants). Virtually all CNS lymphomas in AIDS patients are associated with EBV.

Physical Examination

Pharyngitis may be exudative and confused with streptococcal pharyngitis. Hypertrophy of lymphoid tissue in the tonsils or adenoids can result in upper airway obstruction, as can inflammation and edema of the epiglottis, pharynx, or uvula. Lymphadenopathy is common with EBV infection, particularly swollen occipital lymph nodes.

Rare complications associated with acute EBV infection include fulminant hepatitis, myocarditis or pericarditis, pneumonia with pleural effusion, interstitial nephritis, and vasculitis. EBV was once believed to be a cause of chronic fatigue syndrome (CFS). However, the association has not been proven. Chronic active EBV infection is very rare and is distinct from the chronic fatigue syndrome. Affected patients have an illness lasting more than 6 months with markedly elevated titers of antibody to EBV and evidence of organ involvement, including hepatosplenomegaly, lymphadenopathy, and pneumonitis, uveitis, or neurologic disease.

DIFFERENTIAL DIAGNOSIS

Cytomegalovirus (CMV) is the most common cause of heterophile-negative mononucleosis-like syndrome.

Patients who have CMV mononucleosis are, on average, older and exhibit fever and malaise as the major manifestations; pharyngitis and lymphadenopathy are less common than with EBV-induced IM. Other conditions that may produce a mononucleosis-like illness are presented in Box 37–1. Streptococcal pharyngitis can appear similar to EBV pharyngitis. About 10% of patients with IM have a concomitant streptococcal infection.

DIAGNOSTIC APPROACH

Laboratory Findings

Lymphocytosis and atypical lymphocytes are usually present and peak during the second or third week of illness. Low-grade neutropenia and thrombocytopenia are common during the first month of illness. Hemolytic anemia is a rare complication. Liver function tests are mildly abnormal in more than 90% of cases. Only rarely are enzymes markedly abnormal.

Serologic Testing

The heterophile test is used for the diagnosis of IM in children and adults. The Monospot test is more sensitive and more commonly used than the classic heterophile test. During the first week of illness the test is positive in 40% of patients with IM and in 80 to 90% during the third week. If the initial test is negative, repeat testing may be helpful. Tests usually remain pos-

---

BOX 37–1
Conditions and Infections Producing a Mononucleosis-Like Syndrome
• Epstein-Barr virus
• Cytomegalovirus
• Malignancies
• Adenoviruses
• Toxoplasma
• Rubella
• Human immunodeficiency virus
• Hepatitis A
• Diphtheria

itive for 3 months after the onset of illness, so a positive finding may not indicate active disease. A Monospot test is often falsely negative in children less than 5 years of age, in the elderly, or in patients presenting with symptoms not typical of IM.

EBV-specific antibody testing is used for patients with suspected acute EBV infection who lack heterophile antibodies and for patients with atypical infections. IgM antibody to viral capsid antigen (VCA) is useful for the diagnosis of acute IM during the first 2 months of the disease. In contrast, IgG antibody to VCA persists for life and can assess past EBV infection.

In the absence of a positive Monospot test or serology, the complete blood count (CBC) with differential may be a reliable indicator of IM if it demonstrates lymphocytosis with 10% or more atypical lymphocytes.

TREATMENT

Therapy for IM consists primarily of supportive measures, with rest and analgesia. Excessive physical activity during the first month, especially in patients with splenomegaly, should be avoided to reduce the possibility of splenic rupture, a rare complication. Splenic rupture requires surgery.

Steroids may be useful in patients with severe tonsillar hypertrophy, autoimmune hemolytic anemia, and severe thrombocytopenia. These agents have also been used in a few select patients with severe malaise and fever and in patients with severe CNS or cardiac disease. Glucocorticoid therapy is not indicated for uncomplicated IM, and in fact may predispose to bacterial superinfection.

◆ KEY POINTS ◆

1. The etiologic agent for infectious mononucleosis is Epstein-Barr virus, although other viral agents, most notably cytomegalovirus, can cause a mononucleosis-like syndrome.

2. The classic physical findings of infectious mononucleosis include fever, lymphadenopathy, pharyngitis, and splenomegaly.

3. Although the presence of heterophile antibodies is considered diagnostic of infectious mononucleosis, children younger than 4 years of age develop an antibody response less than 20% of the time.

4. The primary route of transmission for infectious mononucleosis is saliva; it rarely is spread via aerosol or fomites. The isolation of patients with IM is unnecessary.

5. Treatment for infectious mononucleosis is generally supportive.

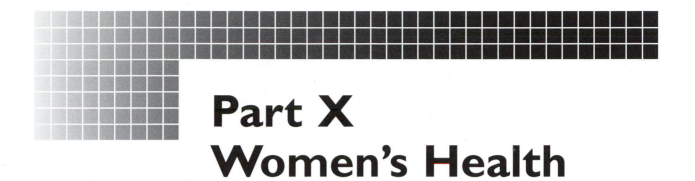

Part X
Women's Health

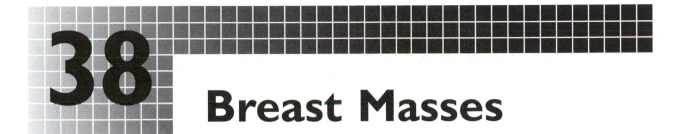

38 Breast Masses

Discovery of a breast mass is a relatively common occurrence. In the U.S., a woman's lifetime risk for developing breast cancer is 8% to 10%, with over 50% of cancers occurring in patients over age 65. Proper evaluation and treatment of breast masses are essential since breast cancer is the most common malignancy in women. Although far less common, 1% of breast cancers occur in men.

PATHOPHYSIOLOGY

Breast tissue contains epithelium, which forms the acini and ducts; fat; and fibrous tissue, which provides structural support. The hormones of the menstrual cycle also cause progression and regression of the ducts and many normal women experience some breast tenderness around their menstrual periods. Under hormonal influence, breast tissue may be overstimulated, leading to development of fibroadenomas, ductal dysplasia, and breast cysts. Cysts result from collections of fluids, such as colostrum or dissolved cellular debris, that result from stricture and fibrosis of the small ductules.

Most breast cancers arise from malignant transformation of ductal or epithelial cells. The exact causes for breast cancer have not been determined for the vast majority of cases. Approximately 5% of cases are thought to be attributable to inheritance of the BRCA1 or BRCA2 genes. Breast cancer is not considered a consequence of fibrocystic disease.

Breast cancers are commonly divided into epithelial or nonepithelial (stromal) malignancies. The epithelial cancers are most common and are further classified as lobular or ductal carcinomas. Lobular carcinomas are more common in younger patients and ductal carcinomas are more frequent in older patients. Ductal carcinomas are more invasive than lobular lesions. The first site of metastases are usually the axillary lymph nodes, although metastases are found in less than 10% of patients with breast tumors less than one centimeter in diameter.

CLINICAL PRESENTATION

History

The history should include questions about how long the mass has been present, how it was discovered, and what has occurred since its discovery. Additional helpful information includes the presence of pain or discharge, weight loss, or bone pain. Past personal or family history of breast cancer, menstrual history, and use of any hormonal therapies should also be obtained.

Physical Examination

Physical examination includes both inspection and palpation of the breast. One should inspect for masses, skin changes such as inflammation or edema, and for skin dimpling or nipple retraction. Palpation of the axillary and supraclavicular regions can be done while the patient is seated, feeling for enlarged lymph nodes. Careful and methodical palpation of each quadrant of the breast should be performed, along with areolar pressure around the nipple to assess for breast discharge.

DIFFERENTIAL DIAGNOSIS

The most common causes for breast masses are fibrocystic breast changes, fibroadenomas, and breast cancer. Less common causes for breast masses include hamartomas, adenomas, abscesses, intraductal papillomas, and fat necrosis. Mastitis and abscess formation are rare in non-lactating women.

Cancer typically presents in a postmenopausal woman as an isolated painless mass discovered on self-examination. The mass often does not have discrete borders, but may be mobile. Over time, cancerous masses will enlarge, become fixed, and may be associated with palpable axillary lymph nodes. Other signs of breast cancer include skin dimpling, nipple inversion, nipple discharge (especially bloody discharge), and skin edema or inflammation.

Fibroadenomas commonly present in younger women as discrete, mobile, painless, rubbery masses. After an initial several month period of growth, fibroadenomas generally stabilize in size, remain mobile, and do not spread to adjacent structures or lymph nodes.

Diffusely lumpy tender breasts may indicate fibrocystic change. Fibrocystic changes will vary with the menstrual cycle and are most commonly found in younger women. Cysts that persist throughout the menstrual cycle, fail to resolve with aspiration or those with a bloody aspirate may be malignant.

DIAGNOSTIC APPROACH

Most women presenting with a breast mass should have a mammogram. The exception is women under age 30 in whom mammograms may be more difficult to interpret due to the density of the breasts. In this case, clinical suspicion will help direct the evaluation. Easy mobility, regular borders, and a soft or cystic feel suggest a benign mass. If the mass is accessible, fine needle aspiration should be performed. If no mass can be palpated after aspiration and the aspirated fluid is not

bloody, then the patient may be followed clinically by re-examination. A persistent mass or bloody fluid mandates excisional biopsy to rule out malignancy. If the mass is not accessible, then ultrasound can determine whether the mass is solid or cystic, and may be used to direct biopsy. Solid masses with no fluid found on fine needle aspiration generally require core needle or excisional biopsy for evaluation.

In postmenopausal women, breast lumps should be regarded as cancer until proven otherwise. Mammography is typically the initial study performed. For best results, the radiologist should be informed of the suspicious area and special views may be obtained to fully evaluate the abnormal area. However, a normal mammogram in a patient with a dominant breast mass on exam does not rule out cancer. Nine to 22% of palpable breast cancers are not seen on mammogram. Therefore any palpable mass in a woman over the age of 40 should be biopsied.

Mammography is still useful since it can help locate the mass, guide needle biopsy or find non-clinically evident lesions in the ipsilateral or contralateral breast. In addition, an initial mammogram provides a baseline for comparison with future mammograms and to help plan the surgical approach if a lesion appears likely to be either benign or malignant. Fine needle aspiration biopsy of a solid breast mass provides adequate specimens in 60% to 85% of cases. Sensitivity is greater than 80% and specificity is greater than 99%. Thus, negative cytology does not preclude breast cancer. Solid lesions that have negative or suspicious cytology and cystic lesions with serosanguinous fluid require excisional biopsy. In lesions that appear to be benign based on examination, mammogram, and a negative needle biopsy, some experts recommend following the lesion with serial mammograms and clinical evaluation. For cysts that are aspirated, resolve, have negative cytology, and do not return on breast examination, mammography or breast examination can be used for follow-up depending upon patient age and risk.

Nipple discharge warrants thorough breast examination. It should be noted whether the discharge is unilateral or bilateral, bloody or milky, spontaneous or expressible, or localized to one duct. Guaiac testing and cytologic testing is helpful. Mammography is essential in evaluating these patients. If nipple discharge is unexplained, a surgeon will need to evaluate the ducts for early ductal cancer.

TREATMENT

Individuals with fibroadenomas may elect to do nothing or to undergo excision of the lesion. Women with fibrocystic change should be informed about the benign nature of the disease and that fibrocystic disease without atypical cells does not increase breast cancer risk. Treatment options include a supportive bra, vitamin E supplements and avoidance of chocolate and caffeinated beverages. More severe cases may be treated with medications such as spironolactone, or short trials of cyclic progesterone, danazol, or tamoxifen.

Management of the patient with breast cancer incorporates a team approach involving the primary care physician along with the surgeon and oncologist. Assessment for metastatic disease initially involves checking a complete blood count, liver enzymes, a chest x-ray, tumor markers (CA15-3), and in some cases a bone scan. A CT scan of the liver is indicated if liver enzymes are elevated. Surgery generally involves either a lumpectomy or modified radical mastectomy and assessment of lymph nodes, commonly with a sentinel node biopsy or axillary dissection. Postoperatively, after the patient has healed, radiation therapy and possibly chemotherapy may be provided depending upon the patient's age, and lymph node and estrogen-receptor status. Coordination of care will require communication and involvement between the various health care team members and the patient to determine the best treatment for the medical and psychological well-being of the patient.

◆ KEY POINTS ◆

1. Fibrocystic change is common in women under 50 years of age and it is hormonally mediated and benign.

2. Fibroadenomas are common benign solid breast masses found in women under age 30.

3. Malignant breast tumors are seen in approximately 20% of all dominant breast masses evaluated.

4. Ultrasonography, mammography, fine needle biopsy, and open biopsy are all methods of evaluating solid breast masses.

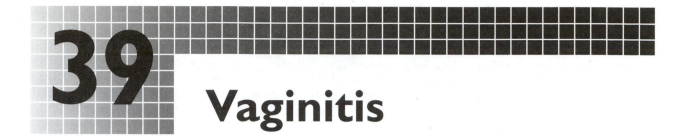

Vaginitis

Vaginitis is characterized by vaginal discharge that is unusual in amount, odor, or symptoms, such as itching or burning.

PATHOPHYSIOLOGY

The normal vaginal environment includes secretions, cellular elements, and microorganisms. Normal physiological vaginal secretions are typically clear to opaque, containing primarily mucus and exfoliated cells. Physiologic vaginal secretions vary with age, stage of the menstrual cycle, pregnancy, and use of oral contraceptives. Normal vaginal flora contains numerous bacteria, with lactobacilli being the most prevalent. The lactobacilli produce hydrogen peroxide, which is toxic to pathogens, and maintains the normal vaginal pH between 3.8 and 4.5. Vaginitis occurs when the vaginal flora is altered by the introduction of pathogens or changes in the vaginal environment.

Antibiotics, contraceptives, sexual intercourse, douching, and the introduction of sexually transmitted organisms are common factors that can disrupt the normal vaginal environment. These events can change the acidic pH of the vagina leading to an overgrowth of different organisms. The most common organisms causing symptoms include Candida, Trichomonas, and Gardnerella, which causes bacterial vaginosis (BV).

CLINICAL MANIFESTATIONS

History

Most women with vaginitis complain of vaginal discharge, itching, or burning. The patient should be asked about the onset and duration of the symptoms, any previous history of vaginitis, and previous treatments and its effects. A general medical review, dermatological review, and contraceptive history can be helpful. Illnesses, such as diabetes and HIV, and medications such as antibiotics or corticosteroids are associated with candidiasis. It is important to inquire about pelvic pain, fever, and possible pregnancy.

A sexual history can help identify patients at risk for sexually transmitted diseases. Inquiry about the use of bubble baths, douches, deodorants, and the use of spermidicide preparations may help identify individuals with irritant or contact vaginitis.

The nature of the discharge, that is, the amount, consistency, color, or odor, may suggest the cause of vaginitis. Candida usually produces itching with a thick, white discharge, sometimes described as cottage cheese-like. Other typical symptoms include vulvar and vaginal itching, burning, dysuria, and dyspareunia. Symptoms of Trichomonas vaginalis also include itching and often a profuse, frothy discharge with an unpleasant odor. The discharge can vary in color and may be yellow, gray, or green. Patients with bacterial vaginosis may be asymptomatic or have a slight increase in discharge. Some patients will complain of profuse discharge, with minimal itching, but often associated with a fishy odor.

Dysuria is also a common symptom of vaginitis. However, dysuria from vaginitis usually occurs when the urine touches the vulva. In contrast, internal dysuria, defined as pain inside the urethra, is usually a sign of cystitis.

Physical Examination

Inspection of the external genitalia for inflammation, masses, lesions, enlarged lymph nodes, and abnormal tissue is important. The pooled vaginal discharge can also be assessed for color, consistency, volume, and adherence to the vaginal wall. Typically, Candida produces a thick discharge that adheres to the vaginal wall while BV or trichomonas causes a thin discharge that pools in the vaginal vault that is easily swabbed off the vaginal wall. A bimanual exam is important to check for uterine or ovarian tenderness or enlargement.

Differential Diagnosis

Approximately 90% of vaginitis cases are secondary to BV, candidiasis, or Trichomonas. Viral infections, such as herpes simplex and human papilloma virus, sometimes cause vaginal irritation and discharge. Cervicitis, related to a chlamydial or gonorrheal infection can also cause a vaginal discharge.

If no infection is identified, other causes of vaginitis that should be considered include an allergic reaction, topical irritation, hormonal changes, and foreign bodies such as a forgotten tampon or condom. Other noninfectious causes of vaginitis include skin conditions such as lichen sclerosis or early vulvar cancer. Atrophic vaginitis is common in menopausal women.

DIAGNOSTIC APPROACH

A speculum exam is necessary to rule out neoplasm and foreign bodies and to determine whether the discharge is from vaginitis or cervicitis. A mucopurulent discharge from the cervix and cervical bleeding induced by swabbing the endocervical mucosa suggest cervicitis. Risk factors for cervicitis include age less than 24 years and a new sexual partner within the past 2 months. If cervicitis is suspected, tests for *Chlamydia* and *Neisseria gonorrhoeae* should be obtained.

If the history and physical are consistent with vaginitis, a sample of the discharge should be obtained. Standard office examinations include a wet mount preparation, a "whiff" test to detect amines and a slide prepared with 10% potassium hydroxide (KOH), and a pH measurement. A whiff test results when 10% KOH is added to a slide. The whiff test is positive if a fishy odor is detected, and is helpful in diagnosing BV. The odor results from the liberation of amines and organic acids produced by the alkalinization of anaerobic bacteria. The KOH also dissolves most cellular material except filamentous hyphae and budding forms of yeast, aiding the detection of fungal tangles and spores. A gram stain of vaginal secretions is even more sensitive for identifying yeast infections.

The wet mount is useful for detecting clue cells, Trichomonas, and polymorphonuclear leukocytes. Clue cells are vaginal epithelial cells that are coated with coccobacilli. They have a sensitivity and specificity up to 98% for the detection of bacterial vaginosis. Scanning several microscopic fields for Trichomonas has a 60% sensitivity and a specificity of up to 99%. The Trichomonas protozoon is slightly larger than a white blood cell and has three to five flagella. A wet mount may also detect fungal hyphae, increased numbers of polymorphonuclear cells (seen in Trichomonas) or round parabasilar cells (seen in atrophic vaginitis).

The pH can be determined by placing litmus paper in the pooled vaginal secretions or against the lateral vaginal walls. A pH greater than 4.5 is found in 80% to 90% of patients with bacterial vaginosis and frequently in patients with Trichomonas vaginosis. The pH level is also high in atrophic vaginitis.

A vaginal culture for candidiasis using Saboraud or Nickerson's media is helpful if microscopy is negative and Candida is still suspected. Alternatively, many clinicians will use a trial of antifungal therapy. Culture for Trichomonas increases the sensitivity of diagnosis. Since BV is a polymicrobial infection, culturing vaginal secretions is usually not recommended for cases of suspected bacterial vaginosis.

MANAGEMENT

Treatment for candidal vaginitis includes topical therapy with one of the azole agents, such as miconazole or terconazole. Miconazole (Monistat) is available as an over-the-counter preparation. Nystatin suppositories and gentian violet are also effective. Fluconazole, given as a 150 mg single oral dose, is as effective as a topical regimen. Recurrent yeast infections may respond to ketoconazole for 1 to 2 weeks, or fluconazole weekly.

Trichomonas can be treated with a single 2-gram dose of metronidazole or with 250 mg TID for 7 days. Metronidazole has the potential for an antabuse-like reaction, so patients should be cautioned about concomitant alcohol usage. Treating the sexual partner is important since 70% of sexual partners will be asymptomatically colonized with Trichomonas. Treatment for BV usually consists of either metronidazole 500 mg BID for 7 days or clindamycin 300 mg TID for 7 days. Single dose therapy with 2 grams of metronidazole is considered when compliance may be a problem. Both clindamycin and metronidazole are available as topical agents and offer an effective alternative.

◆ KEY POINTS ◆

1. Most cases of vaginitis in women of childbearing age are due to infection from Candida, Trichomonas, or bacterial vaginosis.

2. Laboratory evaluation of vaginal discharge consists of a wet mount, KOH preparation, whiff test, and pH determination.

3. A thick cottage-cheese discharge suggests Candida, while a profuse malodorous gray-green frothy discharge is more consistent with Trichomonas.

4. Bacterial vaginosis is a polymicrobial infection.

5. Metronidazole is effective for Trichomonas and bacterial vaginitis.

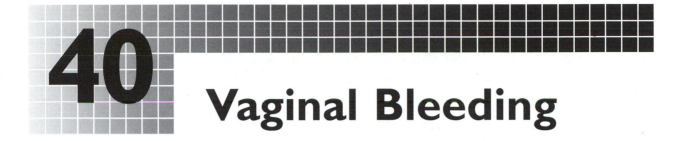

40 Vaginal Bleeding

The normal menstrual cycle ranges from 25 to 35 days. Day 1 of the cycle is the first day of bleeding. The average amount of blood loss is 30 cc; less than 80 cc is considered normal. Women usually flow from 2 to 7 days. Abnormal vaginal bleeding is subdivided into (1) menorrhagia: irregular cycles with either excessive flow, duration or both; (2) metrorrhagia: irregular bleeding between cycles; (3) menometrorrhagia: excessive bleeding either in amount, duration or both; (4) polymenorrhea: regular bleeding at intervals less than 21 days; (5) oligomenorrhea: regular bleeding at intervals greater than 35 days; and (6) intermenstrual bleeding: uterine bleeding between regular cycles.

PATHOPHYSIOLOGY

A normal menstrual cycle consists of proliferative and secretory phases. During the proliferative or follicular phase, FSH released by the pituitary stimulates a primary ovarian follicle to release estrogen, which stimulates the endometrium. At midcycle, a luteinizing hormone (LH) surge triggers ovulation. After ovulation, the luteal or secretory phase begins, the corpus luteum develops, and progesterone levels increase. Normal menstruation occurs if fertilization does not take place and estrogen and progesterone levels drop, resulting in the sloughing off of endometrium. Normally, this cycle recurs with a regular periodicity with menstruation generally occurring 14 days after ovulation. Cycle length variability is primarily due to variability in the time for follicle development during the proliferative phase.

An imbalance between estrogen and progesterone in the proliferative phase, at ovulation, or in the secretory phase causes abnormal vaginal bleeding. Persistently low levels of estrogen are associated with intermittent spotting and light bleeding. Excess estrogen stimulates the proliferation of endometrium, but without sufficient progesterone, the endometrium becomes abnormally thin and vascular. Eventually the endometrium outgrows its hormonal support and becomes friable, sloughing off irregularly, resulting in estrogen breakthrough bleeding. A sudden estrogen withdrawal after ovulation may trigger self-limited vaginal bleeding (midcycle spotting).

The most common form of abnormal vaginal bleeding is dysfunctional uterine bleeding (DUB). DUB is abnormal vaginal bleeding from the uterine endometrium, unrelated to an anatomic lesion of the genital tract, medications, systemic disease, or pregnancy. It is caused by hormonal imbalances from a functionally abnormal hypothalamic-pituitary-ovarian axis and is typically associated with anovulatory periods. In DUB, the vaginal bleeding occurs irregularly (metrorrhagia) because of a progesterone-deficient secretory phase. Progesterone breakthrough bleeding can occur in patients taking high progesterone-to-estrogen ratio oral contraception or IM progesterone. The endometrium is atrophic and ulcerated, which leads to metrorrhagia.

Abnormal vaginal bleeding can be due to structural abnormalities, such as uterine fibroids and polyps, or hyperplasia may cause abnormal shedding of the endometrial lining. Systemic illnesses, such as coagulation disorders, platelet abnormalities and renal or hepatic disease may affect coagulation as well as the metabolism and excretion of estrogen and progesterone. Obesity increases peripheral estrogen production, which interferes with the hypothalamic-pituitary axis. Thyroid disease, adrenal disease, and prolactin disorders alter the normal hormonal feedback mechanisms, thus again leading to alteration of menstrual flow.

CLINICAL MANIFESTATIONS

History

The menstrual history should include onset of menarche, duration, frequency, flow and bleeding pattern. Anovulatory cycles, when compared with ovulatory cycles, lack regular cycle length and a biphasic temperature curve. Women are also less likely to experience premenstrual symptoms, dysmenorrhea, breast tenderness, and a change in cervical mucus. A history of liver, renal, or thyroid disease may suggest a potential etiology. Use of anticoagulants, oral contraception, or hormone replacement therapy is a potential cause for abnormal bleeding. Review of systems, particularly regarding weight change, hirsutism, exercise or increased stress, and presence of galactorrhea or visual changes may help in determining the cause of abnormal bleeding.

Physical Examination

Physical examination should include vital signs, including orthostatic blood pressure and pulse, signs of pregnancy, assessment for systemic disease with a general exam, and a thorough sterile speculum and bimanual exam. Orthostatic changes indicate significant blood loss and a more acute course. Patients with polycystic ovarian syndrome and anovulatory bleeding often have hirsutism in conjunction with irregular menses and obese body habitus. A cushingoid appearance may indicate an adrenal abnormality, whereas presence of a goiter and hyporeflexia may indicate thyroid disease. Characteristics of hyperprolactinemia include visual field change and milky nipple discharge. A bleeding diathesis can present with petechiae, ecchymoses, along with menorrhagia. A thorough sterile speculum exam can identify vaginal or cervical lesions and directly visualize the amount of bleeding. The bimanual exam can assess cervical motion tenderness and detect uterine and adnexal masses.

DIFFERENTIAL DIAGNOSIS

Table 40–1 list some causes of abnormal vaginal bleeding. Establishing the pattern of bleeding as ovulatory or anovulatory helps narrow the differential diagnosis. For example, anovulatory bleeding is common in DUB, obese patients, and those suffering from infertility. Pregnancy-related bleeding can be due to an ectopic pregnancy, miscarriage, threatened abortion, placenta previa or an abruption. Abnormal bleeding can be a side effect of oral contraception or other hormone therapy. Pelvic inflammatory disease, coagulopathies, and anatomic lesions (e.g., cervical erosions) are other causes for premenopausal bleeding. Perimenopausal bleeding is typically irregular. The likelihood of cervical and endometrial cancer and endometrial hyperplasia is greater in those over age 35, particularly in peri- and postmenopausal patients. Fibroids and polyps are benign neoplasms that can cause abnormal bleeding. In postmenopausal women, vaginal bleeding is most commonly associated with endometrial carcinoma or hormone replacement therapy.

DIAGNOSTIC APPROACH

Figure 40–1 outlines the evaluation of the patient with abnormal vaginal bleeding. The initial evaluation should include a Pap smear (unless there is a record of a recent documented normal smear), a complete blood count and in peri- and premenopausal patients a pregnancy test. If a genital lesion is detected, then appropriate treatment or referral for evaluation and treatment should be advised. If the uterus is enlarged, then an ultrasound to assess the uterus should be obtained.

In younger patients with menorrhagia, coagulation disorders should be considered if there are other signs or symptoms of a bleeding disorder. Adolescents and young women with anovulatory patterns should have TSH and prolactin levels checked. Those with suspected polycystic ovarian syndrome (PCOS) may warrant measuring the LH, FSH, DHEAS, and free testosterone levels on the third day of the menstrual

TABLE 40–1

Symptoms Associated with Different Patterns of Vaginal Bleeding

Type	Associations	Causes	Ovulation
Midcycle spotting	pelvic pain (mittelschmerz)	ovulatory bleed	+
Menorrhagia	von Willebrand's dz, platelet disorder, structural lesion	thrombocytopenia, uterine fibroids, adenomyosis, endometrial polyps	+
Metrorrhagia	situational stress, weight loss, exercise training, hypo- or hyperthyroidism, hyperprolactinemia	hypothalamic dysfunction with progesterone-deficient state	−
	infertility, hirsutism, obesity or amenorrhea	polycystic ovarian syndrome	−
Menometrorrhagia	menstrual cramps	uterine fibroids	+
Oligomenorrhea	frequency >35 D	prolonged follicular phase	+
Polymenorrhea	frequency <21 D	inadequate luteal phase or a short follicular phase	+
Intermenstrual bleed		IUD cervical disease	+
Postcoital bleed	cervix ulcerations, spotting b/w menses	cervical cancer	+
		cervical polyps, erosions, vaginal lesions	+
	fever, pelvic pain, cervical discharge	pelvic inflammatory diseases	+
Pregnancy	amenorrhea, vaginal spotting, unilateral pelvic pain	ectopic pregnancy	NA
	painless vaginal bleeding	placenta previa	NA
	vaginal bleed w/ clots, abdominal pain	placenta abruption	NA
Perimenopausal bleed	metrorrhagia, vasomotor symptoms	estrogen-withdrawal	−
Postmenopausal bleed	>40 yo	endometrial cancer cervical cancer cervical or vaginal lesions	−
	continuous combined estrogen w/progesterone cyclic: 3 wk on & 1 wk off	estrogen breakthrough bleed or spotting	−

NA = not applicable.

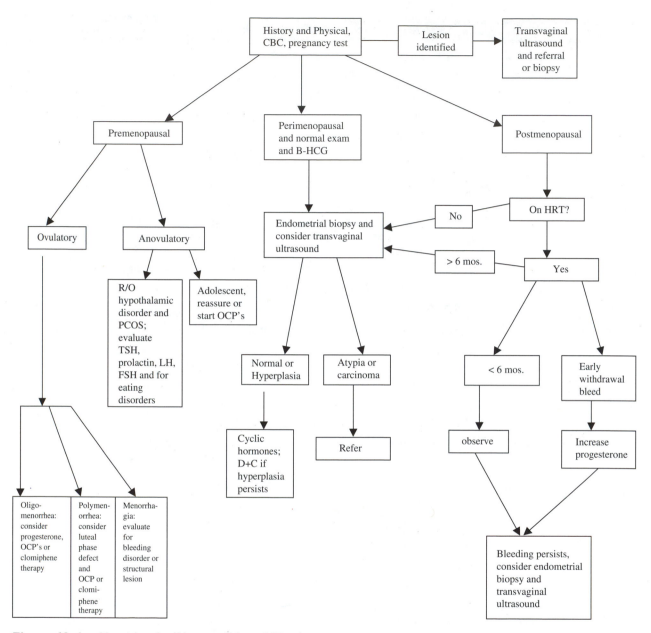

Figure 40–1   Algorithm for Abnormal Vaginal Bleeding.

cycle. A LH:FSH ratio greater than 2:1 is consistent with PCOS.

Women over the age of 35 require an approach that considers the possibility of endometrial cancer. Thus, in this age group ultrasound and endometrial biopsy are recommended. The exception to this may be in those postmenopausal women who have recently been started on hormone replacement therapy. Bleeding occurs com-

monly in the first 6 months of hormone replacement therapy and adjustment of the progesterone dosage followed by observation may be tried. If abnormal bleeding persists, further evaluation is indicated.

Vaginal bleeding more than 12 months after menopause is considered postmenopausal bleeding. Postmenopausal bleeding is abnormal and merits investigation because of the risk of cancer in this age group.

MANAGEMENT

Management depends upon the degree of bleeding, presence of anemia and the results of the evaluation. In hemodynamically unstable patients, hospitalization, transfusion, and stabilization of the bleeding with intravenous estrogen or surgical management are necessary. For patients with DUB who are not anemic, observation may be sufficient or oral contraceptives can be used to regulate menstrual cycles. Supplemental iron is indicated for anemic or iron deficient individuals. Patients with DUB unresponsive to medical therapy warrant referral.

In oligomenorrhea and polycystic ovarian syndrome, induction of menses at least every 3 months with progesterone is indicated to prevent endometrial hyperplasia and its risk for progression to cancer. Progesterone used in this manner will not prevent pregnancy and oral contraceptives are indicated for those patients with oligomenorrhea desiring contraception. Clomiphene is useful for those desiring pregnancy.

Perimenopausal and postmenopausal women without surgical conditions can be treated with cyclic hormonal therapy or adjustment of previously prescribed doses of hormones. Lesions of the vulva and vagina should be biopsied. Those with surgical causes or who are not responding to medical therapy warrant gynecology referral.

◆ KEY POINTS ◆

1. The most common cause of abnormal vaginal bleeding in a premenopausal patient is dysfunctional uterine bleeding (DUB) secondary to anovulation; in a perimenopausal patient endometrial hyperplasia and carcinoma; and in a postmenopausal patient, endometrial carcinoma and hormone replacement therapy.

2. Dysfunctional uterine bleeding (DUB) is not associated with pelvic pathology, medications, systemic disease, or pregnancy.

3. Because of the high likelihood of cancer in peri- or postmenopausal patients, endometrial biopsy and transvaginal ultrasound ought to be done early in the investigation.

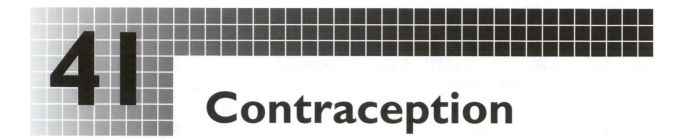

41 Contraception

More than half of all pregnancies in the United States are unintentional. About half of these pregnancies end in abortion and the other half in live births. Contraceptive methods have been developed in order to limit the number of unintended pregnancies. Methods of birth control include natural family planning, barrier methods, intrauterine devices, steroid medications, and surgical sterilization. Each birth control method has its disadvantages and advantages. In order to decide upon a method of contraception, the patient needs education about the different available options and their effectiveness. The theoretical efficacy rate of a birth control method is the number of unintended pregnancies per 100 women when the method is used exactly as instructed. Actual efficacy rates reflect the rate of women actually using the method for a year. Table 41–1 lists the efficacy rates of common forms of birth control. Birth control methods that require minimal patient involvement, such as surgical sterilization, have actual rates that approach theoretical rates, while actual rates may be much lower than theoretical rates for methods such as barrier contraception that require active patient involvement.

NATURAL FAMILY PLANNING

This form of birth control includes several different methods based upon abstinence or abstinence at selected times during the menstrual cycle. With natural family planning one must keep track of the normal menstrual cycle and abstain from sexual intercourse during the period (7–10 days) surrounding ovulation. Measuring cycle length (calendar method), cervical mucus changes and temperature changes can accomplish this. With the calendar method, ovulation is targeted as occurring 14 days before the onset of menses and requires that women abstain from sexual relations for several days before and after ovulation. When assessing cervical mucus, the woman inserts her fingers into the vagina to determine the amount and consistency of the mucus. Intercourse should be avoided when the mucus is thin and copious. The temperature method involves the woman measuring her temperature first thing in the morning before getting out of bed. At ovulation, the temperature will rise by 0.4 to 0.8 degrees centigrade. Again, sexual intercourse should be avoided during the period surrounding ovulation. The recent availability of home hormonal assays has also come to play a part in natural family planning. Some couples combine barrier methods with natural planning.

Natural methods are not effective directly after childbirth because it may take several months for the resumption of normal menstrual cycles especially if the mother is breastfeeding. Natural methods should not be recommended in women with irregular menses. Candidates for this type of contraception must be highly motivated, since prolonged periods of abstinence are necessary. Studies have found the failure rate for this

TABLE 41–1

Failure Rates for Various Contraceptive Methods

Method	Percent of Women who Become Pregnant	
	Theoretical Failure Rate	Actual Failure Rate
No method	85.0	85.0
Periodic abstinence	—	20.0
Calendar	9.0	
Ovulation method	3.0	
Symptothermal	2.0	
Postovulation	1.0	
Withdrawal	4.0	18.0
Lactational amenorrhea	2.0	15.0–55.0
Condom		
Male condom	2.0	12.0
Female condom	6.0	21.0–26.0
Diaphragm with spermicide	6.0	18.0
Cervical cap	6.0	18.0
Sponge		
Parous women	9.0	28.0
Nulliparous women	6.0	18.0
Spermicide alone	3.0	21.0
IUDs		
Progestasert	2.0	2.0
Paraguard copper T	0.8	0.7
Combination pill	0.1	3.0
Progestin only pill	0.5	3.0–6.0
Norplant	0.09	0.09
Depo-Provera	0.3	0.3
Tubal ligation	0.2	0.4
Vasectomy	0.1	0.15

Adapted from Speroff L and Darney P, A clinical guide for contraception, 2nd ed. Baltimore: Williams & Wilkins, 1996:136.

form of contraception to be approximately 20% per year.

BARRIER METHODS

Commonly used barrier methods are diaphragms and condoms. Since both methods require active patient participation, patient motivation must be taken into account when choosing this method.

Diaphragm use requires instruction and experience and is more effective in older women who are familiar with its use. The failure rate is estimated at 2.4 to 19.6 per 100 women years. In users over 25 years old and with at least 5 months experience the failure rate was 2.4 per 100 women years. The diaphragm is placed into the vagina along the anterior vaginal wall and should cover the entire cervix, thus preventing passage of semen into the cervix. Diaphragms come in different sizes. After an initial fitting, patients need to be refitted after pregnancy, pelvic surgery, or a weight change of more than 10 pounds. The diaphragm must be used together with spermicidal lubricants containing nonoxynol-9. It must be inserted no longer than 6 hours prior to coitus and left in the vagina at least 6 hours but not longer than 24 hours after coitus. Additional spermicide should be placed intravaginally without removing the diaphragm for each episode of intercourse. Women using this form of contraception may be more prone to urinary tract infections.

There are two general types of condoms—one for the male and one for the female. The male condom is a sleeve made of latex or lambskin that prevents passage of semen into the vagina. The condom must be placed on the erect penis before penetration. The female condom is placed in the vagina before intercourse and also prevents passage of semen into the vagina. Condoms can be used with other forms of contraception (e.g., spermicides) and latex condoms are recommended to prevent transmission of sexually transmitted diseases. The pregnancy rate for condoms is approximately 1.6 to 12 per 100 women years depending on age and motivation of the patient.

STEROID CONTRACEPTIVE MEDICATIONS

Oral contraceptives, specifically estrogen and progestin preparations, are among the most reliable form of birth control. Pregnancy rates are less than 0.5 per 100 women years with good compliance. Oral contraceptives containing estrogen (most frequently ethinyl estradiol) together with one of several different progestin components inhibit gonadotropin secretion and ovarian function and induce changes in the cervical mucus and endometrial lining that inhibit sperm passage and ovum implantation.

Box 41–1 lists some non-contraceptive benefits of oral contraceptives. Women with a history of ovarian cysts or dysmenorrhea will benefit from the effects of oral contraceptives in ovarian suppression and thinning the endometrium.

Oral contraceptive use is contraindicated in women 35 years and older who smoke secondary to the increased risk of venous thrombosis and cardiovascular complications. Additional contraindications for oral contraceptive use include venous thromboembolic disease, known cardiovascular disease, undiagnosed vaginal bleeding, breast cancer, and active liver disease. Relative contraindications include depression, diabetes, gallbladder disease, lactation, and obesity. Side effects include weight gain, nausea, headache, breast tenderness, acne, and depression.

Women desiring pregnancy after discontinuation of the pill should be counseled that there might be a several month delay in resumption of ovulation. Postpartum oral contraceptives can be started as early as 2 to 3 weeks in nonbreastfeeding individuals. Lactation can be suppressed by oral contraceptives containing more than 50 mg of ethinyl estradiol or mestranol.

Progestin-only hormonal contraception is available orally, by injection, and as subdermal implants. These agents may be used in patients unable to tolerate estrogenic side effects or with contraindications to estrogens (e.g., cardiovascular disease, venous thromboembolic disease). The oral progestin-only contraceptives, also known as the "mini-pill," are slightly less effective than the combination pills. The injectable form of steroid contraception, depot medroxyprogesterone acetate, is 99% effective in preventing conception. It is given as 150 mg intramuscularly every 3 months. Levonorgestrel subdermal implants are the most effective form of reversible contraception. The major disadvantages are the expense and occasional difficulty in removing the implants that are placed underneath the skin. An etonogestrel single rod implant is available and effective for 3 years. Side effects of progestin-only contraception include acne, headache, weight gain, and irregular bleeding. Spotting and bleeding are the most common and troublesome side effect of these agents. Progestin-only agents do not affect lactation.

A recent addition to the steroid contraceptive medications is the monthly injectable combination of medroxyprogesterone acetate and estradiol cypionate, which has a 1 year cumulative pregnancy rate of 0.2%. Return to fertility is rapid when injections are stopped. Ovulation occurs during the third month post treatment. The most frequent reasons for discontinuation are weight gain, excessive bleeding, breast pain, menorrhagia, and dysmenorrhea.

Hormone releasing vaginal rings provide low-dose release of 120 mcg etonogestrel and 15 mcg of ethinyl estradiol per day. The ring is one-size-fits-all, stays in place for 3 weeks, and is taken out for the fourth week. Limited data for efficacy is available at present. Disadvantages include the fear of a foreign body in the vagina and fear of expulsion.

BOX 41–1

Non-contraceptive Benefits of Oral Contraceptives

Reduce the risk of the following conditions

- Ovarian Cancer
- Endometrial Cancer
- Ectopic Pregnancy
- Pelvic Inflammatory Disease
- Anemia
- Dysmenorrhea
- Functional Ovarian Cysts
- Benign Breast Disease
- Osteoporosis

INTRAUTERINE DEVICES

The intrauterine device (IUD) works by interfering with sperm mobility and fertilization. IUDs have an efficacy rate of 2 to 3 pregnancies per 100 women years. This form of contraception is independent of the act of intercourse, highly effective, inexpensive, and reversible. Thus, women who use IUDs are among the most satisfied of all contraceptive users.

Two main types of IUDs are the copper-containing T-shaped devices and the progesterone-releasing devices. Copper-containing IUDs can remain in place for 10 years, whereas progesterone-releasing devices must be changed after 5 years. The copper-containing IUDs may cause irregular uterine bleeding, an effect that is less prevalent with the progesterone IUDs. The Levonorgestrel Intrauterine System releases low doses of levonorgestrel at 20 mcg/day in the uterine cavity for 5 years. The 5-year cumulative failure rate is 0.71 per 100 women, nearly equal to that of sterilization.

IUDs must be inserted under sterile conditions. It is recommended that an IUD should be placed within 5 days of the menstrual cycle, but may be inserted any time the patient is not pregnant. Contraindications to IUD insertion are pregnancy, undiagnosed vaginal bleeding, and pelvic inflammatory disease. Relative contraindications include nulliparity, prior ectopic pregnancy, history of multiple sexual partners, history of a previous sexually transmitted disease, abnormal Pap smear that has not been fully evaluated, and uterine anomalies.

Complications of IUDs include pelvic inflammatory disease, ectopic pregnancy, spontaneous abortion, increased menstrual flow and pain, and uterine perforation. The risk of PID associated with IUD users is correlated to ascending contamination at the time of insertion. Nonetheless, IUDs are usually contraindicated in women at high risk of cervical sexually transmitted diseases.

STERILIZATION

There are approximately one million sterilizations performed in the United States per year. The two forms of sterilization performed are vasectomies and tubal ligations. Of these two procedures, tubal ligation is performed more commonly than vasectomy and is the most commonly used birth control method in the world. In order to avoid postprocedure regret, it is extremely important to stress the irreversibility of these procedures. Risk factors for regret include: depression, young age, low parity, unstable marriage, and having the procedure at the time of C-section.

Tubal ligation is an invasive procedure that can be performed laparoscopically or at the time of a cesarean section. Tubal continuity is interrupted surgically, thus preventing passage of the sperm or ovum. Vasectomies

can be performed as an outpatient procedure under local anesthesia with less time away from work and a more rapid recovery. The procedure involves incising the scrotum, identifying the vas deferens, and then surgically removing a portion of each vas, thus preventing passage of sperm. Vasectomy does not result in immediate sterility. Clearance of sperm occurs after about 25 ejaculations and must be confirmed by semen analysis. Complications from either procedure are uncommon. Vasectomy failures can be picked up by postoperative semen analysis, whereas failures of tubal ligation are detected when the patient becomes pregnant. Each of these procedures are potentially reversible, despite their labeling as "permanent" sterilization. Tubal ligations can be reversed with a success rate of 40% to 85%. Success rates for reversal of vasectomy range from 37% to 90%.

POST-COITAL CONTRACEPTION

Post-coital hormonal approaches include the use of Ovral or Lo-Ovral, with a dose of 2 Ovral pills taken within 72 hours of unprotected intercourse, followed by 2 more taken 12 hours later. Emergency contraception prevents at least 3 of 4 pregnancies that would have occurred. Post-coital IUD insertion within 5 days after intercourse is also effective.

◆ KEY POINTS ◆

1. More than half of pregnancies in the United States are unintended.

2. Natural family planning methods focus on abstinence around the time of ovulation, but have a 20% failure rate.

3. Barrier methods require significant patient motivation, but can be effective.

4. Condoms can be combined with other methods of contraception and can help prevent sexually transmitted disease.

5. The most effective methods of contraception are intrauterine devices, hormonal contraception and surgical sterilization.

6. The method of contraception should be tailored to the individual patient.

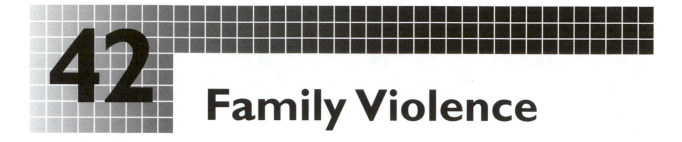

42 Family Violence

Family violence poses serious public health risks, and manifests itself in various forms including child abuse (CA), domestic violence (DV) between intimate partners, and elder abuse (EA) or neglect. Abuse may be physical, sexual or emotional, with the abuser exerting control over the victim.

DV causes a spectrum of health risks particularly for women, ranging from minor injuries to death. Recent studies estimate that 2 to 4 million women each year suffer injuries from DV, and more than 1 million seek medical attention for such injuries. Approximately 30% of all female homicides in the United States are the result of domestic violence.

CA has been reported to occur in over 1 million children in the U.S. (about 14/1000 children), and many cases are unreported. Intentional injury is the number one cause of injury-related death in children under 1 year of age. Children who have been abused physically or sexually are significantly more likely to be sexually active as teens, abuse tobacco and alcohol, attempt suicide, and exhibit violent or criminal behavior.

The exact EA incidence is not well established, and it is estimated that only 1 in 5 cases are ever reported. The abuser is usually a relative, and is most commonly the patient's spouse or caregiver.

RISK FACTORS

Victims of DV are more likely to be young women between the ages of 12 and 35 years, from a lower income group, single, separated, or divorced; to have not attended college; to have experienced abuse as a child; and to have a partner abusing alcohol or drugs. The single most common risk factor in DV is whether the victim witnessed parental violence as a child or adolescent. This risk factor is consistently associated with being a victim of DV from a spouse.

DV is associated with poorer pregnancy outcomes. Up to a third of pregnant women are abused during pregnancy, making battery far more common than the combined incidence of rubella, Rh and ABO incompatibility, hepatitis, and gestational diabetes. Pregnant women who are battered are more likely to register for late prenatal care, suffer preterm labor or miscarriage, and have low birth-weight infants. Box 42–1 lists various factors that increase the risk for domestic violence.

PATHOPHYSIOLOGY

Domestic violence often results from one partner's need to achieve dominance and control. The abuser learns that violence is an effective way to maintain control. Abusers tend to blame family stress and unfulfilled expectation in their partners. Typically there is a cycle of violence in which an assault is followed by a time when the batterer is remorseful and often loving. Following this is a tension-building period, which then culminates in another episode. Over time, the episodes become more frequent and severe.

BOX 42–1

Risk Factors for Domestic Violence

Medical:
- Alcoholism/substance abuse
- Mental or physical disability

Relationships:
- Past history of abusive relationships
- Witness to parental violence as a child or adolescent
- Rigid family rules or conflicted roles
- Social isolation

External Stressors:
- Poverty, financial struggle
- Losses
- Work stress
- Life cycle changes

BOX 42–2

Clues to Child Abuse

- The story given by the parents does not seem to explain the injury.
- The explanation given by the parent or caretaker is inconsistent or contradictory.
- There is a long interval between the injury and seeking care.
- The parent's reaction to the injury is inappropriate.
- The parent's interaction with the child seems inappropriate.

CLINICAL MANIFESTATIONS

History

Identifying victims of abuse is challenging in all but the most obvious cases. The chief complaint can be related to an injury or extend to any organ system. In many cases, abused patients may present with non-traumatic diagnoses, like upper respiratory tract symptoms and bronchitis.

Many studies have identified provider barriers to the identification of battered women, which include lack of knowledge or training, time limitations, inability to offer lasting solutions, and fear of offending the patient. Health care providers may have personal experiences that contribute to their reluctance to broach the issue of abuse. Class elitism, racial prejudice, and sexism may also serve as barriers against properly identifying and treating victims of DV.

Domestic Violence Screening

Studies have shown that direct questioning of patients at risk for DV yields better information than written questionnaires. Three important questions to ask are:

1. "Have you been hit, kicked, punched or otherwise hurt by someone within the past year? If so, by whom?"

2. "Do you feel safe in your current relationship?"

3. "Is there a partner from a previous relationship making you feel unsafe now?"

The first question regarding physical violence is nearly as sensitive and specific as the combination of all three questions. Thus, the problem of identifying women involved in abusive relationships may be simplified by the use of routine screening tools as above.

Child Abuse Screening

Screening for child abuse during the interview is difficult, and standardized questions have not been shown to be sensitive or specific in detecting child abuse. Open-ended questions about parenting and discipline may be useful, however, in eliciting evidence of CA. For example, the health care provider may ask, "What do you do when he or she misbehaves? Have you ever been worried that someone was going to hurt your child?" Box 42–2 lists clues for suspecting an injury is due to abuse. Neglect is another type of abuse and can consist of medical, physical, or emotional neglect. Poor supervision, such as leaving a young child alone without adequate adult oversight, is another type of abuse.

Elder Abuse Screening

Screening for elder abuse has not been studied as well as DV or CA. The value of screening the patient for EA is limited if the abuser is present because he or she is often the primary caregiver to the victim.

Physical Examination

Certain types of injury patterns suggest family violence. These include injuries to the face, abdomen, and genitals. Also multiple injuries in various stages of healing suggest possible abuse. Since many women seen in the emergency room for trauma are victims of abuse, there should be a high index of suspicion for any acute injury that does not have a clear cause. Burns in children are often a tip-off for abuse, particularly burn patterns that suggest an immersion injury or a cigarette burn.

MANAGEMENT AND INTERVENTION

The most important and most easily provided intervention is the simple message that no one deserves to be hurt and that the victim is not to blame for the behavior of the perpetrator.

Domestic Violence Intervention

Battered women report that the most desirable behaviors by physicians with whom they interact include listening, providing emotional support, and reassuring the woman that being beaten was not her fault. Women in the same study reported that the most undesirable behaviors include treatment of physical injuries without inquiry as to how they occurred.

Once a patient has been identified as a victim of abuse, it is important to address safety needs, such as ascertaining whether there are guns or other weapons in the house. Simply asking patients if they feel safe to go home can yield valuable information. Questions about the safety of children are crucial, because as many as 70% of batterers also abuse children. Patients should be encouraged to begin to make plans to be safe whether or not they plan to leave the relationship or home situation.

Referral to community services is an important part of treatment for battered women. Shelters provide much more than refuge for victims of DV. Women there can take advantage of child services, counseling, and legal and employment services.

The physician can offer to contact the police unless required by law to do so; in that case, the patient should understand the physician's duty to report. Victims should be informed that battering is a crime throughout the United States and that there is help available from the judicial system. Civil protection orders (*stay-away orders*) are available in every jurisdiction. In addition to barring contact between the perpetrator and victim, these orders can include temporary custody of children and mandate payment of rent or mortgage by the batterer, even if he is not allowed to live in the home.

The worst thing that the physician can do is nothing. Even if the patient refuses any help, it is still critical to acknowledge the patient's disclosure and assign responsibility to the abuser. Supportive statements emphasizing that this is not the patient's fault and that violence is not an acceptable means of conflict resolution can be helpful. It is important to remember that terminating an abusive relationship is often a long process. Continuous support, follow-up, and accessibility are critically important for those individuals who choose to remain in an abusive relationship.

Child Abuse Intervention

Intervention studies in child abuse have concentrated on primary prevention. Home visits to high-risk families have been shown to decrease the rate of CA and the need for medical visits early in life. Unfortunately, most clinicians do not have the option of providing this level of intervention, much less extending this type of treatment for long periods of time. Recurrent abuse despite interventions may occur in up to 60% of cases.

Elder Abuse Intervention

Effective interventions for elder abuse may also be limited, in large part because the abuser is often the primary caregiver. Nursing home placement may be the only alternative, and victims may be reluctant to give up their independence in order to escape abuse. A review of elder physical abuse victims in Illinois reported that most victims received few tangible services from social service agencies other than case management (primarily monitoring).

DOCUMENTATION

Medical records must document abuse accurately and legibly since these records are readily admissible at civil and criminal trials. They can provide objective diagnosis that can substantiate a victim's assertion of harm. These records can be used even when the victim is unable or unwilling to testify. Whenever possible, the patient's own words should be used. The relationship of the perpetrator to the victim also should be clearly stated. If possible, the record should include photographs because these are particularly valuable as evidence. Areas of tenderness, even in the absence of visual injury, should be documented in writing as well as on a body map. Attention to detail is invaluable when attempting to recreate the circumstances of abuse for the criminal justice system. A well-documented medical record improves the likelihood of successful prosecution without testimony from the health care provider.

REPORTING

In all states, suspected cases of child abuse or neglect must be reported to local child protective services agencies. In most states, suspected elder abuse must also be reported. Almost all states mandate reporting injuries that result from the use of a gun, knife, or other deadly weapon. Whether mandatory reporting of domestic violence results in improved outcome for a victim is controversial, however. Nevertheless, health care providers must be familiar and comply with local laws. A few states now require that health care workers report cases of suspected domestic violence. Reporting abuse is not a substitute for proper intervention and management for CA, DV, or EA.

BATTERERS

Information on batterers is limited. This is particularly worrisome because the solution to the problem of abuse lies largely in changing perpetrator behavior. Most studies surrounding batterers have focused on the influence of the criminal justice system on changing behavior. More data are needed to establish which interventions are most helpful with batterers.

◆ KEY POINTS ◆

1. Approximately 30% of all female homicides in the United States are the result of domestic violence.

2. Children who have been abused physically or sexually are significantly more likely to be sexually active as teens, abuse tobacco and alcohol, attempt suicide, and exhibit violent or criminal behavior.

3. The chief complaint can be related to an injury, however, in many cases, abused patients may present with non-traumatic diagnoses, like upper respiratory tract symptoms and bronchitis.

4. The most important and most easily provided intervention is the simple message that no one deserves to be hurt and that the victim is not to blame for the behavior of the perpetrator.

5. More data are needed to establish which interventions are most helpful with batterers.

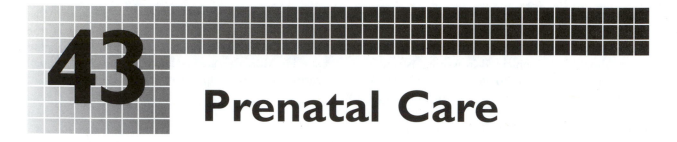

Prenatal Care

Prenatal care is the care and management of the pregnant patient until delivery. The purpose of prenatal care is to identify psychosocial and medical conditions that may lead to a poor pregnancy outcome and to institute medical and support measures to limit the effects of these conditions. Prenatal care should begin as early as possible and should include education of the patient in such matters as nutrition, exercise, common symptoms, danger signs of pregnancy, and signs of labor. The stages of pregnancy are divided into trimesters and the focus of the history, physical, laboratory tests, and patient education vary by trimester.

CLINICAL MANIFESTATIONS—FIRST TRIMESTER (UP TO 14 WEEKS)

The first prenatal visit should include a complete history and physical exam. Goals for this visit are to assess the gestational age and to plan care for the remainder of the pregnancy. Follow-up visits during this time generally are every 4 weeks.

History

The obstetrical history begins with the date of the last menstrual period (LMP). The date of delivery can then be estimated using Naegele's rule: Estimated date of delivery (EDD) = LMP − 3 months + 7 days. A woman's obstetrical history is often described in a shorthand version in terms of gravidity and parity. Gravidity refers to the total number of pregnancies, whereas parity describes the number of pregnancies continuing past 20

weeks of gestation. Further subdivision of parity is often provided using the "TPAL" system where T = number of term deliveries, P = number of premature deliveries, A = number of abortions, and L = number of living infants. For example, a woman who is currently pregnant with one living child who was born prematurely would be described as G2P0101. In documenting the history, the total number of pregnancies should be listed in chronological order with their outcomes. This should include the gender, weight, condition at birth, and any complications during the pregnancy or delivery.

The past medical history should include acute and chronic illnesses such as hypertension, diabetes, seizure disorders, and renal disease as well as any sexually transmitted diseases such as HIV and hepatitis B. History of past surgeries or pelvic fractures should be noted. A medication review, including the use of over-the-counter drugs is important.

In the social history, habits such as smoking, alcohol, and drug use should be noted. If the patient admits to using any such substances, she needs counseling not only regarding the risks to her unborn child but to her health as well. Social issues such as family support and domestic violence should also be noted. A family history can identify individuals at risk for genetic diseases such as Tay-Sachs or sickle cell anemia.

Physical Examinations

The first prenatal visit should include a complete physical exam. Weight prior to conception should be noted. A pelvic exam should be done on the first visit to evaluate uterine size and to assess the adequacy of the pelvis. Follow-up visits should note any changes in weight as well as blood pressure (BP). Fetal heart sounds should be monitored every visit starting at 12 weeks of gestation.

Laboratory Testing

The initial prenatal visit should include a Pap smear, complete blood count, urinalysis, blood type (including Rh) and antibody screen (CBC). Rapid plasma reagin (RPR), rubella antibody titer, hepatitis B surface antigen, and chlamydia and gonorrhea cultures are other important screening tests for pregnant patients. Human immunodeficiency virus antibody testing should be offered and if risk factors for tuberculosis are identified, a tuberculin skin test can also be performed.

Patient Education

Nutritional education is an important part of prenatal care. Proper weight gain is essential for both maternal and infant health. The recommended weight gain during pregnancy is between 25 and 35 pounds. The recommended weight gain for a twin pregnancy is 35 to 45 pounds. Much of this weight gain occurs in the second and third trimesters and in the first trimester the patient may gain only 2 to 4 pounds.

Iron requirements during pregnancy increase due to increased maternal red cell production and to meet the needs of the growing fetus. Thirty milligrams of elemental ferrous iron per day is recommended. If the patient has anemia, 60–120 mg/day is required. Folic acid and other prenatal vitamins should also be supplemented.

Nausea and vomiting are common complaints in the first trimester and are due to increased levels of human chorionic gonadotropin. If vomiting is severe and is accompanied by weight loss and ketones in urine, the patient may need to be hospitalized. Milder symptoms can be managed by educating the patient on dietary measures that may decrease the nausea, such as eating dry crackers, cereal, or toast before getting out of bed in the morning, separating fluid intake from solid food by one-half to one hour and eating small frequent meals.

Patients may continue normal exercise and sexual activity during pregnancy unless complications such as vaginal bleeding or preterm contractions occur. Since pregnancy can increase the risk of thromboembolic events, long trips should be avoided as this can cause venous stasis and increase the risks for deep venous thrombosis. If patients must take long trips, then stopping every two hours to walk and increase venous return from the legs is advised. When traveling in automobiles, patients should be encouraged to wear seat belts.

CLINICAL MANIFESTATIONS—SECOND TRIMESTER (14–28 WEEKS)

History

In the second trimester (14–28 weeks) patients generally feel well and do not have many physical complaints. During this time the patient may report fetal movement or quickening which normally occurs between 18 and 20 weeks. Office visits during this time should occur every 4 weeks.

Physical Examination

The physical exam at each visit should include fetal heart tone auscultation, fundal height measurement, and maternal weight and blood pressure measurement. At 20 weeks the uterus should be at the umbilicus. Poor weight gain or lagging uterine enlargement may be signs of intrauterine growth retardation or oligohydramnios and warrant evaluation. Excessive weight gain may suggest pregnancy-induced hypertension (PIH) or gestational diabetes. A weight gain of more than 5 pounds per week should prompt further evaluation.

Laboratory Testing

At each visit a urinalysis for glucosuria and proteinuria should be checked to monitor for PIH and diabetes. In the second trimester at 15 to 20 weeks, a maternal serum alpha-fetoprotein (MSAFP) level should be offered as a screening test for neural tube defects or trisomy. An alternative is the triple marker screen that consists of the MSAFP, estriol, and HCG levels. If the MSAFP is abnormal, an ultrasound should be done. Some causes of an elevated MSAFP include: incorrect pregnancy dates, twin pregnancy, and neural tube defects. Decreased levels of MSAFP are associated with pregnancy dating errors or trisomy 21. In practice, many physicians will order routine ultrasound examinations when ordering the MSAFP to confirm the EDD established by the LMP and to assist in interpreting the MSAFP results.

Patient Education

During the second trimester, patients should be instructed to report any swelling of the face or fingers, headaches, blurring of vision, abdominal pain, persistent vomiting, fever, chills, dysuria, watery vaginal discharge, vaginal bleeding, or change in intensity of fetal movement, all of which may indicate a risk to the pregnancy. During the second trimester, patients should gain weight at a faster rate than in the first trimester. On average, 1 pound per week is recommended. In addition, late in the second trimester, patients can begin attending birthing, breast-feeding and parenting classes.

CLINICAL MANIFESTATIONS—THIRD TRIMESTER (28 WEEKS–DELIVERY)

History

During the third trimester, patients may complain of fatigue and increasing discomfort as the abdomen enlarges. Evaluation of physical complaints and preparing the patient for labor and delivery are the focus of visits at this time. Follow-up visits should be every 2 weeks until the 36th week. After the 36th week patients should be evaluated every week until delivery.

Laboratory Testing

Glucose screening for diabetes is performed at 28 weeks and consists of a 50-gram oral glucose load with measurement of blood glucose levels 1 hour after glucose ingestion. A blood glucose level more than 135 mg/dl is positive and should be confirmed with a 3-hour 100-gram oral glucose tolerance test (OGTT). Additional testing commonly includes a hemoglobin at 28 weeks and a vaginal and rectal culture to detect the presence of Group B streptococci at 28 to 36 weeks. At 28 weeks, Rh-negative patients should receive Rhogam to decrease the likelihood of complications due to maternal-fetal Rh-incompatibility.

Patient Education

In the third trimester, patients often complain of such symptoms as back pain, acid reflux, pelvic pain, and vari-cosities. The back pain is often due to the strain on the lumbar spine from the enlarging uterus. Patients should be instructed to rest and to take acetaminophen for severe pain. The acid reflux is due to the enlarging uterus compressing the stomach as well as due to the relaxing effect of progesterone on the smooth muscle. The symptoms may be controlled by informing the patient not to lie down for 2 hours after eating, encouraging the patient to eat smaller quantities of food more frequently, or by use of calcium-containing antacids for acid reflux. Pelvic pain may be due to the stretching of the ligaments in the pelvis. Walking often aggravates this pain. As a result patients should be encouraged to rest and refrain from prolonged standing. This will also help limit symptoms due to varicosities in the lower extremities.

Patients should also be educated on signs of labor, which include rupture of membranes, onset of regular contractions, or vaginal bleeding. Patients should have a number to call where assistance is available 24 hours a day. Any preferences regarding the method of delivery, anesthesia, or other requests should be discussed with the patient during the later stages of their pregnancy.

◆ KEY POINTS ◆

1. Purpose of prenatal care is to identify and treat medical and social problems that may lead to a poor pregnancy outcome.

2. Date of delivery can be estimated using Naegele's rule: EDD = LMP − 3 months + 7 days, where LMP = last menstrual period.

3. Follow-up visits should be every 4 weeks until the 28th week of pregnancy, every 2 weeks until the 36th week of pregnancy and then every week until delivery.

4. Any preferences regarding the method of delivery, anesthesia, or other requests should be discussed with the patient during the later stages of their pregnancy.

Amenorrhea

Amenorrhea is the absence of menstrual periods in a woman of reproductive age. Physiologic amenorrhea occurs when a woman reaches menopause, becomes pregnant, or breast feeds. Primary amenorrhea is defined as the absence of menarche by age 16 years with normal pubertal development, or by age 14 years without the onset of puberty. Secondary amenorrhea is defined as absence of menses for 6 months, or for 3 cycles in a woman who previously had menses. Excluding physiologic causes, secondary amenorrhea has a prevalence rate of about 4%. Primary amenorrhea is less common, with about 99% of women having menses by age 16.

PATHOPHYSIOLOGY

The hypothalamus, anterior pituitary, ovary, and uterus orchestrate the menstrual cycle. The pulsatile release of Gonadotropin Releasing Hormone (GnRH) from the hypothalamus stimulates the anterior pituitary gland to release Luteinizing Hormone (LH) and Follicle-Stimulating Hormone (FSH) into the bloodstream. In the ovary, FSH stimulates the ovarian follicles, which produce estrogen and later progesterone. Estrogen stimulates the endometrial lining. A LH surge and ovulation occurs midcycle, triggered by the positive feedback between FSH and the hypothalamus-pituitary axis. The dominant follicle develops into a corpus luteum and secretes progesterone. If the oocyte fails to be fertilized, the progesterone production of the degenerating corpus luteum decreases, and the endometrial lining of the uterus begins to slough off. If there are no anatomic anomalies that inhibit outflow, menstruation occurs. Amenorrhea reflects an interruption of the mechanisms of normal menstruation and may result from abnormalities in the hypothalamus, anterior pituitary, ovaries, or uterus.

CLINICAL MANIFESTATIONS

History

The history should include a menstrual history (presence of menarche, menstruation duration and flow, dysmenorrhea), a review of development (growth and sexual development), chronic illnesses, and medications. It is also important to discuss a teenager's sexual history and substance abuse while reassuring the confidentiality of the conversation in a private setting. Emotional stress or pronounced weight loss may be a clue to hypothalamic dysfunction. It is useful to ask about visual changes, headache, galactorrhea (CNS cause); presence of goiter, fatigue, palpitations (thyroid disease); presence of abdominal pain, bloating, and normal pubertal changes (vaginal outlet obstructions). In female athletes, discussion of nutrition, physical activity, weight changes, dieting, and body image may give clues to an underlying eating disorder.

Physical Examination

Physical examination begins with vital signs including weight and height, followed by a careful funduscopic examination, thyroid gland palpation, breast exam with attempts to express galactorrhea, abdominal exam and a bimanual pelvic exam. In patients with primary amenorrhea evaluation for signs of virilization and uterine or vaginal abnormalities is important. A pale vaginal mucosa lacking normal rugal folds suggests estrogen deficiency. Short stature (<60 inches) in a patient with primary amenorrhea merits evaluation for Turner's syndrome. Hirsutism, obesity, and acanthosis may be signs of PCOS.

DIFFERENTIAL DIAGNOSIS

Table 44–1 lists common causes for primary and secondary amenorrhea. The causes of primary amenorrhea include hormonal aberrations, congenital defects, chromosomal abnormalities, and hypothalamic and pituitary dysfunction. In patients with primary amenorrhea and normal secondary sexual characteristics, the most likely cause is an anatomic abnormality such as the failure to develop a normal uterus or vagina. In contrast, the lack of secondary sexual characteristics suggests a hormonal problem. The most common hypothalamic etiology is Kallmann's syndrome while a tumor or compression from a Rathke's pouch cyst may cause pituitary gland dysfunction. Ovarian function may be defective due to gonadal dysgenesis as seen in Turner's syndrome.

Many of the causes of secondary amenorrhea overlap with the causes of primary amenorrhea. After pregnancy, the most common causes are hypothalamic amenorrhea from stress or illness, hyperprolactinemia, or PCOS. In a few women, Turner's syndrome may present as premature ovarian failure.

DIAGNOSTIC EVALUATION

The evaluation of a patient with primary amenorrhea is driven by the clinical examination (Figure 44–1). If secondary sexual characteristics such as breast development are present, then anatomic abnormalities or testicular feminization syndrome should be suspected. For patients with a uterus but no breasts, gonadal dysfunction or a hypothalamic-pituitary axis problem is likely. The absence of both a uterus and breasts indicates the need for a chromosomal analysis. Consultation with a specialist is often useful in a patient with primary amenorrhea.

The evaluation for secondary amenorrhea starts with a pregnancy test. If the pregnancy test is negative and no obvious explanation exists for the amenorrhea, a prolactin level and a TSH should be measured. About 20% of cases of secondary amenorrhea are caused by hyperprolactinemia. If these levels are normal, a progesterone challenge test determines if a woman produces estrogen. Medroxyprogesterone acetate (Provera) given in a 10 mg oral daily dose for 5 to 7 days is a commonly used means for a progesterone challenge. Any bleeding, even a small amount, in the week after completing progesterone indicates that the major components of the hypothalamic, pituitary, ovarian, and uterine pathways are at least minimally functioning and that the patient is anovulatory. The most common cause of anovulatory periods is PCOS or a functional abnormality in the hypothalamus. Functional hypothalamic amenorrhea is a diagnosis of exclusion, but a history of anorexia nervosa, stress, or extreme exercise suggests the diagnosis. No bleeding indicates that either an estrogen deficiency or an anatomic abnormality is present. If an estrogen deficiency is suspected, assessing the FSH level is the next step. An elevated FSH level indicates ovarian failure. Patients younger than 30 years old with ovarian failure should undergo karyotyping. If the FSH is low or normal, an MRI scan of the hypothalamus and pituitary is indicated to rule out a CNS lesion such as a craniopharyngioma, meningioma, pituitary adenoma, or granulomatous disease. If an outflow problem is suspected, then a combination of estrogen and progesterone can be given. Estrogen is given daily for 3 weeks and progesterone is added the last 5 days. Failure to bleed after a combined estrogen and progesterone challenge indicates an outflow abnormality. In anovulatory patients with hirsutism, testosterone and dehydroepiandosterone sulfate (DHEA-S) levels should be obtained in patients with signs of virilism. Testosterone levels greater than 200 mg/dl and/or DHEA-S levels greater than 7 mg/dl require a CT scan to rule out an adrenal or ovarian tumor.

MANAGEMENT

Management depends on the underlying cause. Patients with congenital anatomic abnormalities usually require

TABLE 44–1

Causes of Amenorrhea

Primary	Helpful Tests
Physiologic	
Pregnancy	B-HCG
Hypothalamic/Pituitary	
Thyroid disease	TSH
Pituitary adenomas	prolactin, MRI or CT scan
GnRH deficiency (Kallmann's syndrome)	LH, FSH
Polycystic ovarian syndrome	LH, FSH, progesterone challenge
Chronic medical disease	LH, FSH, estradiol, prolactin
Stress, eating disorders	LH, FSH, estradiol, prolactin
Medications	Trial off medication
Ovarian	
Gonadal dysgenesis	LH, FSH, karyotype
Congenital adrenal hyperplasia	17-hydroxyprogesterone
Testicular feminization	karyotype
Outflow tract	
Imperforate hymen	Physical examination
Rokitansky-Kuser-Hauser syndrome	Physical exam, karyotype, pelvic ultrasound

Secondary	
Physiologic	
Pregnancy	B-HCG
Lactation	History
Menopause	History/age, FSH
Hypothalamic/Pituitary	
Thyroid disease	TSH
Pituitary adenoma	Prolactin, MRI/CT scan
Polycystic ovarian syndrome	LH, FSH, progesterone challenge
Sheehan's syndrome	LH, FSH
Stress/eating disorders	LH, FSH, estradiol, prolactin
Chronic medical disease	LH, FSH, estradiol, prolactin
Medications	Trial off medications
Ovarian	
Premature ovarian failure	FSH, estradiol; karyotype <age 30
Uterine	
Asherman's syndrome	hysterosalpingogram, estrogen/progesterone

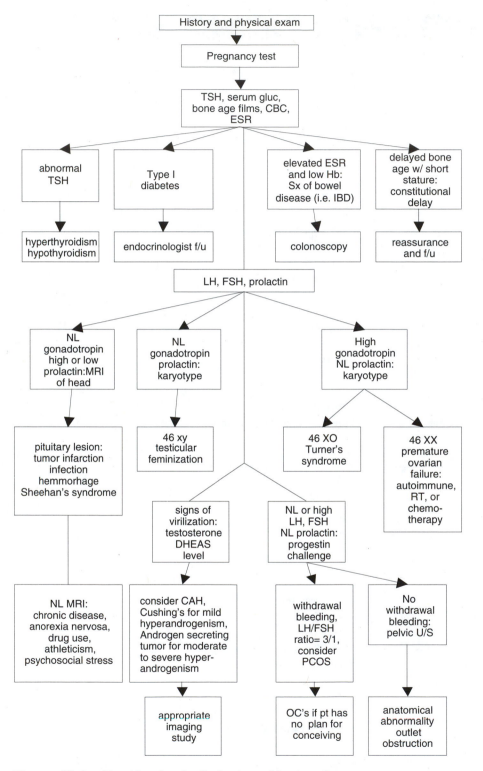

Figure 44-1 Algorithm for the Evaluation of Amenorrhea.

referral for surgery. Patients with primary amenorrhea with an absent uterus and no breast tissue can be treated with estrogens to promote breast development and to prevent osteoporosis. Patients with breast tissue and an absent uterus may not require treatment.

Patients with hypothyroidism need replacement therapy. Those with a pituitary macroadenoma need evaluation for possible surgery, while patients with microadenomas may be treated with bromocriptine and close follow-up.

Management of patients with anovulatory periods depends on whether the patient currently desires pregnancy or contraception. Those patients desiring contraception may elect to take birth control pills. For patients with anovulatory periods desiring pregnancy, drugs such as clomiphene are used to induce ovulation. For patients who do not respond to clomiphene, gonadotropins can be used to stimulate ovulation. If patients are not sexually active or do not want birth control pills, progesterone should be given on a regular basis to induce withdrawal bleeding and to prevent endometrial hyperplasia. Patients with premature ovarian failure need hormone replacement therapy (HRT) to reduce the risks of osteoporosis, bone fractures, and heart disease.

No data supports the usage of HRT in treating amenorrheic female athletes, who are typically treated by the use of OCP initially, proper nutrition, and adjusted training regimens.

◆ KEY POINTS ◆

1. Primary amenorrhea is the absence of menarche by 16 years of age with normal pubertal development, or no puberty development by the age of 14 years. Secondary amenorrhea is the absence of menses for 6 months or 3 previous cycles after establishing normal menses.

2. Concealed pregnancy remains the most likely cause of primary or secondary amenorrhea in an otherwise normal adolescent.

3. History taking should include a careful menstrual and medical history, reviewing all medications, sexual history, and a review of systems and history of drug abuse.

4. Management of amenorrhea depends on the underlying causes. The most common treatment is restoring the menstrual cycle with either progesterone withdrawal method or combined estrogen-progesterone therapy such as OCP.

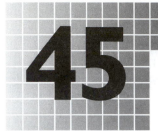

45

Abnormal Papanicolaou Smear

The Papanicolaou (Pap) smear was developed as a screening tool for cervical cancer in the late 1940s. Its widespread use has been associated with a decrease of cervical cancer from 14.2 cases per 100,000 in 1973 to 7.8 cases per 100,000 in 1994. The accepted false negative rates for Pap smears vary between 15% and 45%. Errors occur from poor sampling and fixation technique, and failure of the cytologist to recognize abnormalities. Recently the ThinPrep® method, which collects cells in a fluid medium to minimize background and drying artifact, has been introduced to improve Pap smear results.

Pap smears are not read as simply positive or negative. Over the years, several different reporting systems have been developed attempting to categorize Pap smears according to severity. The Bethesda system (Box 45–1), currently the preferred system, uses the term squamous intraepithelial lesions, which include 2 grades, low-grade squamous intraepithelial lesion (LGIL) and high-grade intraepithelial lesion (HGIL). LGIL is consistent with HPV infection and mild dysplasia. HGIL includes moderate and severe dysplasia.

PATHOPHYSIOLOGY

The cervix is covered by squamous and columnar epithelium. As the cervix matures columnar cells are replaced by squamous cells in a process know as squamous metaplasia. It is the squamocolumnar junction—where squamous metaplasia is most active—that is vulnerable to injury and the area where the development of abnormal cells usually begins.

The observation that the immature squamous cell epithelium at the squamocolumnar junction is particularly sensitive to injury correlates with the epidemiological observation that this is the most common site for cervical cancer. Immature cells are also more common at menarche and during the postpartum period, which may explain why early sexuality and multiple pregnancies place women at high risk for cervical cancer. The natural history of cervical cancer should be viewed as a progression from mild dysplasia to carcinoma in situ to invasive carcinoma. The slow progression of these changes and the availability of acute early treatment make the Pap smear one of the most effective cancer screening tools.

HPV (Human Papillomavirus) is the major cause for most abnormal Pap smear results. DNA fragments of HPV have been found in over 90% of cervical cancer cells. Serotypes 16, 18, and 31 are most closely associated with cervical cancer. Recent improvements in testing for these viral serotypes may prove to be an important adjunct to the traditional Pap smear.

CLINICAL MANIFESTATIONS

History

A good history can identify risk factors for cervical cancer and facilitate decision-making about how frequently to obtain Pap smears. Risk factors include: early age for sexual activity, multiple sexual partners, history of sexually transmitted diseases, smoking, and previously abnormal Pap smears. The frequency of Pap smears is controversial. Since there is a long asymptomatic period and early cervical intraepithelial neoplasia is easily treated when detected, the American Cancer Society (ACS) no longer recommends annual Pap smears for women at low risk for cervical cancer. Starting at age 18 (or younger if the patient is sexually active) the ACS recommends obtaining Pap smears in low-risk women every 3 years after 2 negative smears 1 year apart. Screening may be discontinued after age 65 provided that previous testing has been normal.

Physical Examination

During the 24 hours prior to the examination, the patient should not douche, have sexual relations, or use tampons. Most physicians recommend rescheduling Pap smears if a woman is having menses. To sample the cervix correctly, a cytobrush is rotated in the cervical canal and a wooden or plastic spatula rotated over the cervix at the squamocolumnar junction. The physical examination may be normal, but occasionally genital warts or a lesion may be visible. Bleeding and cervical friability can be a sign of cervical disease or infection. When the cervix appears abnormal, a Pap alone may not be sufficient for evaluation. In other words, a normal

---

BOX 45–1

Bethesda System

Adequacy of specimen
Satisfactory for evaluation
Satisfactory for evaluation but limited by (SBLB): no endocervical cell, inadequate history provided
Unsatisfactory for evaluation, specify reason

Descriptive diagnosis
Within normal limits
Benign cellular changes (BCC):
    Infection: Trichomonas vaginalis, Candida, Coccobacilli c/w shift in vaginal flora, Actinomyces species, HSV
    Inflammatory changes, except cellular changes of HPV infections
    Epithelial cell abnormalities
    Squamous cell
        ASCUS: borderline changes more reactive than definitive.
        LSIL: borderline changes including HPV, mild dysplasia, CIN I
        HSIL: moderate dysplasia or CIN II, severe dysplasia or CIN III, and CIS, +/– HPV changes
        Squamous cell carcinoma: cancer or invasive.
    Glandular cell
        Endometrial cells, cytological benign in a postmenopausal woman—endometrial hyperplasia or cancer
        *AGCUS (atypical glandular cells of undetermined significance): borderline cells between reactive changes to premalignant/malignant process
        ACIS: adenocarcinoma in situ
        Adenocarcinoma: endocervical suggesting adenocarcinoma or ACIS, endometrial suggesting possible endometrial cancer, extrauterine that could be from vagina, ovary, tube or metastatic
Other malignant neoplasms: small cell carcinoma, melanoma, lymphoma, sarcoma, etc.
Hormonal evaluation (vaginal smears only): hormonal pattern compatible or incompatible with age and history
Hormonal pattern incompatible with age and history: specify
Hormonal evaluation not possible due to: specify

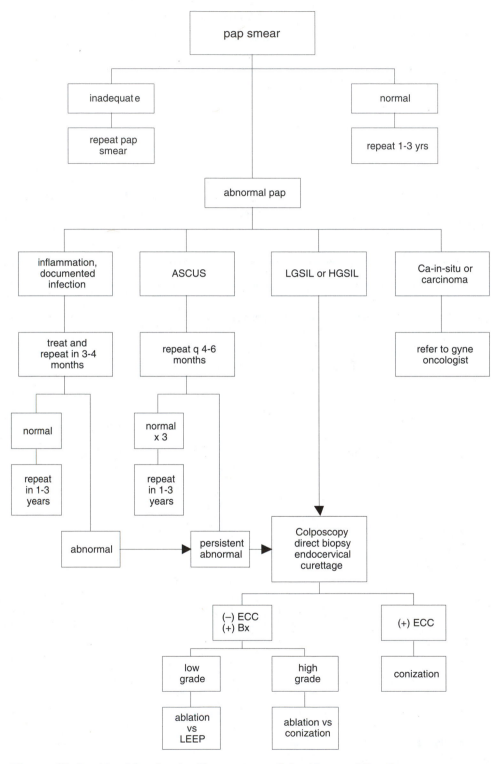

Figure 45–1 Algorithm for the Management of the Abnormal Pap Smear.

Pap smear should not prevent a clinician from proceeding to colposcopy if there is a suspicious lesion.

DIFFERENTIAL DIAGNOSIS

Box 45–1 lists the descriptive changes for Pap smears. In addition to cervical intraepithelial dysplasia and HPV infection, Pap smear abnormalities may be due to infection trauma and hormonal changes.

DIAGNOSTIC APPROACH

The first step is to evaluate the adequacy of the Pap smear. If there are no endocervical cells present, this indicates inadequate sampling of the squamocolumnar junction. Often these smears need to be repeated, unless this is expected (i.e., pregnancy, menopause). However for a low-risk individual with previously normal Pap smears, a physician may exercise discretion and defer a repeat examination for 1 year. Cervical inflammation from infections such as chlamydia or yeast may cause cells to appear abnormal and the Pap smear should be repeated after treating the infection.

Atypical squamous cells of undetermined significance (ASCUS) are changes seen in cells that appear beyond the normal reactive process but lack the criteria for a squamous intraepithelial lesion (SIL). When this occurs, the patient may be followed by repeat Pap smears every 4 to 6 months. A subsequent abnormal smear is an indication for colposcopy. If adherence to more frequent monitoring is a concern or the patient is at high risk, then immediate colposcopy is indicated. Occasionally atypical glandular cells of undetermined significance (AGUS) are noted on a Pap smear. Colposcopy with endocervical curettage (ECC) and evaluation of the upper genital tract with an endometrial biopsy should be considered. If the source for the AGUS Pap remains unclear the patient should be referred to a specialist.

Patients with either a low-grade intraepithelial lesion (LGIL) or a high-grade lesion (HGIL) should usually undergo colposcopy, directed cervical biopsy, and endocervical curettage. If the assessment is inadequate (i.e., the lesion cannot be fully visualized), then conization is indicated.

MANAGEMENT

Since abnormal Pap smears are associated with HPV, other STDs should be considered when evaluating these patients (Figure 45–1). Approximately 60% of Pap smears with ASCUS /LGIL regress spontaneously. Low-risk patients may be followed with repeat Pap smears every 4 to 6 months. Patients at higher risk or with an abnormal smear on follow-up require colposcopy to rule out a high-grade lesion. Most experts recommend that patients with LGIL and HSIL should undergo colposcopy and directed biopsy. Therapy is based on the histologic readings and ECC findings. Since dysplasia is thought to be a precursor to cervical cancer, destruction or excision of the abnormal area of the cervix is usually performed. Higher-grade lesions or positive endocervical curettage generally require conization or a loop electroexcision procedure (LEEP). Lower-grade lesions may be treated with observation, laser, cryotherapy, or by LEEP depending on the size and location of the lesion. Carcinoma in situ is generally referred to a gynecologist and requires conization. After treatment for dysplasia, women need Pap smears every 4 months for 1 year, then every 6 months for another year. If Pap smears remain normal for 2 years, then screening can occur annually. In pregnancy, ASCUS and LSIL should be followed up with colposcopy at 8 to 10 weeks, 28 weeks, and at postpartum. HSIL should be followed up with colposcopy every 8 weeks during pregnancy and postpartum. In either situation, endocervical curettage is always contraindicated during pregnancy.

◆ KEY POINTS ◆

1. HPV virus is the major cause of abnormal Pap smears.

2. ASCUS may be followed with repeat smears in a low-risk individual. Higher-risk individuals or patients whose repeat smear is abnormal should undergo colposcopy.

3. Individuals with LGIL and HGIL on Pap smear should undergo colposcopy, endocervical curettage, and directed cervical biopsy.

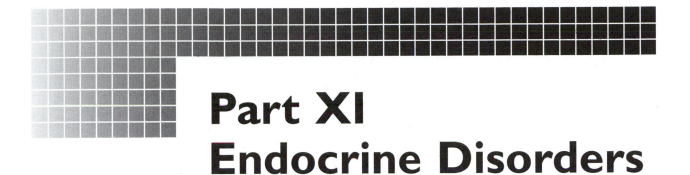

Part XI
Endocrine Disorders

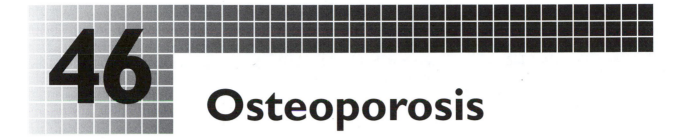

Osteoporosis

Osteoporosis is a reduction in bone mass per unit of volume, and is seen primarily in elderly individuals. As our population has aged, the number of individuals with osteoporosis has grown to over 10 million with an additional 18 million individuals at high risk for developing osteoporosis. The majority of these are women (80%), and by age 75 one out of three white women will suffer an osteoporotic hip fracture. While men have a lower incidence of osteoporosis, it is estimated that 2 million men have osteoporosis and an additional 3 million are at risk for developing the disease. Osteoporosis is responsible for 1.5 million fractures each year with an annual cost of approximately $14 billion. Approximately 20% of patients who suffer a hip fracture die of a medical complication within 1 year after the fracture, and those who survive are often unable to live independently.

PATHOPHYSIOLOGY

The resorption and formation of bone is a continuous process. Under steady state, these processes are equal and linked. At around age 35 bone mass peaks and both genders begin to lose bone mass after age 40. The reason why osteoporosis develops is uncertain. Estrogen receptors are present on osteoblasts, the cells that form bone, which may explain why estrogen deficient states result in bone loss. There also appears to be an uncoupling of osteoblasts from the action of osteoclasts,

the cells that resorb bone. Several different chemical modulators may mediate this uncoupling, but the precise mechanisms have not yet been determined.

Osteoporosis can either be primary or secondary to an underlying disease. Primary osteoporosis is an age-related bone disorder, consisting of two types. Type I, or postmenopausal osteoporosis, affects women approximately 20 years after menopause. It primarily affects trabecular bone and is due to increased osteoclast activity. Trabecular bone is present in the hip, vertebrae, distal radius, and the heel. Type II osteoporosis, or senile osteoporosis, involves loss of both cortical and trabecular bone, and primarily affects individuals over age 70. Type II changes appear to be related to age-related decreases in calcium absorption and decreases in vitamin D absorption and synthesis. The effects of Type I and Type II are additive and most individuals with osteoporosis have elements of both types.

CLINICAL MANIFESTATIONS

History

Patients with osteoporosis are generally asymptomatic. However, chronic pain and tenderness over the affected area may occur, particularly in association with osteoporotic fractures. The bones most commonly affected by osteoporotic fractures are the spine, hip, and distal radius. Eliciting other symptoms that may occur as complications of osteoporosis is important. For example, a vertebral fracture may result in spinal cord compression and neurological findings. Osteoporosis of facet joints may also contribute to back pain.

History is useful to identify those patients with risk factors for osteoporosis. Risk factors for osteoporosis can be grouped into several different categories: 1) genetic: Caucasian or Asian ethnicity, small stature, and a family history of osteoporosis; 2) lifestyle: tobacco, alcohol, caffeine consumption, lack of physical activity; 3) nutritional: low calcium intake; and 4) other risk factors such as older age and postmenopausal.

Physical Examination

In physical examination, height reduction greater than 1.5 inches, dorsal kyphosis (dowager's or widow's hump), exaggerated cervical lordosis, gait deficits, and low body weight are common findings associated with osteoporosis. Dorsal kyphosis is due to wedge-shaped deformity in the mid-dorsal vertebrae. Due to the risk of spinal cord compression, it is important to perform a complete neurological exam to rule out neurological involvement from an osteoporotic fracture.

DIFFERENTIAL DIAGNOSIS

While osteoporosis is commonly age related, other diseases or conditions may secondarily cause osteoporosis. These can be divided into five different categories (Table 46–1). Identification and treatment of these underlying diseases can limit bone loss. When the disease or condition is not modifiable, as in patients requiring chronic corticosteroids, the use of preventative medicines such as a bisphosphonate (e.g., alendronate) may help bone loss.

DIAGNOSTIC APPROACH

Patients at risk for developing osteoporosis are candidates for screening. These include 1) postmenopausal women younger than 65 years old with one or more risk factors besides menopause; 2) all postmenopausal women over 65 years; 3) postmenopausal women with a history of fractures; and 4) those who are on long-term corticosteroid treatments. In addition, those who are considering treatments or preventive measures for osteoporosis may benefit from information gained through screening. Patients being treated for osteo-

TABLE 46–1	
Secondary Causes of Osteoporosis	
Endocrine:	Acromegaly
	Diabetes mellitus
	Cushing's disease
	Hyperparathyroidism
	Hypogonadism
	Hyperthyroidism
Nutritional:	Malabsorption
	Malnutrition
	Anorexia nervosa
	Liver disease
	Vitamin D deficiency
	Alcoholism
Collagen vascular:	Rheumatoid arthritis
	Ehlers-Danlos syndrome
	Marfan syndrome
	Osteoporosis imperfecta
Cancer:	Multiple myeloma
	Bone metastases
	Breast cancer
	Lymphoma
	Leukemia
Medications:	Glucosteroid
	Phenobarbital
	Phenytoin
	Heparin
	Methotrexate
	Excess thyroid hormone replacement

porosis require repeat testing to assess therapy. Measurement of the Bone Mineral Density (BMD) is the standard method for screening and establishing the diagnosis of osteoporosis. Dual-Energy X-ray Absorptiometry (DEXA) is the preferred method for confirming the diagnosis and monitoring therapy because it represents the best combination of sensitivity, technical simplicity, reproducibility, cost, and minimizes radiation exposure. BMD determinations of both the spine and hip provide the best assessments since the degree of osteoporosis can differ between sites.

The BMD report provides a T-score and Z-score. The T-score compares the patient's BMD with that of the normal same sex young adult 25 to 30 years of age of the same sex. The Z-score compares the patient's BMD with that of the same age group and gender. Osteoporosis is defined as a T-score of more than 2.5 standard deviations below the mean (-2.5 SD). Osteopenia, low bone mass, is defined as a T-score between -1.0 and -2.5. Z-scores of -1.5 suggest a secondary cause of osteoporosis. The risk for an osteoporotic fracture increases 2 to 4 fold for every standard deviation in reduced BMD.

In addition to a DEXA scan, blood tests are useful for identifying and managing secondary cases of osteoporosis. Initial tests consist of a CBC, ESR, chemistry panel including calcium, phosphorus, alkaline phosphatase levels, and renal and kidney functions. Calcium and phosphate measurements help detect hyperparathyroidism and vitamin D deficiencies. In patients with anemia and an elevated ESR, multiple myeloma should be considered. Electrolyte abnormalities can identify patients with chronic acidosis or renal tubular acidosis. Serum alkaline phosphatase is a marker of osteoblastic activity, and is elevated in malignancy, hyperparathyroidism, and other high turnover states. More selective tests such as vitamin D levels or PTH levels should be selectively ordered based on history, physical, and preliminary lab findings.

MANAGEMENT

The first line of prevention for osteoporosis is lifestyle changes, while pharmaceutical agents are the first line of treatment of osteoporosis. Smoking cessation, modest alcohol consumption, weight-bearing exercise, and improving dietary habits are helpful in preserving bone mass. It is recommended that calcium intake should be 1000 mg per day for premenopausal women and 1200 mg per day for postmenopausal women. As

TABLE 46–2

General Guidelines for Pharmacological Agents

Agent	Benefits	Contraindications
HRT[a]	Inhibits bone reabsorption in estrogen-deficient patients Controls vasomotor symptoms	Breast cancer Estrogen-dependent neoplasm Undiagnosed vaginal bleeding H/O-thromboembolic disorder H/O migraine
Bisphosphonates	Inhibits bone reabsorption	Gastric ulcer Abnormal esophageal motility Unable to sit upright ×30 min.
Calcitonins	Most effective in spine Analgesic effect in back pain	Allergy to salmon protein Unable to tolerate nasal spray
SERM[b]	Pt. w/ contraindications to HRT use Decrease total & LDL cholesterol	No vasomotor symptom relief H/O thromboembolic disorder

[a] HRT: hormone replacement therapy.
[b] SERM: selective estrogen receptor modulator.

patients age, the risk for falls increases and minimizing falls is another priority for reducing the number of osteoporotic fractures. Improving vision, adjusting sedative medications, and balance exercises are beneficial. Other environmental adjustments such as minimizing clutter, anchoring rugs, adding handrails, and better lighting in dark hallways are helpful in preventing falls.

Pharmaceutical therapy should be considered for individuals with a BMD T-score below −2.0 without risk factors, T-scores below −1.5 with multiple risk factors, women older than 70 years old with multiple risk factors, and patients undergoing long-term corticosteroids. Table 46–2 lists some of the medications available for treatment. The bisphosphonates need to be taken on an empty stomach with a large glass of water with the patient remaining upright without eating for at least 30 minutes. Recently, new formulation allows these medicines to be administered in a single weekly dose, increases the ease of therapy, and improves adherence.

◆ **KEY POINTS** ◆

1. Osteoporosis is a reduction in bone mass per unit of volume that is seen primarily in older individuals.

2. Approximately 20% of patients who suffer a hip fracture die within 1 year after the fracture.

3. Osteoporosis can either be primary or secondary. Secondary causes include medications, cancers, endocrine disorders, collagen vascular disease, or nutritional problems.

4. DEXA is the preferred method for detecting osteoporosis and is reported as a T-score that compares the patient's BMD with peak bone mass, and a Z-score that compares the patient's BMD with age and sex-matched controls.

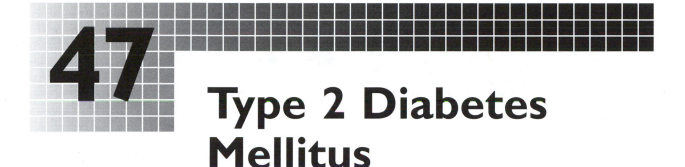

Type 2 Diabetes Mellitus

Diabetes mellitus affects 2% to 4% of the population and is the most common endocrine problem encountered in family medicine. Diabetes is a group of heterogeneous metabolic disorders characterized by the abnormal metabolism of glucose with defects in insulin secretion, insulin action, or both. Diabetes is generally divided into Type 1 diabetes, which is characterized by little or no insulin produced by the pancreas, and Type 2, in which the initial defect appears to be a resistance to the action of insulin. Type 2 diabetes accounts for approximately 90% of individuals with diabetes. Of the 15 million patients with Type 2 diabetes, many have few symptoms and about 5.4 million remain undiagnosed.

PATHOPHYSIOLOGY

Type 1 diabetes is believed to be an autoimmune disorder, with the production of autoimmune antibodies against pancreatic islet cells. The disease typically develops during childhood, possibly triggered by a viral infection. Type 1 patients are prone to ketoacidosis and patients always require exogenous insulin. In Type 2 diabetes, insulin is produced, but cells are resistant to the action of insulin. However, since insulin is produced, individuals with Type 2 diabetes generally do not develop ketoacidosis.

Early in Type 2 diabetes, elevated levels of insulin may be present as the pancreas attempts to compensate

for insulin resistance. Eventually the beta cell can no longer compensate for the insulin resistance and hyperglycemia occurs. In addition to hyperglycemia, lipid metabolism is also affected. Patients with Type 2 diabetes frequently have low levels of high-density lipoproteins (HDL), moderately elevated cholesterol levels, and high triglycerides. Type 2 diabetes develops more commonly in African-Americans, Hispanics, and American Indians. Other risk factors include having a first degree relative with diabetes mellitus, obesity—especially central obesity—and a sedentary lifestyle.

Gestational diabetes mellitus (GDM) affects 1% to 2% of pregnancies, usually during the third trimester. Blood sugars usually return to normal after delivery, but among women with GDM up to 30% develop diabetes mellitus later in life. Acute complications of diabetes include ketoacidosis, hyperosmolar non-ketotic diabetic coma (HNKDC), and hypoglycemic reactions from treatment. HNKDC is a syndrome characterized by severe fluid deficits induced by hyperglycemic diuresis. Generally it develops in debilitated patients such as nursing home residents who are unable to take in adequate fluids.

Most of the morbidity and mortality associated with diabetes mellitus result from long-term complications. These can be divided into microvascular and macrovascular complications. Microvascular complications include retinopathy, neuropathy, and nephropathy. Macrovascular complications are related to the premature atherosclerosis that affects the cardiovascular, cerebrovascular, and peripheral vascular systems. Myocardial infarction is the primary cause of the excess morbidity seen in diabetic individuals.

CLINICAL MANIFESTATIONS

History

Patients with Type 1 usually present with an abrupt illness, often in ketoacidosis caused by an acute stress such as an infection. Other common initial symptoms are nausea, abdominal pain, polyuria, polydipsia, polyphagia, and weight loss.

Patients with Type 2 diabetes present more gradually. Classic symptoms include polyuria, polydipsia, and polyphagia. Patients may initially complain of fatigue, blurred vision, or recurrent infections. Many patients are asymptomatic and are first diagnosed by blood tests that reveal an elevated glucose. Others may present with symptoms related to complications such as burning in the feet from a painful neuropathy. The history should also seek to identify risk factors for cardiovascular disease and ask about symptoms such as chest pain or claudication, which may indicate macrovascular disease.

Physical Examination

The physical examination should focus on weight, body habitus, and for younger individuals, growth. Most findings are not diagnostic, but result from complications of the disease. An eye exam may show evidence of retinopathy such as exudates, hemorrhages, and microaneurysms. A cardiovascular exam, including blood pressure, listening for carotid bruits and assessing peripheral pulses, is important. A skin and foot examination looking for ulceration, deformities, and skin infection should be performed. Neurologic examinations can detect signs of neuropathy such as sensory loss.

DIFFERENTIAL DIAGNOSIS

Hyperglycemia may result from stresses such as an infection or a heart attack that subsequently resolves when the inciting event is under control. Elevated blood sugars may also be related to pancreatic disease from pancreatitis, pancreatic cancer, pancreatic resection, and hemochromatosis, which is often referred to as bronze diabetes. Endocrinopathies such as Cushing's disease,

pheochromocytoma, and acromegaly and medications such as high-dose steroids, beta-blockers, oral contraceptives, phenytoin, and hydrochlorothiazide may cause hyperglycemia.

DIAGNOSTIC APPROACH

The American Diabetes Association (ADA) recommends that high-risk individuals be screened for diabetes with a fasting blood sugar. The ADA also recommends that all patients over age 45 should be screened with a fasting blood sugar every 3 years. The diagnosis of diabetes mellitus can be established by one of three criteria: 1) fasting blood glucose greater than 126 mg/dl on two or more separate occasions; 2) random blood glucose greater than 200 mg/dl with polyuria, polydipsia, and polyphagia; and 3) a 2-hour postprandial glucose greater than 200 mg/dl. Although a HbA1C, or glycosylated hemoglobin level, is not one of the diagnostic criteria, it is a crucial test to assess the degree of blood sugar control. Normally about 4% to 6% of hemoglobin is glycosylated. The percent of glycosylated hemoglobin rises with the average level of blood glucose. Since the average lifespan of a red blood cell is 120 days, the HbA1C reflects the average glucose levels over the past 2 to 3 months.

In addition to establishing the diagnosis of diabetes, the initial evaluation should be aimed at evaluating risk factors and detecting diabetic complications. Routine laboratory testing should include a fasting lipid profile, glycosylated hemoglobin, urine analysis, electrolytes, BUN, creatinine, and an EKG in patients over 40. For patients over 30 years of age or those with diabetes mellitus for more than 5 years duration, screening for microalbuminuria should be performed annually.

MANAGEMENT

This section will focus mainly on Type 2 diabetes, which is more common in the primary care setting. Diet and exercise are the cornerstones of treatment. Eighty to 90% of individuals with Type 2 diabetes are overweight. Even a modest weight loss of 10 to 20 pounds may be sufficient to improve glycemic control. Reducing fat intake is also important since diabetic patients are at risk for developing hyperlipidemia and vascular disease. Exercise is important for controlling weight and may also improve insulin resistance.

If lifestyle modifications fail to control the blood sugar, then pharmacological therapy is the next step. In addition to insulin, there are five classes of oral agents: sulfonylureas, biguanides, thiazolidinediones, repaglinide, and alpha-glucosidase inhibitors. All of these agents need the presence of some endogenous insulin to be effective.

Sulfonylureas stimulate insulin release from pancreatic beta cells. Contraindications include allergy, pregnancy, and significant renal dysfunction. The most common serious side effects of these medications are hypoglycemia and weight gain. About 50% to 70% of patients initially can be controlled solely with a sulfonylurea. As beta cell functions worsen, 5% to 10% of patients per year previously controlled with a sulfonylurea will lose glycemic control. Sulfonylureas generally improve fasting blood sugars by 30 to 60 mg/dl and HbA1C by 1.5% to 2.0%.

Metformin is the only biguanide available in the United States. It works by inhibiting hepatic gluconeogenesis and by increasing glucose uptake in the peripheral tissues. Metformin, when used alone, does not cause hypoglycemia, but can potentiate hypoglycemia when used in conjunction with insulin or sulfonylureas. The most common side effects are nausea, diarrhea, and dyspepsia. A rare but often fatal complication is lactic acidosis. Avoiding the use of metformin in patients with renal dysfunction (creatinine greater than or equal to 1.5 mg/dl in men; 1.4 mg/dl in women), congestive heart failure, acute or chronic acidosis, and hepatic dysfunction reduces the risk of lactic acidosis. Metformin is similar in effectiveness to sulfonylureas.

Thiazolidinediones work by decreasing insulin resistance in the skeletal muscle and liver. They can be used with insulin or other medications. They can cause hepatotoxicity and require monitoring liver enzymes. Repaglinide is a member of a new class of oral medications, the meglinides, that stimulate the pancreas to secrete insulin and have a more rapid onset and short half-life, allowing it to be given with meals. Alpha-glucosidase inhibitors inhibit an enzyme that hydrolyzes disaccharides, thus limiting the rate of carbohydrate absorption and reducing postprandial elevation of glucose. The major side effects are flatulence, diarrhea, and abdominal pain.

Eventually, as the beta cell function worsens over time, about 50% of Type 2 patients will end up taking insulin. Given in sufficient doses, insulin can usually control even the most refractory hyperglycemia. Characteristics of insulin preparations vary in terms of onset of action and duration of action. Patients on insulin usually require self-monitoring at home using a glucometer.

Type 2 diabetes is a progressive disease and a single agent may be ineffective at the outset or lose effectiveness over time. Combination therapy with two or more agents that work by different mechanisms may reduce the blood sugar to an acceptable level. A biguanide with a sulfonylurea is the most widely studied combination. The effect of the two medications is additive; switching from one to another does not improve control.

All individuals with diabetes who receive medication to lower blood sugar need to be warned about the possibility of a hypoglycemic reaction manifested by confusion, loss of consciousness, tachycardia, shakiness, headache, or sweatiness. Persons at risk for hypoglycemia should be instructed about the symptoms of a reaction and should carry either a hard candy or glucose gel to take if hypoglycemic symptoms develop.

Monitoring, preventing, and treating complications are another important element of managing patients with diabetes mellitus. Hypertension and hyperlipidemia should be aggressively treated. Many experts recommend a target blood pressure of 130/85 mm Hg and initiating treatment for an LDL cholesterol over 130 mg/dl with a target of 100 mg/dl or less. The ADA also recommends prophylactic aspirin use in patients age 50 or older of those with cardiovascular risk factors.

The ADA recommends monitoring the HbA1C every 3 to 6 months with a target goal of 7% to prevent microvascular complications. Levels above 8% usually suggest the need to reexamine treatment, either by reemphasizing adherence to current therapy or by changing management. Currently the ADA recommends annual dilated eye exams and screening for microalbuminuria in patients with diabetes. Patients with retinopathy need monitoring by an ophthalmologist. Microalbuminuria is defined as excreting from 30 to 300 mg of urinary protein over 24 hours. The presence of microalbuminuria should prompt a careful retinal evaluation since retinopathy usually precedes nephropathy. Reducing blood pressure to less than 130/85 mm Hg and using an ACE inhibitor are strategies that may slow the progression of nephropathy. For patients who cannot tolerate an ACE inhibitor, an angiotensin receptor-blocking agent is an alternative. Neuropathy is one of the most common diabetic complications. In addition to sensory loss, diabetic neuropathy can cause bladder and bowel problems, impotence, and orthostatic hypotension. Patients with sensory neuropathies frequently also have peripheral vascular disease and are especially prone to foot problems. Painful neuropathies may respond to tricyclic antidepressants or to carbamazepine or gabapentin.

◆ **KEY POINTS** ◆

1. There are two main types of diabetes mellitus, Type 1, characterized by little or no insulin production and Type 2, in which the initial defect is insulin resistance.

2. Many individuals with Type 2 diabetes are asymptomatic and are identified by blood testing.

3. Good glycemic control reduces the risk of developing complications and slows the progression in those who already have established complications.

4. The cornerstone of treatment in Type 2 diabetes mellitus is diet and exercise with pharmacological treatment reserved for those who do not reach treatment goals with diet and exercise alone.

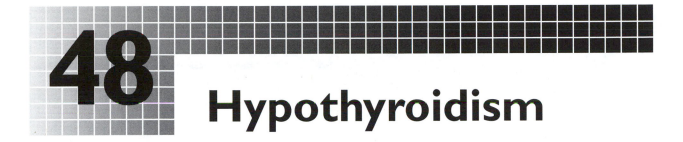

48 Hypothyroidism

Hypothyroidism occurs in about 1% to 3% of the population and affects people of all ages, including newborns and the elderly. The incidence is higher in women than in men (10:1 ratio) and also in elderly individuals. The range of symptoms experienced by those with hypothyroidism extends from mild fatigue to myxedema coma. Family physicians must have a high index of suspicion for considering the diagnosis of hypothyroidism because of its many symptoms.

PATHOPHYSIOLOGY

Thyroid hormone regulates cellular metabolism and affects virtually every cell in the human body. Hypothyroidism may be due to agenesis of the thyroid, failure of the pituitary gland to produce thyroid stimulating hormone (TSH), or inadequate production of thyroid hormone by the thyroid gland. Because iodine is a core constituent of thyroid hormone, geographic areas that lack sufficient iodine have an increased rate of endemic hypothyroidism, cretinism, and goiter. To avoid this, most developed nations currently provide iodine as a dietary supplement. Because thyroid hormone is necessary for normal neurological and physical development, all newborns in the U.S. are screened for congenital hypothyroidism.

Autoimmune destruction of the thyroid gland is the most common cause of non-iatrogenic hypothyroidism. Hashimoto's thyroiditis is the most common autoimmune disease affecting the thyroid and is characterized by elevated levels of antibodies to thyroid peroxidase and thyroglobulin. These antibodies cause inflammation of the thyroid gland, which can result in a goiter and lead to diminished production of thyroid hormone. Hashimoto's is much more common in women, has a genetic predisposition, and is often associated with other autoimmune disorders.

Therapies for hyperthyroidism such as radioactive iodine and surgery are common causes of iatrogenic hypothyroidism. Medications such as lithium, iodine, and interferon may also cause hypothyroidism. Any disorder causing dysfunction of the hypothalamus or pituitary glands, such as pituitary adenoma or postpartum pituitary necrosis, may lead to lower levels of TRH (thyroid releasing hormone) and TSH. This then results in diminished production of thyroid hormone.

Myxedema from severe hypothyroidism causes systemic problems secondary to abnormal cellular metabolism and increased deposition of mucopolysaccharides into subcutaneous tissues. This results in a variety of abnormalities including fluid accumulation in the pericardial sac, firm and tense swelling of the skin, connective tissue abnormalities, and neurological dysfunction.

Rarely, individuals with long-standing hypothyroidism may experience myxedema coma. This life-threatening condition most often occurs after significant cold exposure or infection and results in hypothermia, mental status changes, and respiratory depression.

CLINICAL MANIFESTATIONS

History

Symptoms of hypothyroidism include weakness, fatigue, cold intolerance, constipation, dry skin, headache, and thinning hair. Although very mild weight gain can occur secondary to a slowing metabolism, excessive weight gain is uncommon. Women may complain of altered menstruation and infertility. Patients with long-standing hypothyroidism often experience a delay in mentation, hoarse voice, muscle cramps, and diminished acuity of taste, smell, and hearing.

Congenital hypothyroidism has a subtle presentation that may include feeding problems, a hoarse cry, jaundice, and constipation. Later findings include developmental delay, short stature, and delayed dentition.

Physical Examination

Physical exam findings often vary according to the degree of hypothyroidism. The general appearance often reveals coarse and dry hair, pallor, thin and brittle nails, large tongue, thinning of the outer halves of eyebrows, and facial puffiness. Vital signs may show hypothermia, bradycardia, and normal to low blood pressure. The neck should be evaluated for the presence of goiter, which may or may not be tender. Cardiovascular exam may reveal evidence of a pericardial effusion or cardiac enlargement. Skin is typically hard and doughy while deep tendon reflexes are usually prolonged with a slow return phase. Children who have had hypothyroidism since infancy have a cretin appearance, which includes a large head, short limbs, widely set eyes, and a broad flat nose.

DIFFERENTIAL DIAGNOSIS

Box 48–1 lists the differential diagnosis of hypothyroidism. The two most common causes are thyroid gland failure due to Hashimoto's thyroiditis and hypothyroidism secondary to surgery or radiation therapy. Endemic goiter due to iodine deficiency is rare in the United States due to iodine supplementation of salt, but is fairly common in other parts of the world.

Diagnostic Tests

TSH, which is synthesized and secreted by the pituitary gland, is the most sensitive indicator of hypothyroidism due to thyroid dysfunction. It is elevated in patients with

---

BOX 48–1

Differential Diagnosis of Hypothyroidism

—Iatrogenic hypothyroidism (post-ablative hypothyroidism)
  —Surgery
  —Radioactive iodine
—Hashimoto's thyroiditis (chronic lymphocytic)
—Subacute lymphocytic thyroiditis
—Subclinical hypothyroidism
—Hypothalamic or pituitary dysfunction
—Iodine deficiency (endemic goiter)
—Congenital hypothyroidism (agenesis)
—Tracheotomy
—Medications

---

hypothyroidism except in the rare cases of central hypothyroidism where the pituitary fails to secrete TSH. TSH and free T4 are both low in cases of hypothalamic or pituitary dysfunction. In subclinical hypothyroidism, TSH is elevated while free T4 is often normal. High titers of thyroid antibodies are seen most commonly in those with Hashimoto's, but may be present in other conditions such as subacute lymphocytic thyroiditis. Radioactive iodine uptake scan (RAIU) is often low or low normal in Hashimoto's and shows a variable pattern with goitrous hypothyroidism. Pituitary failure can be confirmed by the failure of TSH to respond to TRH stimulation.

Hypothyroid patients may have elevations of cholesterol, CPK, and liver enzymes. A complete blood count may demonstrate a macrocytic anemia secondary to decreased B12 absorption. Serum electrolytes occasionally show hyponatremia. EKG and chest x-ray may reveal findings consistent with a pericardial effusion. Patients with low TSH and low free T4 should have an MRI to evaluate for abnormalities of the pituitary or hypothalamus.

MANAGEMENT

The main form of therapy for hypothyroidism is levothyroxine. It is widely available, inexpensive, and is converted to T3 in the peripheral tissues at a rate similar to that seen in euthyroid individuals. Most patients require a daily dose between 75 and 150 mcg. Thyroid levels in the hypothyroid newborn need to be quickly corrected and maintained to avoid long-term sequelae. Young adults with mild hypothyroidism are typically given a starting dose of 50 mcg, with increments of 25 to 50 mcg every 3 to 4 weeks. Older patients and those with cardiovascular disease are often very sensitive to thyroid replacement. In order to avoid precipitating an anginal attack or palpitations, these patients should be started on lower doses of levothyroxine such as 25 mcg with gradual incremental increases to therapeutic levels over 4 to 6 months. After therapy is started, serum TSH should normalize, be followed closely, and kept in the normal range.

Patients with an elevated TSH and normal free T4 levels are at much higher risk for subsequently developing hypothyroidism and should be retested every 6 to 12 months. Therapy is initiated if the patient becomes symptomatic, if the TSH levels rise above 10 mU/L, or if free T4 levels fall below normal.

Myxedema coma is a medical emergency and has a high rate of mortality. Intravenous levothyroxine and steroids, warming blankets, and mechanical ventilation in an intensive care unit are the mainstays of treatment.

Once patients have achieved euthyroid status on a maintenance dose of levothyroxine, TSH should be assessed every 6 to 12 months. This ensures that iatrogenic hyperthyroidism and its sequelae (see chapter 49 on hyperthyroidism) do not occur.

◆ **KEY POINTS** ◆

1. Hypothyroidism occurs in about 1% to 3% of the population and affects people of all ages, including newborns and the elderly.

2. Symptoms of hypothyroidism include weakness, fatigue, cold intolerance, constipation, dry skin, headache, and thinning hair.

3. Physical exam findings often reveal coarse and dry hair, pallor, thin and brittle nails, large tongue, thinning of the outer halves of eyebrows, and facial puffiness.

4. The two most common causes are thyroid gland failure due to Hashimoto's thyroiditis and hypothyroidism secondary to surgery or radiation therapy.

5. TSH, which is synthesized and secreted by the pituitary gland, is the most sensitive indicator of hypothyroidism due to thyroid dysfunction.

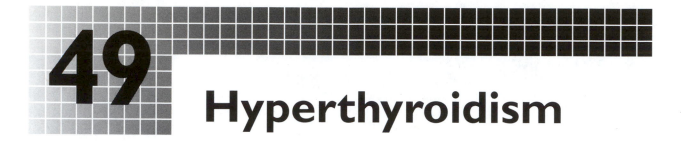

49 Hyperthyroidism

Thyroid diseases are second only to diabetes as the most common endocrine problems encountered in medicine. Thyroid hormone affects virtually every cell in the human body. Primary care physicians need to be aware of the many and varied clinical manifestations of thyroid disease, as well as the different causes and treatment options.

PATHOPHYSIOLOGY

The thyroid gland is derived from pharyngeal epithelium and during development it descends in the neck to its final location just anterior to the larynx, with the thyroglossal duct indicating its path of descent. Thyroid stimulating hormone (TSH) is released by the pituitary gland via stimulation from hypothalamic thyrotropin-releasing hormones (TRH). TSH causes increased trapping of iodine by the thyroid, elevated production and release of T3 and T4, and growth of the gland itself. Thus, elevated levels of TSH may lead to diffuse or nodular enlargement of the thyroid gland (i.e., goiter). Heightening levels of thyroid hormone cause the pituitary gland to be less sensitive to TRH and thus create an effective feedback loop that normally maintains a euthyroid state.

Thyroxine (T4) and T3 are the active thyroid hormones and are 99% protein bound by thyroxine-binding globulin (TBG) and other serum proteins. In the peripheral tissues, T4 gets converted into free T3, which has 40 times the affinity for the cellular receptors of T4. Thus, at the cellular level, T3 is the metabolically active thyroid hormone and principally responsible for the metabolic effects of the thyroid hormone. However, due to extremely low concentrations of serum T3, free T4 is more easily measured.

Many states alter the amount of thyroid binding globulin and thus may affect measured thyroid hormone levels. Circumstances that increase TBG include pregnancy, acute liver disease, the newborn state, and medications such as oral contraceptive pills (OCPs) and tamoxifen. Elevated levels of androgens, chronic liver disease, glucocorticoid excess, severe illness, and nephrotic syndrome all diminish TBG levels.

Conditions such as Grave's disease, in which circulating antibodies mimic the activity of TSH, cause enlargement of the thyroid gland and abnormally elevated levels of circulating thyroid hormone. Thyroid nodules occasionally release T3 and T4 independent of levels of TSH. These autonomously functioning nodules often produce excessive levels of thyroid hormone that result in systemic abnormalities and atrophy of the remaining normal thyroid tissue. Postpartum and autoimmune thyroiditis (Hashimoto's) are inflammatory conditions of the thyroid that can result in hyperthyroidism early in the process as a result of excess release of T3 and T4 associated with thyroid cellular injury.

CLINICAL MANIFESTATIONS

History

Patients with symptomatic hyperthyroidism (a.k.a. thyrotoxicosis) often complain of weight loss despite normal or high caloric intake, nervousness, heat intolerance, fatigue, increased perspiration, more frequent bowel movements, and inability to sleep. Older patients may complain of angina, palpitations, and shortness of breath. Women who are premenopausal often experience irregular vaginal bleeding. Those with Grave's disease may describe a doughy and swollen appearance of their pretibial area (i.e., myxedema), have visual changes secondary to exophthalmos, and are more likely to suffer from other endocrine disorders. In patients with a thyroid nodule, history of head and neck radiation is important because these patients have a higher rate of thyroid carcinoma.

PHYSICAL EXAMINATION

Individuals suffering from hyperthyroidism often appear restless and fidgety. Their skin may be moist and velvety and palmar erythema is often detectable. Patients often have a fine resting tremor and a "frightened" facial appearance secondary to ocular abnormalities that include widened palpebral fissures, infrequent blinking, and lid lag. Cardiovascular exam may reveal atrial fibrillation, sinus tachycardia, widened pulse pressure, and heart failure. Neck exam may demonstrate the presence of a goiter or a nodule. Patients with thyroiditis may have thyroid tenderness in addition to enlargement of the gland. If a goiter is present, auscultation may reveal a bruit or venous hum. Deep tendon reflexes are typically brisk and symmetric.

DIFFERENTIAL DIAGNOSIS

The most common causes for hyperthyroidism are Grave's disease, toxic multinodular goiter, and thyroiditis. Other potential causes are thyroid adenomas (a variant of toxic multinodular goiter) and, rarely, factitious thyrotoxicosis or pituitary disorders. A non-endocrine etiology that may cause hyperthyroidism related to pregnancy or presence of a hydatidiform mole is hypersecretion of human chorionic gonadotropin, which may bind to the TSH receptor and act as a thy-rotropic substance. In areas of the world where there is insufficient iodine, ingestion of iodine or amiodarone may stimulate the thyroid and lead to hyperthyroidism.

Diagnostic Evaluation

The thyroid stimulating hormone (TSH) is often the initial test ordered in evaluating for thyroid disease. The TSH is very sensitive in detecting both hyper- and hypothyroidism. Follow-up testing for abnormal TSH results formerly involved measurement of total serum T4, T3 resin uptake and free thyroxine index. These tests may still be used, but free T4 and free T3 have largely supplanted their use, since the free levels of these hormones define disease activity in hyperthyroidism. TSH is decreased in patients with Grave's disease, toxic multinodular goiter, toxic nodule, and occasionally with thyroiditis. Patients with these conditions have primary hyperthyroidism and will have elevated levels of thyroid hormone (free T4 and T3). A thyroid radioactive iodine uptake scan is useful in the setting of hyperthyroidism to differentiate between a diffuse process (e.g., Grave's disease or thyroiditis) and a nodular disorder. The thyroid scan will show diffusely increased uptake in Grave's disease, nodular hyperfunctioning in toxic multinodular goiter, and decreased uptake in thyroiditis. For patients with a palpable nodule, the thyroid scan also helps differentiate between hot (hyperfunctioning) and cold (hypofunctioning) nodules. Thyroid scanning, ultrasound and fine-needle aspiration are often used to monitor thyroid nodules. Ultrasound is used to determine if the nodule is solid or cystic. Thyroid antibodies are commonly found in patients with thyroiditis (Hashimoto's) and Grave's disease. In hyperthyroid patients with abnormally high levels of TSH, MRI is useful in evaluating for pituitary pathology.

MANAGEMENT

Optimal management of hyperthyroidism must take into account patient age, comorbidities, and underlying cause for the disorder. Initial therapy for hyperthyroidism is targeted towards controlling thyroid hormone production using medications. Definitive treatment will depend upon the underlying disease process as well as the age and preferences of the patient.

Antithyroid medications as definitive therapy are most commonly used in patients less than 40 years old and include propylthiouracil (PTU) and methimazole (tapazole). These medications are relatively safe and inhibit iodine processing during production of thyroid hormone and inhibit the peripheral conversion of T4 to T3. Agranulocytosis is a serious side effect of these medications so complete blood counts should be followed. Other side effects include allergic reactions and elevation in liver function tests. Treatment typically lasts 1 year followed by a gradual taper. Roughly 50% of those with Grave's disease will have no further episodes. In those in whom hyperthyroidism returns, options include retreatment, radioactive iodine, and surgery.

Radioactive iodine (131I) is a very common treatment of thyrotoxicosis but is contraindicated in young children and pregnant women. The main disadvantage is resultant hypothyroidism for which lifelong treatment with thyroid replacement is necessary. Treatment is maximally effective at 3 to 4 months and may be repeated at 6 months if hyperthyroidism returns. Pretreatment with antithyroid medications is often initiated to avoid excess release of thyroid hormone that may occur during radiation.

Surgery is a useful treatment and offers a quick and definitive cure. It is most often performed in younger patients and those with a hyperfunctioning nodule. Post-surgical hypothyroidism occurs but is less common than in those undergoing radioactive iodide treatment. The main risks include those associated with neck surgery and include recurrent laryngeal nerve damage, damage to the parathyroid, infection, bleeding, and hypothyroidism.

Thyroid storm is a rare, life-threatening syndrome of severe thyrotoxicosis. Symptoms include nausea, fever, heart failure, tachycardia, and diaphoresis and usually occur in an individual with unknown or inadequately treated hyperthyroidism. Treatment is similar to, but more aggressive than, that used to treat hyperthyroidism and includes high-dose antithyroid medications, intravenous iodine, intravenous beta-blockers, and high-dose steroids.

The symptomatic treatment of thyrotoxicosis is another important consideration. B-blockers such as propranolol are given and increased until the anxiety, restlessness, and tachycardia are adequately controlled. For patients with thyroiditis, this may be the only therapy required, as these patients typically progress to become euthyroid and ultimately hypothyroid and require thyroid replacement therapy. Definite treatment of other forms of hyperthyroidism is typically achieved by radioactive iodine treatment, antithyroid medications, or surgery.

Patients with Grave's disease and exophthalmos are at risk for corneal ulcers and permanent visual deficits secondary to optic nerve compression and extraocular muscle involvement. To prevent corneal ulcers, eye patches, protective glasses, and artificial tears are often employed. Steroids tapered over several weeks are also commonly used in preventing permanent ocular damage. In severe cases, radiation of the extraocular muscles or orbital decompression is indicated. Treatment of the pretibial myxedema usually consists of a topical steroid.

Patients with thyroid nodules need to be evaluated over time to detect malignancies. Those with hyperfunctioning solitary nodules may be treated surgically or with thyroid suppression using exogenous thyroid hormone. Because roughly 1 out of 20 nodules (functioning and nonfunctioning) are malignant, all thyroid nodules need to be evaluated using ultrasound and biopsy.

◆ KEY POINTS ◆

1. Patients with symptomatic hyperthyroidism (a.k.a. thyrotoxicosis) often complain of weight loss despite normal or high caloric intake, nervousness, heat intolerance, fatigue, increased perspiration, more frequent bowel movements, and inability to sleep.

2. The most common causes for hyperthyroidism are Grave's disease, toxic multinodular goiter, and thyroiditis.

3. The thyroid stimulating hormone (TSH) is often the initial test ordered in evaluating for thyroid disease, and if abnormal is followed by serum free T4 and free T3 to define disease activity in hyperthyroidism.

4. A thyroid radioactive iodine uptake scan is useful to differentiate in the setting of hyperthyroidism, between a diffuse process (e.g., Grave's disease or thyroiditis) and a nodular disorder.

5. Definitive treatment of hyperthyroidism is typically achieved by radioactive iodine treatment, antithyroid medications, or surgery.

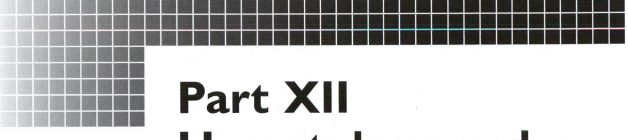

Part XII
Hematology and Oncology

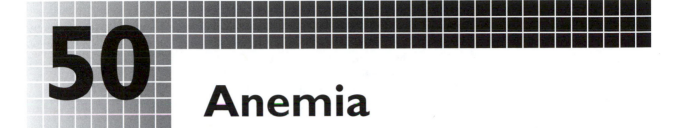

50 Anemia

In adults, anemia is defined as a hematocrit of less than 41% (hemoglobin <13.5 g/dl) in males or 37% (hemoglobin <12 g/dl) in females. In the United States, the most common cause of anemia in elderly individuals is anemia of chronic disease whereas in females of reproductive age, the most common cause is iron deficiency. The most common cause of anemia worldwide is iron deficiency.

PATHOPHYSIOLOGY

Anemia can result from blood loss, increased destruction of red blood cells, or inadequate red blood cell production. Individuals with anemia may experience tissue hypoxia, which is detected by the oxygen sensing cells in the area of the juxtaglomerular apparatus of the kidney. As a result, the kidney increases erythropoietin production, the primary regulatory hormone for erythropoiesis. In chronic renal disease, anemia may result from a decrease in renal production of erythropoietin. In chronic illnesses, impaired incorporation of iron into hemoglobin can cause an anemia of chronic disease. Chronic blood loss, hemolysis, malabsorption, malnutrition, inflammatory states, or bone marrow suppression by infection or drugs may also contribute to the pathogenesis of anemia of chronic disease.

For normal erythropoiesis, an adequate supply of iron is needed. Normally, the circulating red blood cell (erythrocyte) has a life span of approximately 120 days and iron is primarily supplied by the recycling of iron from senescent red cells destroyed by the reticuloendothelial system. In a healthy non-menstruating person, the daily loss of iron is minimal and as a result only 1–2 mg of iron are required per day. Iron is primarily absorbed from the duodenum, transported to the bone marrow, and used to form hemoglobin. Excess iron is converted to ferritin and stored in the liver and bone marrow. When the stores of iron are inadequate due to blood loss or chronic dietary inadequacy, normal hemoglobin synthesis in disrupted and a microcytic, hypochromic anemia results.

Deficiencies in vitamins B12 (cobalamine) and folate result in impaired DNA synthesis. Although DNA synthesis is slowed, cytoplasmic development continues and there is more cytoplasm than normal, resulting in larger cells or a megaloblastic anemia. Folate deficiency generally results from inadequate dietary intake. In addition to inadequate intake, causes of B12 deficiency include malabsorption and lack of intrinsic factor. In order for vitamin B12 to be absorbed, it must first bind with intrinsic factor (IF), which is secreted by the parietal cells of the stomach. Conditions such as gastric atrophy or gastrectomy can result in a vitamin B12 deficiency due to lack of IF. Since the cobalamine-IF complex is absorbed in the ileum, intestinal disease involving the terminal ileum, such as Crohn's disease, may also lead to lack of absorption of the cobalamine-IF complex.

Genetic factors can cause abnormal hemoglobin synthesis. The normal hemoglobin molecule consists of

2 alpha chains and 2 beta chains. An abnormality in the synthesis of alpha or beta chains can result in low hemoglobin or abnormal hemoglobin consisting of only alpha or beta chains. The abnormal hemoglobin may aggregate and form insoluble cytoplasmic inclusion bodies that damage the cells, leading to premature destruction of these cells by the spleen and liver.

CLINICAL MANIFESTATIONS

History

Anemia can result in an inadequate supply of oxygen to the tissues, causing symptoms in vulnerable organ systems. For example, patients with heart disease may present with angina pectoris or decompensated congestive heart failure. However, many patients are asymptomatic until their hemoglobin level falls below 8 gm/dl. General symptoms include dizziness and fatigue or weakness, either at rest or brought on by exertion.

The history should focus on potential sources of blood loss. The gastrointestinal tract is the most common source of blood loss and the presence of melena, hematochezia and hematemesis indicate gastrointestinal bleeding. Premenopausal females should be assessed for abnormal vaginal bleeding since this is a common cause of iron deficiency anemia. In the elderly population, inquiring about chronic illnesses such as hepatic, renal, inflammatory, malignancies, and infectious diseases is important since these conditions are associated with anemia of chronic disease. A family history of anemia may point to an inherited cause such as thalassemia. Alcohol consumption should be determined in all patients, since excess alcohol can suppress the bone marrow, cause chronic liver disease, and is associated with folate and other vitamin deficiencies. If the patient reports a history of jaundice, pruritus, and history of gallstones, hemolytic anemia should be suspected.

Physical Examination

Physical findings include pallor, tachycardia, and dyspnea. A systolic ejection murmur may be heard due to hyperdynamic circulation. Abdominal and rectal examinations can detect organomegaly and occult blood. Signs of iron deficiency include cheilosis (scaling at the corner of the mouth), koilonychia (spoon shaped nails), and brittle nails.

Patients with B12 deficiency may have neurologic deficits such as abnormal reflexes, ataxia, Babinski's sign, and poor position and vibration sense. These neurologic findings are not found with folate deficiency.

Differential Diagnosis

Anemias can be classified based on the mean corpuscular volume (MCV) into three categories: microcytic, macrocytic, or normocytic. Microcytic anemia is defined as a mean corpuscular volume (MCV) less than 80 fL, a macrocytic anemia with an MCV greater than 100 fL, and normocytic anemias with MCVs between 80 and 100 fL. The differential diagnosis varies by cell size. For example, the three major causes of microcytic anemia are iron deficiency, thalassemia, and anemia of chronic disease, whereas the most common causes of macrocytic anemia are B12 or folate deficiency. A full review of the many causes of normocytic anemia is beyond the scope of this book.

After classifying the anemia, identifying the underlying disease is important. Most iron deficiency is caused by gastrointestinal or menstrual blood loss. Iron deficiency due to a nutritional deficiency is common in children. Anemia of chronic disease is associated with chronic infections, neoplastic diseases, renal disease, connective tissue disease, or endocrine disorders.

Macrocytic anemia from B12 and folate deficiency may be secondary to autoimmune disease, nutritional deficits, infections, gastrectomy, or ileal resection surgery. Since B12 is found only in foods of animal origin, vegetarians are at an increased risk of developing B12 deficiency. The most common cause of B12 deficiency is pernicious anemia, an autoimmune disease where the parietal cells that make intrinsic factor are destroyed.

The most common cause of folate deficiency is decreased dietary intake. Alcoholics often present with folate deficiency. Drugs such as phenytoin, trimethoprim-sulfamethoxazole or sulfasalazine may also impair the absorption of folate.

Causes of normocytic anemia are many, and include acute blood loss as well as the hemolytic anemias, which may be inherited or acquired.

DIAGNOSTIC APPROACH

The classification of an anemia as microcytic, macrocytic, or normocytic helps direct the work-up. A reticulocyte count can help to differentiate whether an anemia is due to underproduction, blood loss, or hemolysis.

The serum iron level should be checked in cases of microcytic anemia. Decreased serum iron level suggests either iron deficiency or anemia of chronic disease. In iron deficiency, the total iron binding capacity (TIBC) is elevated and the percent saturation low, while the TIBC is low and the percent saturation is normal or increased in anemia of chronic disease. Also the ferritin level is decreased in iron deficiency but elevated or normal in anemia of chronic disease. Typically in anemia of chronic disease, the hemoglobin does not fall below 8 gm/dl, the MCV is usually only mildly decreased, and the reticulocyte count is low and does not respond to iron therapy. Although rarely needed, a bone marrow aspiration and staining for iron stores is the definitive test for iron deficiency. If the serum iron is increased, a sideroblastic anemia should be suspected. If the serum iron level is normal, hemoglobin electrophoresis should be performed to evaluate the possibility of a hemoglobinopathy, such as thalassemia, as the cause of anemia.

B12 and folate levels should be measured if there is a macrocytic anemia. RBC folate levels are more accurate than serum folate levels. Another useful test to differentiate between B12 and folate deficiency is to measure the serum methylmalonic acid and homocysteine (HC) levels. Both methylmalonic acid and HC are elevated in B12 deficiency, whereas only HC is elevated in folate deficiency.

Examining the peripheral blood smear is important. Finding sickled cells requires a hemoglobin electrophoresis to rule out sickle cell anemia. Spherocytes suggest a hemolytic process causing the anemia. Basophilic stippling with microcytic anemia is seen in lead poisoning and thalassemia. In thalassemia, liver disease, and hemolysis, target cells are also found in the peripheral smear. Teardrop cells seen in myelofibrosis and abnormal types of circulating cells such as blast cells suggest a malignancy. Howell-Jolly bodies are common in post-splenectomy patients and sickle cell anemia. Hypersegmented neutrophils may indicate presence of a megaloblastic anemia.

In a normocytic anemia, the reticulocyte count is the most important test because it helps to differentiate between hemolytic anemias, blood loss, and bone marrow disorders. The reticulocyte count must be corrected for the level of anemia. (Corrected reticulocyte count = retic count × patient hct/expected hct.) A corrected reticulocyte count of 2% or less suggests decreased production. If the reticulocyte count is greater than 3%, blood loss or hemolytic anemia should be suspected. A low haptoglobin, elevated lactate dehydrogenase, and an increase in unconjugated bilirubin can confirm hemolysis. A Coombs test helps distinguish between immune and non-immune hemolysis. A normal or low reticulocyte count indicates a hypoproliferative bone marrow. Follow-up tests should screen for renal, hepatic, and endocrine etiologies and may also include examination of the bone marrow. A hypoproliferative state may also be seen in hematinic deficiencies such as low iron or B12.

TREATMENT

Management of anemia depends on an accurate diagnosis. Oral ferrous sulfate (FeSO4) is preferred for iron therapy since it is soluble, inexpensive, and easily administered. The required amount of elemental iron is 150–200 mg per day, which can be achieved by taking 325 mg of $FeSO_4$ two to three times daily. Although food can impair iron absorption, side effects such as nausea, constipation, and heartburn may require giving $FeSO_4$ with meals. Other iron preparations such as ferrous gluconate and ferrous fumarate may be better tolerated than ferrous sulfate, but are more expensive. Indications for parenteral iron therapy are an inability to tolerate oral therapy, malabsorption or inflammatory bowel disease, severe iron deficiency, and ongoing blood loss. Iron deficiency anemia responds to treatment within 7 to 10 days, evidenced by an elevated reticulocyte count. Hemoglobin levels should return to normal within 1 to 2 months unless there is continued blood loss, and iron supplements continued for 6 months or until ferritin is greater than or equal to 50 ng/liter. Definitive therapy of iron deficiency anemia involves identifying and treating the underlying cause. Most men and women older than 35 to 40 years of age or without a history of significant menstrual bleeding require an evaluation for gastrointestinal bleeding.

Patients with renal failure, AIDS, or undergoing chemotherapy may benefit from recombinant erythropoietin. In thalassemia major, only symptomatic therapy is available and patients may need multiple transfusions. Since this can lead to iron overdose, chelation therapy with deferoxamine may be required. Other therapies include splenectomy and bone marrow transplant.

For patients with B12 deficiency from IF deficiency, parenteral replacement of B12 is indicated. If folate deficiency is suspected, 1 mg/day of folate along with B12 should be given since the neurologic symptoms of B12 deficiency can be worsened or become permanent if folate is not replaced. In normocytic anemias the underlying process causing the anemia should be treated.

◆ KEY POINTS ◆

1. Anemia can result from blood loss, increased destruction of red blood cells, or inadequate red blood cell production.

2. Anemia can result in an inadequate supply of oxygen to the tissues, causing symptoms in vulnerable organ systems. Most individuals do not experience symptoms unless their hemoglobin is less than 8 gm/dl or there is an acute drop in hemoglobin.

3. The classification of an anemia as microcytic, macrocytic, or normocytic helps direct the work-up.

4. The three major causes of microcytic anemia are iron deficiency, thalassemia, and anemia of chronic disease, whereas the most common causes of macrocytic anemia are B12 or folate deficiency.

5. In a normocytic anemia, the reticulocyte count is the most important test because it helps to differentiate between hemolytic anemias, blood loss, and bone marrow disorders.

6. Oral ferrous sulfate ($FeSO_4$) is preferred for iron therapy since it is soluble, inexpensive, and easily administered.

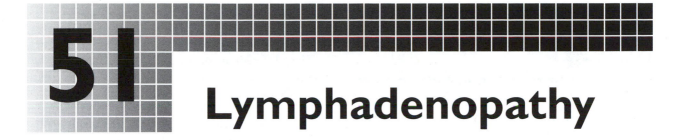

Lymphadenopathy

Lymphadenopathy is the enlargement of the lymph glands, usually greater than 1 cm. Two exceptions are inguinal lymph nodes (LN), which are considered normal up to 1.5 cm, and epitrochlear lymph nodes, which are enlarged if greater than 0.5 cm. Generalized lymphadenopathy is defined as enlargement of three or more noncontiguous areas. Regional lymphadenopathy exists when the swelling is limited to a specific region, such as cervical lymph nodes.

PATHOPHYSIOLOGY

Three mechanisms can produce enlarged LN. First LN can increase in size if cells within the gland respond to an antigen or from reactive hyperplasia from inflammation. They also enlarge if primary cells within the lymph gland transform into neoplastic cells and enlarge the gland as they proliferate. Finally, lymph nodes may enlarge if there is an invasion of cells from outside the node, such as malignant cells from a metastatic cancer or from a benign infiltrating disorder, such as sarcoidosis.

CLINICAL MANIFESTATIONS

History

Lymphadenopathy usually causes no symptoms unless the nodes are acutely inflamed or large enough to cause lymphatic obstruction or press on a nerve. If symptoms are present, they usually relate to the underlying disease. Regional lymphadenopathy can be caused by a local infection or immunization in the area drained by the lymph node. The history should focus on the area in question. For example, in cases of cervical lymphadenopathy, asking about pharyngeal symptoms, dental problems, and hoarseness is appropriate.

Generalized lymphadenopathy requires a thorough history since it is seen in a wide spectrum of diseases, including infections, immunological, metabolic, and malignant disorders. Onset is important since acute infection becomes a less likely cause as time progresses. Constitutional symptoms such as fever and weight loss suggest cancer, systemic infection, or connective tissue disease. Recent rashes, arthralgias, pharyngeal symptoms, or pet exposure may suggest a specific diagnosis, such as connective tissue disease, viral illness, or cat scratch fever. Syphilis and AIDS should be considered in patients at risk for these infections.

Risk factors for less common infections include sheep contact (brucellosis), geographic locale (coccidioidomycosis or histoplasmosis), and animal bites (tularemia or Pasteurella).

Physical Examination

All lymph nodes should be characterized by size, tenderness, texture, and consistency. Small, palpable cervical lymph nodes (less than 1 cm) are common in children. Mild inguinal bilateral lymphadenopathy (less

---

BOX 51–1

Lymphadenopathy Characteristics and Findings

Lymph Node Characteristics

Malignant: hard, matted, fixed, non-tender, and usually greater than 3 cm

Infectious: warm, erythematous, fluctuant

Reactive: discrete, rubbery, and freely mobile

Key Findings of Associated Disorders

Thyromegaly: hyperthyroidism

Arthritis: connective tissue disease and leukemia

Splenomegaly: cancer, infectious mononucleosis, storage diseases, leukemia and lymphoma

Skin rash: viral exanthem, connective tissue disease, and Kawasaki disease

---

than 1.5 cm) is common throughout life. Box 51–1 lists characteristics associated with different etiologies and other clues on physical examination that may suggest a specific etiology.

Generalized lymphadenopathy is usually characterized by multiple small discrete lymph nodes often associated with splenomegaly.

DIFFERENTIAL DIAGNOSIS

Generalized lymphadenopathy can be caused by infection, immunological disorder, metabolic disease, malignancy, and miscellaneous inflammatory conditions. Common viral infections causing lymphadenopathy include infectious mononucleosis, CMV virus, and HIV. Less common infections include tuberculosis, syphilis, histoplasmosis, and toxoplasmosis. Immunological disorders include connective tissue disease such as systemic lupus erythematosus or rheumatoid arthritis and immunologic reactions such as a drug reaction or serum sickness. Metabolic disorders include hyperthyroidism and, rarely, storage diseases such as Gaucher's and Niemann-Pick disease. Malignant causes of generalized lymphadenopathy include leukemia, lymphomas,

metastatic carcinoma, and malignant histiocytosis. Miscellaneous causes include disorders such as Kawasaki disease and IV drug use.

The differential diagnosis of localized lymphadenopathy depends on the involved region. Cervical lymphadenopathy is the most commonly encountered form and is usually caused by infections, primarily upper respiratory infections. Box 51–2 lists the differential diagnoses of lymphadenopathy by region.

DIAGNOSTIC EVALUATION

Lymphadenopathy is common and usually indicates benign self-limited disease. This is particularly true in children and young adults who are prone to reactive lymphadenopathy. Localized lymphadenopathy usually represents disease from the area of drainage. If it appears that the patient has a benign cause of lymphadenopathy, close observation or limited testing (e.g., monospot or strep screen) is indicated to confirm the suspected diagnosis. In contrast, in individuals whose initial assessment suggests a malignant disorder, more extensive testing and consideration of a lymph node biopsy is indicated.

If the diagnosis is uncertain, stepwise testing with a CBC and serology is appropriate. A markedly abnormal CBC revealing a severe anemia or malignant cells implies cancer and an urgent need for more complete evaluation, including bone marrow or lymph node biopsy. A CBC may also suggest infectious mononucleosis or a viral infection (atypical lymphocytes), pyogenic infection (granulocytes), or hypersensitivity states (eosinophilia). Serologic testing may be helpful, including a monospot or Epstein-Barr virus titers. Other serological tests that may be helpful are those for CMV or toxoplasmosis titers, HIV antibodies, ANA, and rheumatoid factor. A chest x-ray is indicated in the presence of pulmonary symptoms, in severely ill patients, or those individuals with supraclavicular lymphadenopathy. A CXR is also useful as a second level of evaluation for persistent undiagnosed lymphadenopathy. The presence of hilar lymphadenopathy suggests sarcoidosis, lymphoma, fungal infection, tuberculosis, or metastatic cancer. A positive tuberculosis skin test suggests mycobacterial infection. Urethral and cervical cultures can be helpful for determining the cause of inguinal lymphadenopathy. Culturing LN tissue or aspirated fluid may also be of value. Special stains can detect cat scratch disease and mycobacteria. Rarely, blood

BOX 51–2

Differential Diagnosis of Lymphadenopathy by Region

Cervical:

- Upper respiratory infection
- Bacterial infection of head and neck
- Mononucleosis
- CMV
- Toxoplasmosis
- Mycobacterial infection
- Neoplasm—primary and metastatic
- Kawasaki disease
- Sarcoidosis
- Reactive hyperplasia

Supraclavicular Lymphadenopathy:

- Tuberculosis
- Histoplasmosis
- Sarcoid
- Lymphoma
- Metastatic disease, particularly lung and gastrointestinal

Axillary:

- Upper extremity infection
- Connective tissue disease
- Cat scratch disease
- Neoplasm

Epitrochlear:

- Hand infection
- Secondary syphilis

Inguinal:

- Local or lower extremity infection
- Localized skin rash
- Syphilis
- Lymphogranularum venereum
- Genital herpes
- Chancroid

- Cat scratch disease
- Neoplastic disorders

Mediastinal Lymphadenopathy:

- Sarcoidosis
- Tuberculosis
- Histoplasmosis
- Coccidioidomycosis
- Lymphoma
- Metastatic cancer

cultures are required in cases of suspected bacteremia or unusual diseases such as tularemia, plague, or brucellosis.

Imaging studies such as ultrasounds, CT, or MRI of the involved area may be useful to differentiate lymphadenopathy from non-lymphatic enlargement. A CT is used for evaluating hilar lymph nodes or to demonstrate the presence of abdominal lymph nodes. Imaging may also identify a primary lesion accounting for regional lymphadenopathy. A bone marrow examination is indicated for patients with severe anemia, thrombocytopenia, or the presence of malignant cells on peripheral smear.

Lymph node biopsy should be considered when there is a failure to establish a diagnosis, if there is a clinical suspicion of a neoplasm or an illness such as tuberculosis or sarcoidosis. Clinical factors such as lymph node size and irregularity, the presence of weight loss, or enlarged liver or spleen suggest a need for an early biopsy. Supraclavicular lymph nodes have a high incidence of serious underlying disease and usually require early biopsy. During follow-up for undiagnosed lymphadenopathy, lymph nodes that remain constant in size for 4 to 8 weeks or fail to resolve in 8 to 12 weeks should be biopsied.

MANAGEMENT

Management is directed at the underlying cause. Treatment for viral infections is largely symptomatic. Cat scratch disease may benefit from antibiotics such as trimethoprim sulfamethoxazole. Nodes affected by atypical mycobacterium may need surgical excision. Active TB should be treated with three antituberculosis drugs such as isoniazid, rifampin, and ethambutol. Initial therapy for acute lymphadenitis consists of antibiotics active against streptococcal and staphylococcus such as a cephalosporin, erythromycin, or a semisynthetic penicillin, such as dicloxacillin. Neoplastic disease should be referred to an oncologist for treatment.

◆ KEY POINTS ◆

1. Generalized lymphadenopathy is defined as enlargement of three or more noncontiguous areas. Regional lymphadenopathy exists when the swelling is limited to a specific region, such as cervical lymph nodes.

2. Lymphadenopathy usually causes no symptoms unless the nodes are acutely inflamed or large enough to cause lymphatic obstruction or press on a nerve.

3. Infection, immunological disorder, metabolic disease, malignancy, and miscellaneous inflammatory conditions can cause generalized lymphadenopathy.

4. Localized lymphadenopathy usually represents disease from the area of drainage.

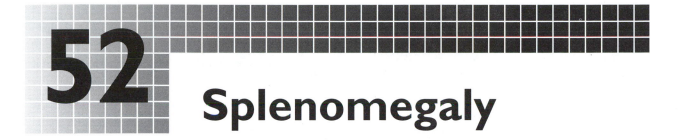

52 Splenomegaly

A palpable spleen is an abnormal finding in adults, however 15% of normal neonates, 10% of normal children, and 5% of normal adolescents may have a palpable spleen on examination.

PATHOPHYSIOLOGY

The basic functions of the spleen are (1) filtration of unwanted elements from the blood by phagocytosis in the splenic cords; (2) acting as an organ in the immune system; (3) generating lymphoreticular cells and sometimes hematopoietic cells; and (4) serving as a reserve pool and storage site of blood. A normal human spleen harbors 30 to 40 ml of erythrocytes, and stores 30% to 40% of the total platelet mass in the body. When the spleen is involved in a disease process affecting one of the functions mentioned above, splenic enlargement may result.

Several mechanisms can cause splenic enlargement. Splenomegaly may result from hypertrophy due to an increased demand for splenic function (e.g., hemolytic anemias where there is a need to remove damaged red blood cells) or in response to a systemic infection.

Congestion due to portal hypertension (e.g., from chronic liver disease or congestive heart failure) may also lead to splenic enlargement. Finally, infiltration with malignant cells, lipids, or glycogen rich macrophages may also cause the spleen to increase in size.

CLINICAL MANIFESTATIONS

History

Patients with splenomegaly may complain of a feeling of fullness in the left upper quadrant. Other symptoms are generally related to the underlying condition. It is important to seek clues in the history for an underlying disease such as a hemolytic anemia or an autoimmune disorder. Sometimes patients will give a history of having a chronic illness associated with splenomegaly. A general review of systems is important to assess general health and to identify symptoms such as fever, weight loss or sweats. In addition, eliciting information about alcohol intake and hepatitis may help identify patients with portal hypertension. A history of foreign travel to an endemic area can increase the suspicion for malaria.

Physical Examination

The physical exam of the spleen should include inspection, percussion, auscultation and palpation. Normally, the spleen is located between the sixth and tenth ribs, posterior to the midclavicular line and is not palpable. Palpation of the spleen below the rib margins indicates possible splenic enlargement. Percussion may assist in delineating the splenic margin. Inspection should note any signs of other contributing disease processes, such as the dilated venous collaterals of portal hypertension. Auscultation of the left upper quadrant may reveal a murmur or bruit signifying increased blood flow through the enlarged spleen. A complete physical examination, including examination for lymphadenopathy, should be performed looking for signs of the underlying etiology for the splenomegaly.

DIFFERENTIAL DIAGNOSIS

Conditions causing splenomegaly are listed in Table 52–1. These conditions may be grouped by the underlying mechanisms of splenomegaly:

1. Congestion from portal hypertension or venous outflow obstruction, for example, congestive heart failure or chronic liver disease
2. Reactive hyperplasia from infection, immune disorders, or hemolytic anemias
3. Infiltrative disease, both neoplastic and non-neoplastic

DIAGNOSTIC APPROACH

The initial approach is to search for a systemic disease, such as a connective tissue disorder, that could explain the splenomegaly. In young adults, infections (e.g., mononucleosis), hemolytic anemia, and Hodgkin's disease need to be considered. A middle-aged individual most commonly has primary liver disease. Lymphomas or a myeloproliferative disorder are other diagnostic possibilities. An elderly person is more likely to have a lymphoproliferative disorder such as a lymphoma, chronic lymphocytic leukemia or a myeloproliferative disorder. A history of an enlarged spleen since childhood usually indicates a congenital disease such as a hereditary hemolytic anemia or a storage disease such a Gaucher's disease. Massive splenomegaly is most common with malignancies such as polycythemia vera or late stage chronic myelogenous leukemia.

Lab tests such as a CBC and a peripheral smear can help to identify infection, mononucleosis, or a hemolytic anemia. The peripheral smear detects premature or abnormal blood cells seen in malignancy, anemias, and rouleaux formation associated with Waldenström's macroglobulinemia. Howell-Jolly bodies sometimes can be seen peripherally due to a non-functioning spleen. Imaging with CT or ultrasound can confirm splenomegaly and may identify tumors,

TABLE 52–1
Causes of Splenomegaly

Congestive
  CHF
  Portal Hypertension (cirrhosis)
  Portal or Splenic Vein Thrombosis

Reactive Hyperplasia
  Chronic Hemolytic Anemias
    Hereditary
      (e.g., spherocytosis)
    Acquired
      (e.g., autoimmune hemolytic anemia)
  Infections
    Bacterial
      (e.g., subacute bacterial endocarditis, brucellosis)
    Mycobacterial
      (e.g., tuberculosis)
    Viral (e.g., infectious mononucleosis, cytomegalovirus, HIV, hepatitis)
    Fungal
      (e.g., histoplasmosis)
    Parasitic
      (e.g., malaria, toxoplasmosis)
  Autoimmune Disorders
    Connective tissue disease
      (e.g., rheumatoid arthritis, lupus erythematosis)

Infiltrative Disease
  Non-neoplastic (e.g., amyloidosis, Gaucher's disease, sarcoidosis)
  Neoplastic (e.g., leukemias, Hodgkin's disease, non-Hodgkin's lymphoma, polycythemia vera, myelofribrosis with myeloid metaplasia)
  Metastatic tumors (very rare)

cysts, or abscesses. A liver-spleen scan can help identify chronic liver disease as the cause for an enlarged spleen. Liver function tests and serologic testing for hepatitis are important in searching for liver disease.

Other laboratory tests may be indicated based on family history or ethnic background. For example, electrophoresis is indicated for patients with a family history or ethnic background that places them at risk for sickle cell anemia or thalassemia; ophthalmic exam, skeletal survey, urinary mucopolysaccharides, enzyme assays or skin biopsies may be indicated for those at risk for Gaucher's and Niemann-Pick disease. A chest x-ray, liver function tests, angiotensin converting enzyme levels, serum calcium, and a 24-hour urinary calcium level may be helpful in diagnosis of sarcoidosis.

MANAGEMENT

If the patient has a known illness that causes splenomegaly such as infectious mononucleosis, then the condition should be treated if possible and the splenomegaly monitored. Clues from the history, physical examination, and initial lab tests may suggest conditions such as bacterial endocarditis or an autoimmune disorder. If a malignancy is suspected and there is no other source for biopsy such as an accessible lymph node, a splenectomy may be indicated. If the diagnosis is uncertain and serious disease appears unlikely, following the patient until the splenomegaly resolves or the diagnosis becomes apparent is appropriate. Splenectomy may be indicated in patients with severe hemolytic anemias, with ITP, for traumatic injury, and in some neoplastic conditions. In young children, partial splenectomy may be beneficial since preserving the spleen can provide immunity against capsular pathogens such as

Streptococcal pneumoniae. In general, the mortality and morbidity of splenectomy is about 5% to 20%. Complications following splenectomy include: postsplenectomy thrombocytosis and thrombosis, respiratory complaints such as atelectasis, pneumonia, subphrenic abscess (more likely in the age group less than 6 years old), injury to other organs (pancreatic injury is most common), post-splenectomy sepsis, and hemorrhage. Vaccinations against *Streptococcal pneumoniae* and *Haemophilus influenzae* should be administered before the splenectomy, if possible, to help confer immunity. Long-term antibiotic prophylaxis may be indicated in immunocompromised patients, in those receiving chemotherapy, and in patients less than 6 years old.

◆ KEY POINTS ◆

1. Fifteen percent of normal neonates, 10% of normal children and 5% of normal adolescents can present with a soft, thin, palpable spleen. However, a palpable spleen in adults is usually abnormal.

2. Several different mechanisms have been described for splenomegaly. They include congestion, reactive hyperplasia, and infiltrative disease—both neoplastic and non-neoplastic.

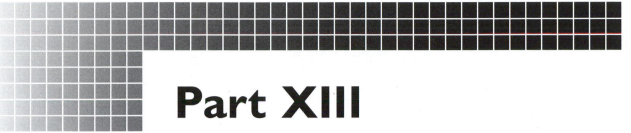

Part XIII
Musculoskeletal Disorders

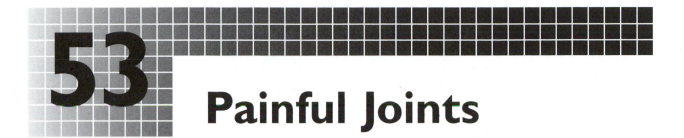

53 Painful Joints

The key to evaluating joint pain involves three issues: 1) if the symptoms are related to the joint or to the periarticular structures, 2) if the problem is monoarticular or polyarticular, and 3) if the process is inflammatory or non-inflammatory.

PATHOPHYSIOLOGY

Arthritis can result from degenerative processes or inflammatory disease. A non-inflammatory disease, such as osteoarthritis, usually stems from the breakdown of cartilage and can eventually cause mechanical joint problems.

Inflammatory disease is mediated by cellular and humoral factors, such as prostaglandins, leukotrienes, interleukin-1, and tumor necrosis factor. Neutrophils, macrophages, lymphocytes, and other cellular mediators of inflammation are involved. Infection, crystalline arthritis, and the autoimmune diseases (e.g., rheumatoid arthritis) are examples of inflammatory arthritis. Periarticular symptoms involve tendons and muscles but may also present as joint pain.

CLINICAL MANIFESTATIONS

History

The number of individual joints involved is important. Monoarticular complaints make infection, gout,

pseudogout, trauma, or toxic synovitis more likely. Multiple joint involvement suggests a connective tissue disease, osteoarthritis or rheumatoid arthritis. Symmetrical polyarthritis is consistent with rheumatoid arthritis. Acute onset joint pain is most consistent with trauma or infection while a more prolonged course suggests osteoarthritis, rheumatoid arthritis, connective tissue disease, or fibromyalgia.

Factors affecting the pain are also important. Nocturnal pain in a younger individual in a single joint raises the possibility of a tumor. Pain that increases with use is consistent with osteoarthritis and tendonitis. Pain that decreases with use is more consistent with rheumatoid arthritis. Morning stiffness that lasts greater than 45 minutes suggests an inflammatory arthritis. Migratory patterns raise the possibility of rheumatic fever, disseminated gonococcemia, Reiter's syndrome, and Lyme disease. Non-articular pain usually does not produce loss of joint function, and may cause pain only with movement in certain directions. In contrast, arthritic pain usually causes discomfort with all joint motions.

Medications such as procainamide and isoniazid can cause a lupus-like syndrome. Table 53–1 lists clues from the history that suggest certain diagnoses.

Physical Examination

Many causes of arthritis have systemic manifestations. Skin manifestations of lupus erythematosis include malar rash or mouth ulcers. Other skin lesions and associated illnesses include: nail pitting and psoriatic

TABLE 53–1

Diagnostic Clues for Arthritis

Historical Clues	Associated Disease
Recent URI	Toxic synovitis
Recent sore throat	Rheumatic fever
Deer tick bite	Lyme disease
Recent Rubella immunization	Immunologic related arthritis
Diarrhea	Inflammatory bowel disease
Podagra	Gout
Urethral discharge	Reiter's disease or gonococcal arthritis
Dry mouth/dry eyes	Sjögren's syndrome
Muscle weakness	Myositis
Photosensitivity	Lupus
Heliotropic rash	Polymyositis/dermatomyositis
Low back pain	Ankylosing spondylitis
Conjunctivitis	Reiter's syndrome
Uveitis	Inflammatory bowel disease
Older age	Gout, pseudogout
Younger age	Rheumatoid arthritis, SLE
Male	Gout, ankylosing spondylitis, Reiter's disease, and hemochromatosis

TABLE 53–2

Differential Diagnosis of Polyarthritis

Inflammatory	Non-inflammatory
Rheumatoid arthritis	Osteoarthritis
SLE	Amyloidosis
Gout	Sickle cell disease
Pseudogout	Hypertrophic pulmonary osteoarthropathy
Septic arthritis	
Reiter's syndrome	Myxedema
Sarcoidosis	Hemochromatosis
Lyme disease	Paget's disease
Gonococcemia	
Viremia	
Subacute bacterial endocarditis	
Psoriatic arthritis	
Scleroderma	

arthritis, erythema migrans and Lyme disease, papillovesicular pustular lesions and disseminated gonococcemia, tophi and gout, heliotropic eyelid rash and dermatomyositis, and SLE, and rheumatoid nodules and rheumatoid arthritis. Fingertip atrophy or ulcers along with calcinosis, and telangiectasia are signs of scleroderma. Keratoderma blenorrhagia, a hyperkeratotic lesion on the palms and soles, and balanitis circinate, a shallow, painless ulcer on the penis, are signs of Reiter's syndrome. Conjunctivitis and uveitis are suggestive of joint diseases associated with inflammatory bowel disease. The cardiopulmonary exam may reveal signs of an effusion, pleuritis, or pericarditis, which can be seen in rheumatoid arthritis and SLE. Splenomegaly can also be found in individuals with rheumatoid arthritis and SLE.

An inflamed joint is usually diffusely tender and there is often increased warmth, redness, and joint effusion. Non-inflammatory joint disease usually has more focal tenderness and few signs of inflammation. Range of motion and joint deformity should be noted. Irregular bony enlargements in the proximal and distal interphalangeal joints (Bouchard's and Heberden's nodes) are signs of osteoarthritis. A tender bony mass near a joint may be a sign of a tumor.

Examination of the periarticular tissues is important since tendonitis, bursitis, and myositis can mimic joint pain.

DIFFERENTIAL DIAGNOSIS

The differential diagnosis can be approached by the number of joints involved and whether the process is inflammatory or not. Table 53–2 lists the differential diagnosis of polyarticular arthritis.

The differential diagnosis of monoarthritis includes infection, crystal-induced arthropathies (gout and pseudogout), trauma, and osteoarthritis. Gonorrhea is the most common infection causing septic arthritis. Another cause of monoarticular arthritis is solitary joint involvement of the polyarticular arthritis, such as rheumatoid arthritis presenting in a single joint. Reiter's syndrome, ankylosing spondylitis, psoriatic arthritis, colitis-associated arthritis and viral synovitis often present with monoarticular arthritis.

DIAGNOSTIC APPROACH

Arthrocentesis is the definitive diagnostic procedure for patients with monoarticular arthritis and joint effusion. Cloudy fluid suggests infection or crystalline disease while bloody joint fluid following trauma suggests internal derangement. Joint fluid examination should include leukocyte count, gram stain, culture, glucose, and an examination for crystals using polarized microscopy. Calcium pyrophosphate crystals, which cause pseudogout, are positively biorefringent while uric acid crystals, which cause gout, are negatively biorefringent. Table 53–3 shows guidelines for determining if the fluid is inflammatory.

Early in the course of arthritis, x-rays may be normal. Radiographic changes in osteoarthritis include joint space narrowing, changes in the subchondral bone, and osteophytes. Osteoarthritic changes may be seen in the absence of symptoms and the severity of the x-ray does not correlate with the degree of symptoms. Bony erosions on x-ray are common in rheumatoid arthritis, but can be seen in septic arthritis and gout. Periarticular osteopenia also implies inflammatory disease. MRI scanning is useful for diagnosing periarticular soft tissue injury.

In suspected inflammatory disease, an ESR is a useful, but non-specific, measure of inflammation. A leukocytosis is common in patients with septic arthritis. Although rheumatoid arthritis is a clinical diagnosis, a rheumatoid factor is positive in about 75% of patients. Generally, the higher the rheumatoid factor titer the more likely the patient has rheumatoid arthritis. Up to 5% to 15% of normals are rheumatoid factor positive, but usually in lower titers. Box 53–1 lists the criteria for diagnosing rheumatoid arthritis.

ANA testing is sensitive for SLE, but lacks specificity and low titers are often falsely positive. Titers greater than 1:160 or more are falsely negative in only about 5% of individuals. If an ANA is positive, testing for antibodies to double-stranded DNA (dsDNA) and for extractable nuclear antigens is indicated. Antibodies to dsDNA are present in about 70% of SLE patients and are very specific. Antibodies to the Smith antigen are also very specific for SLE, but positive in only 30% of patients.

Routine chemistries are useful in assessing renal function and uric acid. A urinalysis can screen for glomerular injury associated with connective tissue disease.

MANAGEMENT

Management depends on the underlying cause. Regardless of the cause, physical therapy is often helpful for

---

TABLE 53–3

Joint Fluid Analysis

WBC (cells/mm^3)	Interpretation
<2000	Non-inflammatory (e.g., osteoarthritis)
2000–50,000	Mild to moderate inflammation (rheumatoid arthritis, crystalline arthritis)
50,000–100,000	Severe inflammation (sepsis or gout)
>100,000	Septic joint until proven otherwise

BOX 53–1

Diagnostic Criteria for Rheumatoid Arthritis

Morning stiffness greater than 1 hour

Arthritis in three or more joints

Involvement of the wrist, MCP, or PIP joints

Symmetric arthritis

Rheumatoid nodules

Positive rheumatoid factor

Bony erosions on hand or wrist films

(Four or more criteria are needed for diagnosing rheumatoid arthritis)

TABLE 53–4

Disease Modifying Drugs for RA

Disease Modifying Drugs	Side Effects
Methotrexate	Bone marrow toxicity, hepatitis, and stomatitis
Sulfasalazine	Rash
Hydroxychloroquine	Retinopathy
Gold	Glomerular toxicity, proteinuria, rash
Penicillamine	Bone marrow toxicity, proteinuria, rash
Azathioprine	Immunosuppression

maintaining joint function, muscle strength, and mobility. In acute flares, it is important to protect the joint (e.g., splinting) to reduce pain and prevent future damage.

Septic arthritis requires appropriate antibiotics and drainage. The first line of pharmacological therapy of osteoarthritis is acetaminophen. NSAIDs are effective, but have more side effects. The symptoms of rheumatoid arthritis are treated with NSAIDs. Most experts recommend consulting with a rheumatologist and starting disease modifying (Table 53–4) drugs such as methotrexate early in the course of rheumatoid arthritis. Corticosteroids in rheumatoid arthritis may be used as bridge therapy until other medicines take effect or given in the form of a single-joint injection. SLE is treated with NSAIDs, corticosteroids, antimalarials, or azathioprine. Gout may be treated with NSAIDs or colchicine. For patients with frequent attacks, allopurinol or uricosuric agents, such as probenecid, are helpful.

◆ KEY POINTS ◆

1. The key to evaluating joint pain involves three issues: 1) if the symptoms are related to the joint or to the periarticular structures, 2) if the problem is monoarticular or polyarticular, and 3) if the process is inflammatory or non-inflammatory.

2. Morning stiffness that lasts greater than 45 minutes suggests an inflammatory arthritis.

3. The differential diagnosis of monoarthritis includes infection, crystal-induced arthropathies (gout and pseudogout), trauma, and osteoarthritis.

4. Although rheumatoid arthritis is a clinical diagnosis, a rheumatoid factor is positive in about 75% of patients. Generally, the higher the rheumatoid factor titer the more likely the patient has rheumatoid arthritis.

5. Regardless of the cause, physical therapy is often helpful for maintaining joint function, muscle strength, and mobility.

6. The first line of pharmacological therapy of osteoarthritis is acetaminophen. NSAIDs are effective, but may have more side effects.

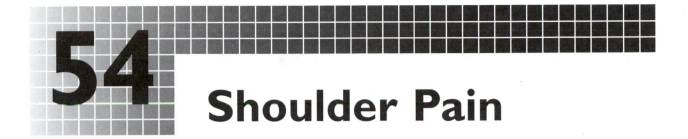

54 Shoulder Pain

Shoulder pain affects people of many ages, but is most prevalent in individuals of middle to older age.

PATHOPHYSIOLOGY

Normal shoulder motion requires smooth articulations between the glenohumeral, acromioclavicular, sterno-clavicular, and scapulothoracic joints. The head of the humerus articulates with the glenoid labrum in a "dish and saucer" fashion (versus the "ball and socket" articulation of the hip). The shallow articulation allows for a wide range of shoulder motion, but also explains why the shoulder is the most commonly dislocated joint. The four muscles of the rotator cuff (supraspinatus, infraspinatus, teres minor, and sub-scapularis) help stabilize the joint by holding the head of the humerus firmly against the glenoid. The subdeltoid and subacromial bursa are located above the muscles and tendons of the rotator cuff and facilitate fluid movement between the muscular layers. Superficial to these bursa are the trapezius, serratus anterior, and rhomboid muscles which aid in scapular stability. All of these structures need to function in concert to create smooth motion of the shoulder. Trauma or chronic stress to any single structure can lead to global dysfunction and pain.

The degenerative process that results in bursitis, tendonitis, and rotator cuff syndromes often begins in the supraspinatus or bicipital tendons that have a poor blood supply and are often under stress. The rotator cuff tendons can become inflamed from impingement between the humeral head and the acromion. Degenerative changes usually occur in individuals over 50 to 60 years of age and can ultimately involve other tendons, bursa, and sometimes the entire capsule.

CLINICAL MANIFESTATIONS

History

A complete history includes age, dominant hand, medications, past medical history, type of work and activity level. Determining if the pain is acute or chronic and inquiring about associated swelling, redness, stiffness, laxity, catching, and decreased range of motion is important.

Patients with rotator cuff problems usually present with an aching shoulder, limited abduction of the arm, and pain when rotating the shoulder. Pain occurring when the patient attempts to sleep with his arm overhead is characteristic of rotator cuff tendonitis. Full tears usually follow trauma, such as a fall, and rarely occur before middle age.

Bicipital tendonitis often occurs in combination with rotator cuff tendonitis and is less common as an isolated condition. Isolated bicipital tendonitis typically results from repetitive stress such as overhead painting or ball throwing. The pain can be severe and often radiates down the arm.

Determining what activities increase or decrease the pain can provide clues to the underlying problem. For example, pain with activities such as throwing, swimming, or serving tennis balls suggests subluxation or dislocation, whereas chronic pain and stiffness with limited motion suggests adhesive capsulitis (frozen shoulder) or rotator cuff injury. A frozen shoulder is most common during middle age and is often more prevalent in women than in men. It generally follows a period of immobilization that results from trauma to the shoulder or from medical conditions such as a myocardial infarction, or stroke.

Most dislocations and sprains occur following trauma. Reflex sympathetic dystrophy (shoulder-hand syndrome) is an uncommon disorder that can cause shoulder pain and swelling as well as pain in the upper extremity, atrophy of the nails, skin atrophy, and signs of vasomotor instability.

Pain from cervical radiculopathy can also radiate to the shoulder. Referred pain to the shoulder can occur in a variety of conditions, such as gallbladder disease, subdiaphragmatic inflammation, pulmonary infarction, and ruptured viscus.

Physical Examination

Physical exam should include inspection of the shoulder for asymmetry, surgical scars, deformity, or muscle atrophy. Palpation should be performed to pinpoint the areas of tenderness, such as in the clavicle, insertions of the rotator cuff or the bicipital groove. A deformity may be evident in acromioclavicular (AC) separations, fractures, and dislocations. Sometimes, if it is not visually evident, palpation may reveal a fracture or an AC separation.

Range of motion testing is critical in evaluating shoulder pain and should be done for both shoulders to allow for comparison. Pain with both active range of motion (AROM) and passive range of motion (PROM) suggests joint or ligament involvement, whereas pain with AROM, but not PROM suggests muscular and/or tendon injury. Performing range of motion movements against resistance helps to determine the etiology of the pain. For example, patients with rotator cuff injury often have pain accompanied by weakness when they abduct the fully extended arm against resistance with the thumbs pointing down. This maneuver compresses the tendons of the rotator cuff against the coracoacromial arch and elicits pain when there is inflammation of the rotator cuff or subacromial bursa. Pain with this maneuver is often called a positive "empty can" sign and indicates pathology of the compressed structures.

Another method for examining the rotator cuff is via the "drop-off" test. This test is performed by passively abducting the patient's shoulder and then observing the patient lower the hand to the waist level. A sudden drop of the arm towards the waist indicates a rotator cuff tear.

Cross arm testing is performed by having the patient raise the arm to 90 degrees and then actively abducting the arm (thus bringing the tested arm across the body). Pain with this maneuver at the acromioclavicular joint suggests pathology in that region and is therefore useful in differentiating between impingement and acromioclavicular injury.

Patients with a suspected shoulder dislocation or subluxation should have instability testing of the shoulder performed. The apprehension test measures anterior instability, which is performed by abducting the arm to 90 degrees, externally rotating it, and then applying pressure to the humerus. Any pain or apprehension by the patient indicates anterior glenohumeral instability. Pushing the humeral head posteriorly and feeling for increased laxity when the arm is 90 degrees abducted and the elbow is flexed to 90 degrees assesses posterior instability of the glenohumeral joint.

Tenderness over the top of the shoulder suggests subacromial bursitis. Cervical root compression can sometimes be differentiated from intrinsic shoulder pain by reproducing the pain with neck movement. The abdomen and chest should be examined to identify any effusions or subdiaphragmatic processes that may be causing referred shoulder pain.

DIFFERENTIAL DIAGNOSIS

Extrinsic disease can sometimes present as shoulder pain. Examples include cervical disease, cervical radiculopathy, diaphragmatic irritation, and myocardial infarction. Box 54–1 lists causes of shoulder pain.

Intrinsic shoulder pain is far more common and includes disorders such as osteoarthritis, fractures, dislocation, rheumatoid arthritis, gout, or osteonecrosis. In the absence of trauma, soft tissue disease such as rotator cuff tendonitis, bursitis, and bicipital tendonitis are the most common causes of shoulder pain. Less common

---

BOX 54–1

Causes of Shoulder Pain

Extrinsic
 Cervical disc disease
 Thoracic outlet syndrome
 Gallbladder disease
 Myocardial infarction
 Diaphragmatic irritation

Intrinsic

Bone/Joint abnormalities
 Dislocation/Subluxation
 Arthritis
 Infection
 AC joint sprain
 Fractures
 Osteonecrosis

Soft tissue abnormalities
 Bicipital tendonitis
 Impingement syndrome
 Bursitis (subacromial)
 Rotator cuff tendonitis/tear
 Adhesive capsulitis (frozen shoulder)
 Subdeltoid bursitis

---

are rotator cuff tears, biceps tendon rupture, and adhesive capsulitis.

DIAGNOSTIC EVALUATION

The history and physical are often sufficient to suggest the diagnosis. In patients with bursitis, tendonitis, and rotator cuff syndromes, no diagnostic work-up is indicated unless the pain persists for more than four to six weeks. If the clinical evaluation suggests cervical disease, C-spine films and possibly a CT or MRI are indicated. The history and physical are usually sufficient to indicate whether evaluation is necessary to rule out conditions causing referred pain.

In patients with trauma or persistent shoulder pain, radiographs can detect conditions such as fracture, dislocation, arthritis, metastatic disease, or avascular necrosis. In soft tissue syndromes, x-rays are usually unremarkable except in cases with calcific tendonitis. Calcium deposits in the areas of the bicipital tendon or calcium deposits in the supraspinatus tendon where it inserts in the greater tuberosity of the humerus may be present. Arthroscopy, which requires a dye injection, may be used to identify a suspected rotator cuff tear. MRI is becoming more popular as a non-invasive means of assessing the soft tissue of the shoulder and rotator cuff tendonitis or tears. However, it is expensive and is not indicated unless there is persistent pain or suggestion of a rotator cuff tear.

MANAGEMENT

The mainstay of treatment for soft tissue inflammation is NSAIDs, combined with ice or heat, and brief periods of rest followed by physical therapy. Physical therapy helps preserve normal motor function before severe weakness and stiffness compound the problem. Basic principles of physical therapy include maintaining range of motion, flexibility, and strength. Treatment progresses from passive range of motion exercises to assisted active exercises, isometrics, and finally active strength building. Most inflammatory conditions resolve with conservative care in six to eight weeks. In cases where the inflammation of the tendons is very severe or in cases of acute calcific tendonitis, a cortisone injection is often helpful.

A torn rotator cuff usually does not heal spontaneously. However, many people with partial or small tears respond to symptomatic care and an exercise program. Large rotator cuff tears usually require surgery.

Adhesive capsulitis is difficult and frustrating to treat. Active exercise to increase range of motion is the cornerstone of non-operative therapy. Occasionally, surgery may be indicated. Therapy for arthritis consists primarily of NSAIDs and exercise. Cortisone injections may also provide some relief. Acromioclavicular sprains are treated with NSAIDs and a sling until the pain resolves. Third degree separations or those involving significant displacement of the clavicle should be referred to an orthopedist. Fractures, rotator cuff tears, advanced arthritis, dislocations, or joint instability and persistent symptoms without improvement are other common indications for orthopedic referral.

◆ KEY POINTS ◆

1. Rotator cuff tendonitis, bursitis, and bicipital tendonitis are the most common causes for shoulder pain.

2. Traumatic causes for shoulder pain include AC separation, dislocation, and fractures.

3. X-ray testing should be reserved for patients with a history of traumatic injury or persisting pain despite therapy.

4. Management for soft tissue etiologies of shoulder pain commonly involves use of NSAIDs along with physical therapy.

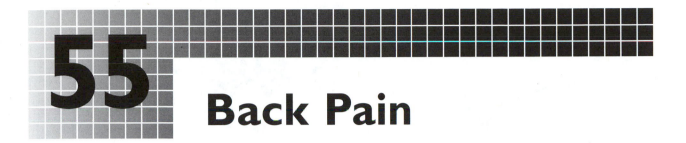

Back Pain

Approximately three-fourths of all adults experience back pain at some time in their life.

PATHOPHYSIOLOGY

Ligaments, vertebral bones, facet joints, intervertebral disks, nerve roots, and muscles are structures that can be a source of back pain. The most common causes of back pain are muscular injuries and age-related degenerative processes in the intervertebral disks and facet joints (Figure 55–1). Muscle fibers of the paraspinal muscles may tear under strenuous activity, such as twisting or heavy lifting. This results in bleeding and spasm that cause local swelling and tenderness. Obesity and poor conditioning contribute to the problem. Age-related degenerated changes in the intervertebral disks and facet joints are the result of chronic stress placed on the lumbosacral spine. Weakening of the fibrous capsule can cause the disk to bulge or herniate beyond the interspace. Disk herniation is responsible for 95% of cases of nerve root impingement. The most common level of disk herniation is at the L5-S1 level, followed by L4–5. Table 55–1 reviews the symptoms and deficits associated with the different levels of nerve impingement. Back pain may also result from visceral structures near the spine such as the aorta, kidneys, pancreas, and gallbladder.

CLINICAL MANIFESTATIONS

History

The history should elicit the onset of pain, severity, location, character of pain, aggravating and relieving factors, past medical history, previous injuries, and psychosocial stressors. Urinary or fecal incontinence may be signs of cauda equina syndrome, a surgical emergency. Red flags such as fever, night pain, weight loss, and bone pain suggest something other than mechanical low back pain. The presence of sciatica, a sharp pain that radiates down the back or side of the leg past the knee, is often a sign of disk herniation with nerve root irritation.

Spinal stenosis, a degenerative disease of the spine, is usually seen after age 50. Patients typically complain of back pain and may experience pseudoclaudication, or paresthesias of the lower back that worsen with standing or back extension.

Evaluating a child with back pain requires the presence of a parent or caretaker. Sports participation may cause injuries. For example, back handsprings or walkovers in gymnastics and hyperextension in football linemen are associated with spondylolysis and spondylolisthesis, which can cause pain. As a general rule, spondylolysis, spondylolisthesis, Scheuermann's disease, muscle disease, and overuse problems improve with rest. In contrast, tumor, infection or inflammatory diseases can cause nighttime wakening from pain and do not improve with bed rest.

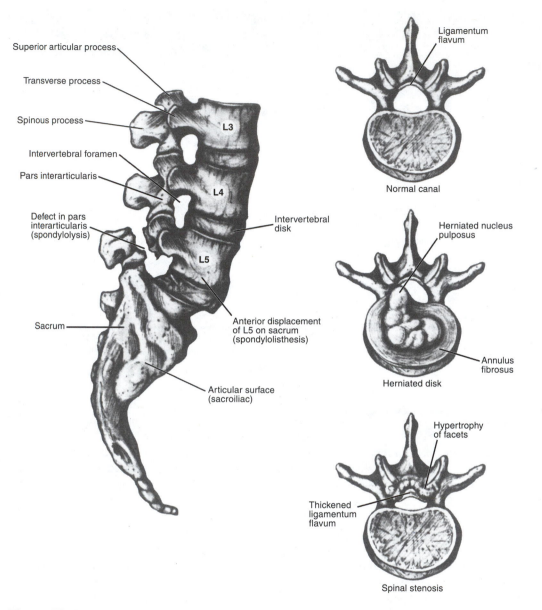

Figure 55–1 Common Pathoanatomical Conditions of the Lumbar Spine.
A superior view of a lumbar vertebra with normal anatomy and canal configuration is shown in the upper right. In the superior view of a lumbar vertebra and intervertebral disk (right center), herniation of the nucleus pulposus into the spinal canal is evident. The usual abnormalities that result in spinal stenosis (lower right) include hypertrophic degenerative changes of the facets and thickening of the ligamentum flavum. Adapted with permission from Deyo RA and Weinstein JN. Low Back Pain. New England Journal of Medicine, February 1, 2001; 344:5: Figure 1, pg. 364.

The clinical manifestations of back pain are summarized in Table 55–2.

Physical Examination

A back examination should include (1) inspecting the back for deformity; (2) checking for leg length discrep-ancy; (3) checking spinal motion; (4) palpating for focal tenderness suggestive of tumor, infection, fracture, or disk herniation; (5) performing a neurological examination to identify motor or sensory deficits; (6) testing straight leg raising (SLR). SLR is positive if sciatica is reproduced with elevations of the leg less than 60

TABLE 55–1

Impingement of Nerve Roots and Symptoms

Level	Nerve Root	Deficits	Sciatica
L3–4	L4	patellar jerk (reflex) dorsiflexion of foot (motor) medial aspects of tibia (sensory)	uncommon
L4–5	L5	extensor of great toe (motor) dorsum of foot/base of first toe (sensory)	common
L5-S1	S1	ankle jerk (reflex) plantar flexion (motor) buttock, post thigh, calf, lateral ankle and foot (sensory)	common

degrees. Ipsilateral SLR is more sensitive for a herniated disk; whereas contralateral SLR (with the symptoms of sciatica in the leg opposite the examining leg) is more specific for a herniated disk.

Examining the abdomen, rectum, groin, pelvis, and the peripheral pulses is also important in patients with back pain. Other signs of systemic diseases are fever, breast mass, pleural effusion, enlarged prostate nodule, lymphadenopathy, and joint inflammation.

DIFFERENTIAL DIAGNOSIS

Box 55–1 lists the differential diagnosis of back pain. Unfortunately a large percentage of patients cannot be given a definitive diagnosis and are often classified as having a lumbar strain or mechanical low back pain. Only a small fraction of patients have a serious problem such as a fracture, malignancy, infection, or visceral disease as a cause of low back pain. Systemic disease that may present as back pain includes metastatic cancer, multiple myeloma, and osteoporosis.

DIAGNOSTIC APPROACH

Box 55–2 lists indications for obtaining spinal x-rays. For most patients x-rays are not recommended unless the pain persists beyond 4 weeks. Negative plain films do not rule out the possibility of significant disease.

Both MRI and CT are more sensitive than plain films for detecting spinal infections, cancers, herniated disks and spinal stenosis and have largely replaced myelography. Because these two tests are highly sensitive and frequently demonstrate "abnormalities" in normal individuals, they should only be ordered if there is strong suspicion of disease to avoid overdiagnosis. Electromyography and measurement of somatosensory evoked potentials may help to define the extent of neurological involvement.

Blood tests are not necessary for most patients with back pain. A CBC, U/A, calcium, phosphorus, ESR, and alkaline phosphatase may be considered in patients with suspected systemic disease, older individuals, and those who fail conservative treatment. A CBC screens for infection or an anemia associated with multiple myeloma or an occult malignancy. An ESR may be elevated in patients with malignancy, infection or a connective tissue disease. Patients who may require long-term NSAIDs may need baseline renal and liver function tests.

MANAGEMENT

Serious non-mechanical causes of lower back pain such as infection, malignancy, or fracture require treatment for the underlying problem. Patients with a progressive neurological finding need hospital admission and prompt consultation.

Most patients with mechanical lower back pain will get better with conservative treatment consisting of pain control, education, reassurance and appropriate activity. About 80% to 90% of patients will recover

TABLE 55–2

Clinical Manifestations of Back Pains

Type	Onset	Trigger	Symptoms
Muscular	acute	heavy lifting	Lateralized back pain, pain in buttock, posterior upper thigh
Disk herniation	recurrent	trivial stress	nerve root L5, S1 impingements, frequent sciatica
Spinal stenosis	old age or congenital	OA* or congenital	pseudoclaudication*
Spondylolisthesis+	chronic	OA, Spondylolysis	nerve root L5, S1 impingement, hyperextension activities
Compression fracture	acute	osteoporosis	pain limited in middle to lower spine, steroid use or h/o mycloma
Neoplasms	insidious	neoplasms^	night pain, not relieved w/ supine position
Cauda equina Syndrome	old age	massive disk herniation	overflow incontinence (90%), saddle anesthesia $ (75%), decreased anal sphincter tone
Osteomyelitis	acute	back procedure	fever, spinal tenderness
Inflammatory Diskitis	young age	S. aureus	refusal to walk, fever, signs of sepsis; disk space narrowing, sclerosis per radiographic
Ankylosing Spondylitis	young age	HLA-B27	morning spinal stiffness, h/o inflammatory bowel disease, sacroiliitis, chest expansion less than 2.5 cm, "bamboo-spine" in radiographic
Spondylolysis	>10 yo	hyperextension	back, buttock pain with activity, tight hamstrings, lordosis
Scheuermann's disease	young age	fatigue	round back; vertebral wedging, end plate irregularity per radiographic

*OA (osteoarthritis); pseudoclaudication is pain in the lower extremity worsened by walking and relieved by sitting down that mimicks vascular insufficiency.
+Spondylolisthesis is forward subluxation of a vertebral body, usually in L4–5 or L5-S1.
^Neoplasms includes primary (i.e. multiple myeloma, spinal cord tumor) or metastatic to the spine (i.e. breast, lung, prostate, gastrointestinal, genitourinary neoplasms).
$Saddle anesthesia is reduction in sensation over the buttocks, upper posterior thighs and perineum.

within 6 weeks. Bed rest is generally not recommended unless the pain is severe enough to preclude normal activities and even then should be limited to 2 to 3 days. Longer periods of bed rest result in deconditioning. During the acute phase of back pain, the patient should be encouraged to continue normal activities including work as tolerated, but told to avoid heavy lifting (>25 lbs.), twisting, prolonged sitting, driving for long periods, and heavy vibration. Traction and analgesic injection are usually not helpful in the acute stage. Although there are no well-controlled studies demonstrating the value of heat, ice, or massage, many clinicians and patients feel these treatments are helpful and have little risk.

Medications are important for relieving pain. Acetaminophen is safe and inexpensive. It is a good first choice alone or in combination with an NSAID or opioid pain reliever. NSAIDs can relieve pain and

have an anti-inflammatory effect. However, they should be used with caution in patients with a history of gastritis, ulcers, hypertension, chronic renal failure, or CHF. For patients who cannot tolerate traditional NSAIDs, the newer COX-2 inhibitors have fewer GI side effects although they still have the same adverse effects on the kidneys and fluid balance. Narcotic pain relievers may be useful in the first few days of treatment, but are not generally indicated for longer treatment courses.

Muscle relaxants are occasionally helpful for individuals in whom spasm plays a major role. However they frequently cause drowsiness and may inhibit a return to normal activities. Surgical treatment is indicated for cauda equina syndrome and for patients with intractable pain and worsening of neurological deficits. For patients with a herniated disk not responding after 4–6 weeks of conservative therapy, diskectomy may be considered. For spinal stenosis, surgery may be of benefit to those who do not respond to conservative care and have disabling symptoms.

Those patients with persistent or frequent recurrences of back pain merit referral. Physical therapy or epidural steroid injections benefit some patients. If the pain persists for greater than 6 months, it is considered chronic and requires a different approach. Consultation with a physiatrist or chronic pain management specialist is often helpful and ensures that no remediable cause of back pain has been overlooked. Individuals who have not returned to work after 6 months of back pain have only a 50% chance of ever being employed again.

BOX 55–1

Differential Diagnosis of Acute Low Back Pain

Mechanical low back pain (97%)
lumbar strain (70%), degenerative processes in the intervertebral disks and facet joints (10%), herniated disk (4%), compression fx (4%), spinal stenosis (3%), spondylolisthesis (2%), spondylolysis, trauma, congenital diseases

Nonmechanical spinal conditions (1%)
neoplasia (0.7%), infections (0.01%), inflammatory arthritis (0.3%), Scheuermann's disease, Paget's disease

Visceral diseases (2%)
diseases of pelvic organs (prostatitis, endometriosis, chronic PID), renal diseases (nephrolithiasis, pyelonephritis, perinephritic abscess), aortic aneurysm, gastrointestinal disease (pancreatitis, cholecystitis, penetrating ulcer)

BOX 55–2

Indications for X-rays in Patients with Back Pain

Age >50
History of significant trauma
Neurological deficit
Systemic symptoms
Chronic steroid use
Possible hereditary condition
History of drug or alcohol abuse
History of osteoporosis
Immunodeficient state
Pain persisting >6 weeks

◆ KEY POINTS ◆

1. As a general rule, spondylolysis, spondylolisthesis, Scheuermann's disease, muscle disease, and overuse problems are better with rest. On the contrary, tumor, infection or inflammatory diseases can present with nighttime wakening from pain and not improve with bed rest.

2. SLR is positive if sciatica (not tightened hamstring) is reproduced with elevations of leg less than 60 degrees.

3. Surgical treatments are indicated for cauda equina syndrome and patients with intractable pain with worsening of neurological deficits.

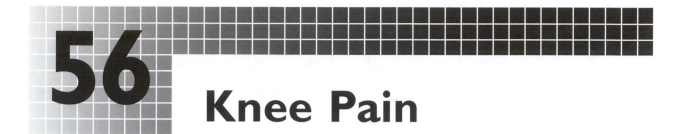

56

Knee Pain

Knee pain is most often due to acute trauma or overuse but can also be the result of degenerative disease, inflammatory arthritis, and crystalline arthropathies. Knowledge of the function and anatomy of the knee is essential in diagnosing and treating knee pain.

PATHOPHYSIOLOGY

The knee is the largest joint in the body and performs a hinge-like motion. The lateral and medial tibiofemoral articulations are the weight-bearing portions of the knee, whereas the patellofemoral articulation acts as a fulcrum for added quadriceps strength. The meniscal cartilage provides cushioning between the bones and provides a smooth surface for movement. The lateral and medial collateral ligaments provide lateral and medial stability to the knee joint while the anterior and posterior cruciate ligaments, located inside the joint, provide anterior to posterior stability. The knee also has multiple bursal that provide lubrication for the many dynamic components of the knee and allow for fluid movement.

Injury or inflammation to the either the soft tissue or bony structures of the knee may cause pain. For example, inflammation of the bursa from either direct trauma or microtrauma associated with overuse can cause pain. Patellar tendonitis is another common cause of pain that results from overuse with activities such as running or jumping. Twisting injuries place stress on the cartilage and may result in a meniscal tear, while sprains of the medial and lateral collateral ligaments usually result from a direct blow to the knee while the foot is planted.

Patellofemoral syndrome occurs with overuse, in combination with biomechanical factors such as muscle imbalance. These factors cause maltracking of the patella, which normally rests in the patellofemoral groove of the femur. Overuse and repeated weight-bearing impact lead to increased pressure in this groove and to subsequent pain.

Osgood-Schlatter's disease is a common cause of knee pain in adolescents. The pain is located on the tibial tubercle and is thought to be due to activities that increase traction on the patellar tendon. This stress leads to micro-avulsions of the growth plate on the tibial tubercle where the patellar tendon inserts.

CLINICAL MANIFESTATIONS

History

Depending on the cause of the knee pain, patients may complain of swelling, erythema, limited range of motion, bruising, and decreased activity. If an injury caused the knee pain, the mechanism of injury (e.g., direct impact to lateral knee during full extension), occurrence of a "popping" sensation, degree of swelling, and ability to ambulate after the event are all relevant pieces of information. The sensation of an unstable knee (the feeling of giving way) suggests ligament damage. Locking of the knee is more consistent with a torn meniscus or bone fragment that becomes trapped. Further useful history includes recent trauma, initiation of new exercise regimen, duration of the knee pain, and any activities or positions which aggravate or alleviate the pain.

Sudden onset of severe knee pain and effusion in a middle-aged man without a history of trauma is most commonly due to gout. Often there is a previous history of a gout attack. Although patients with gout may have a fever, an elevated temperature with a swollen red joint is more consistent with septic arthritis. In younger individuals, gonorrhea is the most common infection and inquiring about genitourinary symptoms, such as a vaginal or penile discharge, is important.

Up to 10% of the population over age 65 suffer from symptomatic osteoarthritis of the knee. Obesity is a major risk factor. The pain is chronic, often starting in the anterior and medial portions of the knee but it can involve the whole knee joint. Mild stiffness in the morning is common, which usually loosens up on moving about. Prolonged standing or walking may precipitate or worsen symptoms.

Prolonged morning stiffness and pain that is worse in the morning, improves with motion, and is associated with systemic symptoms such as fever suggests an inflammatory arthritis. In rheumatoid arthritis, multiple symmetric joint involvement is the rule, although patients may develop pain only in the knee. Pain behind the kneecap that is worsened by standing up or climbing stairs is consistent with chondromalacia.

Physical Examination

Examination should be performed with the patient lying down in the supine position with both legs fully exposed. During general inspection asymmetry, bruising, bony deformities, effusions, and erythema of the knee should be noted. The feet and hips should be examined for abnormalities contributing to or causing the knee pain. A key part of the exam is to determine if the pain is intra-articular or extra-articular. Pain on both active and passive range of motion suggests an intra-articular problem, while pain on active but not passive motion of the joint suggests extra-articular disease. Palpating along the joint line and bony landmarks is followed by determining the degree of flexion and extension of both the healthy and injured knee. Pain with any segment of the exam provides clues as to which components of the knee may be injured. Varus and valgus stress while maneuvering the knee between full flexion and full extension are used to assess the medial and lateral collateral ligaments. Anterior to posterior laxity is assessed via the Lachman test. This maneuver is performed by flexing the knee at 20 to 30 degrees, holding the femur stable, and moving the tibia forwards and backwards. The degree of laxity is assessed by comparison with the healthy knee and determines the competency of the cruciate ligaments. The McMurray test is used to evaluate the meniscus. This test is performed with the knee fully flexed and the foot rotated outward to test medial meniscus and inward to test lateral meniscus. The knee is then fully extended while rotating the foot in the opposite direction. A painful "click" is considered a positive test and indicates a possible meniscal injury.

DIFFERENTIAL DIAGNOSIS

Common diagnoses of knee pain include ligamentous injuries, meniscal injuries, bursitis (patellar, anserine), fractures, patello-femoral dysfunction, Osgood-Schlatter's disease, iliotibial band fasciitis, Baker's cyst, osteoarthritis, rheumatoid or other inflammatory arthritis, gout, pseudogout, and septic arthritis.

DIAGNOSTIC APPROACH

Many patients can be diagnosed by history and physical exam alone. However, x-rays should be obtained in all patients who are thought to have a possible fracture. Magnetic resonance imaging (MRI) is used to diagnose rupture of the anterior cruciate ligament (ACL) and can often detect injury to the meniscus and collateral ligaments.

Laboratory testing may be helpful in evaluating patients with fever, rash or involvement of other joints. An elevated erythrocyte sedimentation rate can be a clue for a systemic process. A rheumatoid factor and an antinuclear antibody (ANA) can screen for rheumatoid arthritis and lupus. A complete blood cell count and uric acid level may also be helpful.

Acute isolated knee pain with an effusion should usually be evaluated with an arthrocentesis. The fluid should be sent for determination of cell count, glucose, gram stain, culture, and examination for crystals. Uric acid crystals (negatively biorefringent under polarized light) in the joint fluid are diagnostic of gout, while calcium pyrophosphate crystals (weakly positively biorefringent) are seen in pseudogout. A bloody aspirate following trauma suggests a significant injury to the knee, and the rare finding of fat globules indicate a fracture. Diagnostic arthroscopy may be helpful in patients with persistent pain despite x-ray and laboratory testing.

MANAGEMENT

Rest, nonsteroidal anti-inflammatory medications (NSAIDs) or acetaminophen are sufficient to manage the majority of patients with knee pain. In patients with mild to moderate degenerative joint disease (DJD), weight loss, judicious use of exercise and rest, physical therapy and medications control most symptoms. In severe DJD, unresponsive to conservative therapy, referral to an orthopedist for possible arthroscopy or surgery is indicated.

Following a knee injury, acute pain usually responds to rest, ice, and NSAIDs. A knee immobilizer may provide support, reduce pain by restricting mobility, and prevent further injury. If there is suspicion of a more severe injury such as a meniscus or ligament tear, orthopedic referral is appropriate.

Treatment of patellofemoral syndrome is geared towards the perceived causes. In patients with overpronation, orthotics are often beneficial. Physical therapy may help strengthen quadriceps muscles and stretch a tight iliotibial band. Rest, non-impact activities, ice, and NSAIDs all benefit patients who deal with this disorder. Taping and knee braces may benefit those patients with obvious lateral subluxation. Rarely, surgery (i.e. iliotibial band release) may be an option for patients refractory to medical management.

NSAIDs usually improve the pain of inflammatory arthritis. Most primary care physicians will co-manage an individual with rheumatoid arthritis along with a rheumatologist, especially in those patients requiring disease-modifying medications (e.g., methotrexate). Joint infection is a medical emergency and merits hospitalization, drainage, and intravenous antibiotics. Gout usually responds to NSAIDs. Patient with multiple attacks may benefit from prophylactic therapy with allopurinol, probenecid, or colchicine. Colchicine or prednisone may be used for acute attacks in patients unable to take NSAIDs.

Treatment of Osgood-Schlatter's disease and soft tissue inflammatory conditions such as patellar tendonitis usually respond to treatment consisting of relative rest from activities that exacerbate the pain, application of ice, occasional use of NSAIDs, and range of motion and stretching exercises. Rarely, referral for surgical consultation and care is necessary.

A tear of the anterior cruciate ligament (ACL) is a more serious injury with long-term implications. Patients often report a "popping" sensation inside the knee related to a sudden change in direction or direct trauma. Patients will experience immediate pain and within a few hours a significant effusion typically develops. In patients who want to remain active, surgical reconstruction is the preferred therapy. However, in older, less active patients, physical therapy and use of a brace may suffice.

Tears of the medial and lateral meniscus typically result from a twisting motion, but a clear event causing the injury may not always occur. Treatment of meniscal tears is symptomatic with rest, ice, compression, and elevation. Many patients with persistent symptoms benefit from arthroscopic knee surgery to remove the torn piece, thus allowing for smooth tracking between the articulated surfaces.

◆ KEY POINTS ◆

1. The feeling of the knee giving way suggests ligament damage. Locking of the knee is more consistent with a torn meniscus or bone fragment that becomes trapped.

2. Sudden onset of severe knee pain and effusion in a middle-aged man in the absence of trauma is most commonly due to gout.

3. Up to 10% of the population over age 65 suffers from symptomatic osteoarthritis of the knee. X-rays should be obtained in all patients who are thought to have a possible fracture. Acute isolated knee pain with an effusion should usually be evaluated with an arthrocentesis.

4. Magnetic resonance imaging (MRI) is used to diagnose rupture of the anterior cruciate ligament (ACL) and can often detect injury to the meniscus and collateral ligaments.

5. A knee injury usually responds to rest, ice, and NSAIDs. A knee immobilizer may provide support, reduce pain by restricting mobility, and prevent further injury.

6. NSAIDs usually improve the pain of inflammatory arthritis.

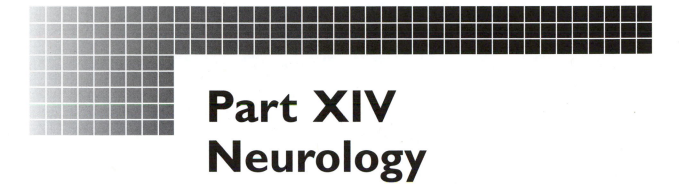

Part XIV
Neurology

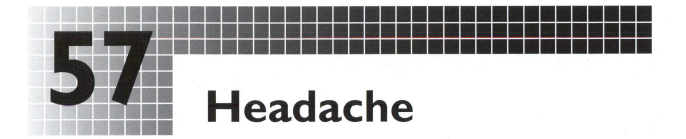

Headache

More than 90% of adults will experience headaches over a one-year period and over 15% of these will consult their physician because of it. Although the majority of headaches seen in the outpatient setting are benign, it is important to remember that in rare instances headache may be secondary to a life-threatening illness.

PATHOPHYSIOLOGY

Headache pain originates in either intracranial or extracranial structures. Intracranial pain sensitive structures include the trigeminal, glossopharyngeal, vagus and the first three cervical nerves. Additionally, the dura, arteries and the venous sinuses but not the brain parenchyma are pain sensitive. Disease processes that cause pressure or inflammation of pain sensitive structures, distention of blood vessels, and obstruction of CSF fluid can cause pain. For example, a mass lesion can cause headache pain by displacing a pain sensitive structure while a ruptured aneurysm can inflame the meninges.

The neurogenic inflammatory hypothesis is the most accepted theory explaining migraine headache. This theory views migraine as a primary neuronal event with subsequent changes resulting from the activity of neurotransmitters on the vasculature and the blood flow. Neuropeptides trigger the release of kinins and bioactive substances that lead to more inflammation and vasodilation. Serotonin receptors are believed to be an important part of this process, which explains why serotonin analogs or agonists benefit patients with migraine.

Extracranial sources of headache pain include the skin, muscles, blood vessels, periosteum of the skull, sinuses, and teeth. Clinical problems affecting the eyes, sinuses, C-spine, trimandibular joint, and cranial nerves can all cause headache pain.

Tension headaches traditionally are thought to originate from scalp muscles. However, myographic recordings show that many, but not all, individuals with tension headaches have muscle contraction. Recent studies suggest that migraine and tension headaches may have similar pathophysiologic mechanisms but with different expression of symptoms. This overlap explains why some patients with tension headaches experience migraine-like symptoms.

CLINICAL MANIFESTATIONS

History

The history provides the most useful information and the physical exam helps exclude organic pathology. Relevant history includes location (unilateral vs. bilateral), severity (worst headache of life), quality (throbbing, squeezing), duration, frequency, associated neurological symptoms, aggravating or alleviating factors (foods, rest, menstruation, OTC medications), and associated symptoms (nausea, emesis, fever, visual changes). Other relevant information includes whether the headache awakens the patient from sleep and caffeine intake since caffeine withdrawal is a known cause of headaches. Foods such as chocolate, alcohol, nuts, and aged cheese may trigger migraines. Reviewing medications is important because a number of drugs such as indomethacin, nifedipine, cimetidine, captopril, nitrates, and oral contraceptives can trigger headaches.

Migraine headaches typically start between ages 15 and 45 years. Seventy-five percent occur in females. Migraine headaches are usually severe, unilateral, throbbing, and often accompanied by nausea, vomiting and photo- or phonophobia. Migraines last between 4 and 72 hours and may be accompanied by an aura. A migraine associated with an aura is called a classic migraine whereas headaches without an aura are labeled common migraines. Auras include flashing lights, shimmering lines, and blind spots. Some individuals may experience paresthesias, numbness, strange odors, and speech disturbances. A family history of migraine is present in over 80% of those who suffer from migraines and is a useful diagnostic criterion. Common triggers include lack of or irregular sleep, hunger, alcohol, certain foods, humidity, and emotional stress.

Tension headache pain is typically of mild to moderate intensity and located in the bilateral occipital-frontal areas. The headache is usually described as dull or band-like, often lasts for hours, and is often associated with stress. Tension headaches usually do not awaken patients from sleep and are not generally associated with vomiting or neurological symptoms.

Cluster headaches are severe, unilateral, localized to the periorbital/temporal area, and are usually accompanied by one of the following symptoms: lacrimation, rhinorrhea, ptosis, miosis, nasal congestion, and eyelid edema. These headaches occur in "clusters" with one to eight daily attacks, lasting 15 to 90 minutes for a period of four to six weeks. These episodes are then followed by pain-free intervals lasting three to six months. Cluster headaches are most common in middle-aged men who smoke but overall are much less frequent than tension or migraine headaches.

New onset headaches merit close attention. A subarachnoid hemorrhage should be considered in any patient who does not usually have headaches and presents with the worst headache of their life. An acute headache with ataxia, profuse nausea and vomiting is consistent with a cerebral hemorrhage. Fever with frontal or maxillary tenderness is suggestive of acute sinusitis.

Physical Examination

Physical exam should include vital signs, funduscopic and cardiovascular assessment, palpation of the head and neck, and a thorough neurological evaluation. A neurological examination is essential because a neurological deficit is an important sign for intracranial pathology. Patients with muscle contraction headaches may demonstrate muscle tightness or trigger points over the posterior occiput in several areas. Temporal artery tenderness in an elderly patient raises the possibility of temporal arteritis, while sinus tenderness, congestion and fever is most consistent with sinusitis. Headache accompanied by a stiff neck may indicate a subarachnoid hemorrhage or meningitis. Headache with abnormal physical signs such as a high blood pressure, a focal neurological deficit, or papilledema may indicate the presence of a mass lesion or malignant hypertension.

DIFFERENTIAL DIAGNOSIS

Headaches may be classified as primary or secondary. Primary headaches have no underlying organic disease and include migraine, tension, and cluster headaches. Secondary headaches result from an underlying disorder such as intracranial mass, infection, CVA, head trauma, drug withdrawal, or metabolic disorders (Box 57–1 gives a complete list). Although primary headaches are not life threatening, they are often very debilitating to patients.

DIAGNOSTIC EVALUATION

The objectives when evaluating a headache patient are to 1) identify patients with life-threatening conditions, 2) identify those with secondary headaches such as sinusitis, and 3) to provide symptom relief to those with primary headache.

Patients presenting with acute onset of severe headache, especially in the presence of meningeal signs, high fever, or evidence of increased intracranial pressure need urgent evaluation. A CT scan is helpful in detecting a subarachnoid hemorrhage (SAH) or intracerebral bleed. If the CT scan is negative when evaluating for a SAH, a lumbar puncture is indicated since a CT will be normal in one out of every ten of those with SAH. A lumbar puncture can also detect the presence of significant disease in patients with meningeal signs and

---

BOX 57–1

Causes of Secondary Headaches

- subarachnoid hemorrhage (SAH)
- intracranial mass
- post-traumatic
- infection
- glaucoma
- sinus disease
- drug withdrawal
- benign intracranial hypertension (pseudotumor cerebri)
- hypoxia
- hypercapnia
- post lumbar puncture
- neuralgias

BOX 57–2

Indications for Neuroimaging

- Headache of recent onset (<6 months)
- Headache beginning after 50 years of age
- Worsening headaches
- Headache that does not fit primary headache pattern
- Associated seizure
- Focal neurological signs or symptoms
- Personality change
- Severe headaches unresponsive to therapy
- History of significant trauma
- New headache in a cancer patient

---

provide fluid for identifying the cause of meningitis. A lumbar puncture is contraindicated when increased intracranial pressure is suspected due to risk of brainstem herniation.

In general, blood tests play a limited role when evaluating headache patients. A CBC may be helpful in assessing a patient with suspected meningitis and a normal ESR is helpful for ruling out temporal arteritis.

The role of CT and MRI scans in patients with chronic headaches is controversial. The probability of finding a significant abnormality in a patient with a history of chronic headaches and a normal physical examination is extremely low. However imaging may still be helpful in certain instances such as when there is a change in symptoms associated with chronic headaches. Box 57–2 lists indications for neuroimaging.

MANAGEMENT

Treatment for tension headaches includes avoidance or improved management of the stress commonly associated with these headaches. Biofeedback, relaxation, and deep-breathing exercises in a quiet environment are often effective. In addition, non-narcotic analgesics such as NSAIDs (e.g., ibuprofen 400–600 mg tid) or acetaminophen (650 mg qid) will usually alleviate symptoms and are therapeutic mainstays. Low doses of antidepressants such as amitriptyline (10–75 mg po qd) can be effective for reducing the number and severity of chronic tension headaches. If these measures fail to improve the headache significantly or if it is associated with neurological symptoms, the diagnosis of tension headache should be questioned and further evaluation is warranted.

Primary treatment of migraine headaches includes avoiding headache triggers, withdrawal from stressful environments (often into a dark, quiet bedroom, placing a cool washcloth to the forehead), and rest. Serotonin receptor agonists are available in a variety of forms and are the primary medications used to abort an attack. The triptans are the most commonly used abortive agents. Triptans are available as injections, nasal sprays, and tablets and may be given in multiple doses until the patient's symptoms resolve. Due to vasoconstrictive properties, the triptans are contraindicated in patients with CAD, PVD, and uncontrolled hypertension.

Ergotamine is another serotonin receptor agonist. It is available as an oral, sublingual, or suppository medication and is maximally effective when given early in the course of a migraine. Because it has vasoconstrictive properties, ergotamine is contraindicated in patients with coronary artery disease or peripheral vascular disease.

Depending on patients' symptoms, NSAIDs, acetaminophen, anti-emetics, narcotics, and caffeine are frequently prescribed. Physicians must use caution when using mild analgesics alone to treat migraines as their limited duration of effectiveness may result in "rebound" symptoms. As a result, patients may take higher than recommended doses. In patients who suffer from migraines more than two times per week, beta-blockers, calcium channel blockers, anti-depressants, and anti-seizure medications are often effective prophylactic therapy. Prophylactic therapy is selected according to patient's age and co-morbidities.

Patients with cluster headaches should be counseled to avoid known precipitants. Breathing 100% oxygen at 7–10 L/min for 10 to 15 minutes via a tight-fitting mask may abort an acute attack. If the patient has no cardiac risk factors, Sumatriptan 6 mg SC with an additional 6 mg given one hour later is helpful. Alternately, dihydro-ergotamine mesylate 1 mg IM or IV may improve symptoms. Prednisone starting with 60–80 mg/day followed by a 2 to 4 week taper has been shown to shorten the duration of episodes and diminish the frequency and intensity of symptoms. Other medications commonly used to treat or prevent cluster headache include verapamil, NSAIDs, propranolol, amitriptyline, and lithium. Patients in whom the above therapies do not help may benefit from referral to a neurologist or major headache center.

Temporal arteritis needs to be considered in older patients who have pain upon palpation of the temporal artery. Although these patients often have an elevated ESR, definitive diagnosis requires biopsy of the temporal artery. Patients with temporal arteritis need to be started on steroids promptly as a delay in treatment may result in blindness.

◆ KEY POINTS ◆

1. Headache pain originates in either intracranial or extracranial structures. Intracranial pain sensitive structures include the trigeminal, glossopharyngeal, vagus and the first three cervical nerves.

2. The neurogenic inflammatory hypothesis is the most accepted theory explaining migraine headache. This theory views migraine as a primary neuronal event with subsequent changes resulting from the activity of neurotransmitters on the vasculature and the blood flow.

3. Headache accompanied by a stiff neck may indicate a subarachnoid hemorrhage or meningitis.

4. The objectives when evaluating a headache patient are to 1) identify patients with life-threatening conditions; 2) identify those with secondary headaches such as sinusitis; and 3) to provide symptom relief to those with primary headache.

5. Serotonin receptor agonists are available in a variety of forms and are the primary medications used to abort a migraine headache.

6. Temporal arteritis needs to be considered in older patients who have pain upon palpation of the temporal artery.

Dementia

Dementia is a progressive decline in memory accompanied by a loss of intellectual capabilities severe enough to interfere with social or occupational function. In addition to memory loss, cognitive impairment can affect language, judgment, cognition, visual-spatial skills and personality.

The prevalence of dementia increases significantly with age, with roughly 1% affected by age 60 and almost 50% after the age of 85. Given that by the year 2030 nearly 20% of the population will be over the age of 65, the societal burden of dementia will become an even greater health care concern in the future. Although the majority of cases of dementia are irreversible, primary care doctors must be aware of the reversible causes, methods of diagnosing the various causes of dementia, and treatment options for both the patients and their families.

PATHOPHYSIOLOGY

Alzheimer's disease (AD) is the most common cause of dementia and accounts for over half of all cases. Post-mortem analysis of patients with Alzheimer's disease demonstrates brain atrophy, enlarged ventricles, and minimal evidence of vascular disease. Histological findings include intracellular neurofibrillary tangles comprised of tau proteins and extra cellular plaques consisting of beta-amyloid protein. This leads to neuronal loss and subsequent disturbances in the cholinergic system, which accounts for the progressive cognitive decline. Although there is an autosomal dominant form of the disease involving the gene for the amyloid protein, most cases are sporadic. Risk factors for Alzheimer's disease include advanced age, female gender, and a family history of the disease. The apolipoprotein, APO-E4, on chromosome 19 is associated with an increased risk for AD. However testing for APO-E4 is neither sensitive nor specific enough to justify using it as a screening test.

Vascular dementia is the second most common cause of dementia and results from tissue damage due to cerebral ischemia and hypoxia. Patients with hypertension, diabetes, a history of smoking and known arterial disease are at risk. Multi-infarct dementia due to a series of small-vessel infarctions known as lacunar strokes is one type of vascular dementia. The multiple infarcts typically cause patients to experience discrete episodes of worsening cognition that occur in a step-wise manner. Especially in older patients, Alzheimer's disease and vascular dementia may occur together.

Severely depressed patients may present with cognitive slowing and poor memory, a condition termed pseudodementia, which mimics dementia. These individuals usually improve once treatment is initiated. Depression is also common in patients with an underlying dementia, particularly early in the course of the disease.

Lewy body dementia is characterized by the presence of Lewy bodies, which are intracytoplasmic inclusions, and by decreased neuronal density in the hippocampus, amygdala, cortex, and other portions of the brain. Patients with Lewy body dementia have a rapid clinical decline, visual hallucinations, episodic delirium, and extrapyramidal motor signs.

Space-occupying lesions such as subdural hematoma and tumor, infections such as syphilis and HIV, and other neurological disorders such as multiple sclerosis, Parkinson's disease, and Huntington's disease may disrupt neural pathways involved with cognition and memory. Normal pressure hydrocephalus is the result of diminished absorption of cerebrospinal fluid, which compresses neural pathways resulting in ataxia, incontinence, and dementia. Medical disorders such as hypothyroidism, hypercalcemia, vitamin B12 or folate deficiency, and acute intoxication can lead to memory impairment. Medications such as sedatives, opiates, anti-hypertensives, and neuroleptics may cause or exacerbate dementia.

CLINICAL MANIFESTATIONS

History

Because most patients with dementia lack objective insight into their condition, the history is often best obtained through family members, friends, and caregivers. Dementia may also be suspected during a routine evaluation if a patient has difficulty recalling medications, recent events, and medical history. Questions should be asked about patient orientation, episodes of forgetfulness, activities of daily living, and job duties. Examples include instances of patients getting lost, forgetting words, names, or recipes, neglecting personal hygiene, and not knowing common facts such as address and current events. Episodes of social withdrawal, frustration with emotional outbursts, and difficulty driving are common in patients with Alzheimer's disease and should be ascertained. The time course of symptoms (e.g., abrupt versus gradual), duration, and course (e.g., continuous, fluctuating, or stepwise), are helpful in determining the type of dementia.

Past surgical and medical history should focus on episodes of head trauma, previous vascular surgery, meningitis, and other neurological diseases. A family history of a first-degree relative with dementia and being female increase the risk for dementia.

All medications need to be reviewed and alcohol intake and nutritional adequacy determined. Sexual history determines risk for HIV and syphilis. Review of systems should focus on signs of depression, thyroid disorder, and other neurological disorders.

Physical Examination

The physical examination should include mental status, neurological examination, and a general examination aimed at identifying illness, which may be contributing to the patient's cognitive decline. A general assessment also provides information about hygiene, nutritional status, and attentiveness. The physical can also identify problems such as hearing or vision loss and orthopedic problems that may be interfering with activities of daily living.

Mini-Mental State Examination (MMSE) is a standardized test that is useful in determining the presence of dementia. Specifically, MMSE provides insight into patient orientation, recall, attention, language ability, visual spatial ability, and executive functioning. The score can be corrected for the level of education and followed over time.

Complete neurological exam can detect abnormalities suggesting prior stroke, a mass, or evidence of Parkinson's disease. Abstract reasoning can be assessed via asking the meaning of phrases such as, "people in glass houses should not throw stones." Psychiatric assessment determines the presence of depression and other psychiatric disorders.

DIFFERENTIAL DIAGNOSIS

Box 58–1 lists causes of dementia. AD accounts for about 50% of cases and about 15% have a vascular dementia. Other patients may have a mixed dementia which is caused by a combination of AD and vascular disease. Dementia must also be distinguished from other causes of mental confusion such as depression and delirium.

Delirium, referred to as an acute confusional state, affects memory and cognition. Delirium typically occurs over hours to days and is often reversible, associated with a clouding of consciousness and disruption of the sleep cycle. Patients with dementia are at increased risk of developing delirium. Acute mental status changes merit ruling out a toxic reaction to medicine, and physical illnesses such as infection, dehydration,

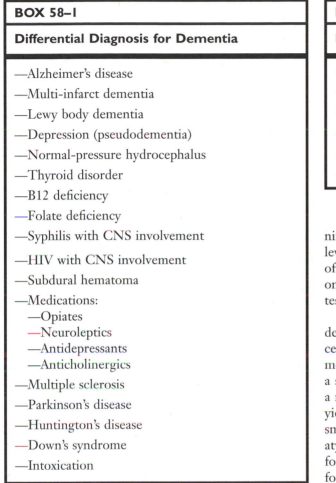

BOX 58–1

Differential Diagnosis for Dementia

—Alzheimer's disease
—Multi-infarct dementia
—Lewy body dementia
—Depression (pseudodementia)
—Normal-pressure hydrocephalus
—Thyroid disorder
—B12 deficiency
—Folate deficiency
—Syphilis with CNS involvement
—HIV with CNS involvement
—Subdural hematoma
—Medications:
  —Opiates
  —Neuroleptics
  —Antidepressants
  —Anticholinergics
—Multiple sclerosis
—Parkinson's disease
—Huntington's disease
—Down's syndrome
—Intoxication

BOX 58–2

Indications for Neuroimaging

• Recent onset dementia
• Rapid progression
• History of head trauma
• Younger age
• Urinary incontinence and gait disorders
• Focal abnormalities on neurological examination

nine, liver function tests, TSH, vitamin B12 and folate levels, and urinalysis. Hearing and vision screening are often useful. A chest x-ray and EKG are commonly recommended and if the patient has risk factors, HIV testing is indicated.

There is controversy about whether all patients with dementia should have some type of neuro-imaging procedure such as a CT or MRI. Some authorities recommend testing all patients to rule out conditions such as a subdural hematoma, normal pressure hydrocephalus, a mass lesion or to detect vascular dementia. Since the yield for finding conditions that change management is small, others advocate limiting imaging to those with atypical presentations. Box 58–2 lists some indications for imaging. A lumbar puncture is useful in evaluating for vasculitis, CNS infection, and multiple sclerosis and may improve symptoms in those with normal-pressure hydrocephalus. Formal neuropsychological testing determines more precisely the extent of cognitive impairment and may be useful in patients with atypical deficits or only mild cognitive decline.

hypoxia, electrolyte imbalance, anemia, and hepatic failure. Depression may mimic dementia. Typically depression symptoms precede memory loss and the patient appears apathetic.

DIAGNOSTIC EVALUATION

The diagnostic evaluation should focus on recognizing potentially treatable causes of dementia and identifying treatable co-existing illnesses that may be contributing to impaired cognition. History, physical, and laboratory testing to rule out conditions that mimic AD identify most patients with AD. Appropriate tests include a complete blood count, sedimentation rate, serum electrolytes, calcium, albumin, blood urea nitrogen, creati-

MANAGEMENT

Patients found to have reversible causes of dementia should receive prompt and appropriate treatment. For example, those with depression should be started on antidepressants and re-evaluated for cognitive improvement. However, because dementia is most often irreversible, the focus is to maintain quality of life and maximize function. Patients and their caregivers should be educated about creating a safe, familiar and nurturing environment for the patient, learning how to manage behavioral problems, and optimally treating comorbid conditions that may exacerbate the patient's cognitive decline. Psychoactive drugs such as phenothiazines (e.g., haloperidol, resperidone), and anticonvulsants are occasionally needed to control disruptive behavior. These medications should be used cautiously with careful dosage titration to avoid worsening a patient's confusion.

Patients with multi-infarct dementia should have optimal control of hypertension, diabetes, hyperlipidemia, and should stop smoking. If not contraindicated, they should receive anti-platelet medications such as aspirin or plavix. Serial lumbar punctures or ventricular shunt placement may provide benefit for patients with normal-pressure hydrocephalus. Medications thought to be contributing to or exacerbating the dementia should be changed or discontinued.

Patients with suspected Alzheimer's disease may benefit from the use of reversible acetylcholinesterase inhibitors. Tacrine (Cognex) or donepezil (Aricept) appear to slow the progression of AD. Caregivers of those with Alzheimer's need education regarding home safety, long-term care options, and the importance of a living will. Caregivers may also benefit from joining support groups, since they are at high risk for burnout.

◆ KEY POINTS ◆

1. Dementia is a progressive decline in memory and a loss of intellectual capabilities severe enough to interfere with social or occupational function. In addition to memory loss, cognitive impairment can affect language, judgment, cognition, visual-spatial skills and personality.

2. Multi-infarct dementia due to a series of small-vessel infarctions known as lacunar strokes is one type of vascular dementia. The multiple infarcts typically cause patients to experience discrete episodes of worsening cognition, which occur in a step-like manner.

3. Most patients with AD are diagnosed by history, physical, and laboratory testing to rule out conditions that mimic AD. Appropriate tests include a complete blood count, sedimentation rate, serum electrolytes, calcium, albumin, blood urea nitrogen, creatinine, liver function tests, TSH, vitamin B12 and folate levels, and urinalysis.

4. Patients with suspected Alzheimer's disease may benefit from the use of reversible acetylcholinesterase inhibitors.

59 Vertigo

Vertigo is a sensation of movement experienced by the patient due to disease in the central or peripheral vestibular system.

PATHOPHYSIOLOGY

Patients that experience true vertigo have a problem affecting either the peripheral or central vestibular systems. The peripheral vestibular apparatus is located bilaterally in the semicircular canals. Peripherally, inflammation, stimulation or destruction of the hair cells of the eighth cranial nerve may cause vertigo. For example, in benign positional vertigo, particulate matter or otoliths may form in the semicircular canal (analogous to renal stone formation). When these otoliths become dislodged and stimulate the sensory hair cells in the semicircular canals, vertigo results. In acute labyrinthitis or vestibular neuronitis, viral infection of the semicircular apparatus causes vestibular dysfunction and vertigo. Meniere's disease, a disease of undetermined etiology, occurs when endolymphatic hydrops results in increased pressure within the semicircular canals and damage to the sensory hair cells. Finally, direct damage to the eighth cranial nerve may result from ototoxic medications or from an acoustic neuroma. An acoustic neuroma is a tumor (schwannoma) of the eighth cranial nerve that will gradually grow and compress the eighth cranial nerve and eventually the brainstem.

Vascular insufficiency, demyelination or medications may affect the brainstem vestibular pathways. Centrally, the vestibular pathways are located in the brainstem and communicate and allow coordination of position with the cerebellum and cerebral cortex. Typically, patients with central vertigo will have other brainstem or cranial nerve findings in association with the vertigo. Vertigo may rarely occur in association with migraine as a result of vascular spasm in the vertebrobasilar artery system. Multiple sclerosis is a demyelinating disease that may affect the brainstem and disrupt the vestibular pathways. Finally, medications, such as phenytoin, may affect the brainstem nuclei and cause vertigo.

CLINICAL MANIFESTATIONS

History

The patient's description of the symptoms helps distinguish vertigo from dizziness. True vertigo is suggested when the patient uses terms such as spinning, weaving or rocking to describe the sensation they are experiencing. Vertigo is commonly associated with head movements, can occur in the supine or upright position and is often accompanied by nausea and vomiting. Symptoms that occur only in association with change in position from the supine to upright positions suggest another etiology, such as dehydration or anemia.

Benign positional vertigo (BPV) generally occurs as an isolated symptom and is short-lived, recurrent and associated with particular head movements. Vertigo, tinnitus and hearing loss are the cardinal features of Meniere's disease. The vertigo and hearing loss are initially fluctuating in nature. The vertigo may last from 30 minutes to 12 hours. Untreated the hearing loss may become permanent.

The presence of other cranial nerve symptoms, cerebral, or cerebellar neurological symptoms suggests vertebrobasilar insufficiency, neoplasm, multiple sclerosis or acoustic neuroma as a cause. Vertebrobasilar insufficiency may present acutely as a transient ischemic attack or stroke. Vertigo from multiple sclerosis may present as a flare of the underlying disease. Acoustic neuromas generally have an insidious onset. Vertigo in association with a viral illness is termed vestibular neuronitis and when accompanied by hearing loss is called labyrinthitis. Vertigo in association with a viral illness generally resolves in 2 to 10 days.

Past medical history should note prior occurrence of similar symptoms, the presence of other medical diseases, and medication use. Benign positional vertigo recurs in up to 30% of patients in the 2 to 3 years following an episode. Multiple sclerosis patients may have symptoms that wax and wane with disease activity, but typically have other symptoms in association with vertigo. Hypertensive patients and those who smoke are at risk for atherosclerotic disease, which may suggest vertebrobasilar insufficiency as a cause. Medication use may reveal a cause for vertigo. Loop diuretics and aminoglycoside antibiotics are drugs associated with vertigo from eighth cranial nerve damage. Diuretics and antihypertensive medications may lead to orthostatic symptoms through volume depletion or blood pressure lowering effects. High dose salicylates may also cause vertigo.

Physical Examination

The physical examination should include assessment of orthostatic blood pressure and pulse as well as cardiovascular, ear and neurological examinations. Carotid bruits should be noted. The neurological examination should include a hearing assessment and an examination of the cranial nerves. The presence and direction of nystagmus should be noted. Bi-directional or vertical nystagmus suggests a brainstem origin for the vertigo. Provocative maneuvers for the symptoms should be included in the examination. For example, true vertigo will be brought on by head movement and by the Barany maneuver. During the Barany maneuver the patient is seated with the head turned to the right and is quickly lowered to the supine position with the head over the edge of the exam table 30 degrees below horizontal. The test is then repeated with the head turned to the left. The test is positive if symptoms are reproduced. Nystagmus is also typically seen during this maneuver. Orthostatic positional changes that bring on symptoms suggest dehydration, anemia, or cardiac causes. Symptoms brought on by hyperventilation suggest anxiety or other psychogenic causes.

DIFFERENTIAL DIAGNOSIS

The differential diagnosis for vertigo includes the many different diseases that cause dizziness. True vertigo is due to either central or peripheral vestibular disease and has a narrower differential diagnosis. In assessing for central versus peripheral causes for vertigo, important distinguishing features are the presence of isolated vertigo with or without hearing loss, which suggests peripheral disease, and associated brainstem or other neurological symptoms, which suggest a central disease (Box 59–1).

BOX 59–1

Differential Diagnosis for Vertigo

Peripheral Vestibular Disease
Benign positional vertigo
Acute labyrinthitis
Vestibular neuronitis
Meniere's disease
Acoustic neuroma

Central Vestibular Disease
Vertebrobasilar insufficiency
Multiple sclerosis
Neoplasm

Other Medical Diseases
Cerebellar disease (e.g., degeneration, infarcts)
Peripheral neuropathy (e.g., diabetic)
Ophthalmologic disease (e.g., cataracts, macular degeneration)
Hypoglycemia
Psychiatric disease (e.g., panic disorder, anxiety)

DIAGNOSTIC APPROACH

The history and physical examination directs any further evaluation and the treatment approach. For those patients in whom the diagnosis is unclear or if it is uncertain whether the vertigo is central or peripheral, then further testing with electronystagmography and audiometry may be helpful. Audiometry is useful for diagnosing Meniere's disease (low frequency hearing loss) and may suggest the need for further evaluation for acoustic neuroma (asymmetric hearing loss).

Additional testing that may be helpful in identifying central causes for vertigo and to identify acoustic neuromas include magnetic resonance imaging (MRI) and brainstem auditory evoked response (BAER) testing. MRI may reveal scattered areas of demyelination, suggesting multiple sclerosis or may show evidence of prior stroke, suggesting vertebrobasilar insufficiency. BAER testing is able to distinguish cochlear from retrocochlear hearing loss, thus helping to distinguish peripheral from more central disease. To identify posterior circulation atherosclerotic disease, magnetic resonance angiography can be performed.

MANAGEMENT

Peripheral causes for vertigo are usually acute in nature and self-limited although empiric therapy often helps control symptoms. Follow-up to assure resolution of symptoms and to assess the need for further work-up should be part of the care provided.

The Epley maneuver for BPV is performed by rotating the patients through a series of positions in an attempt to relocate the debris in the semicircular canal into the vestibule of the labyrinth. It is reported to have a success rate approaching 80%. Vestibular exercises where a patient performs a Barany maneuver to reproduce their symptoms and holds the position until the symptoms are extinguished are also useful. This exercise is repeated several times daily and the time to extinction of symptoms should progressively get shorter the more the exercise is performed. Medications used to treat labyrinthitis, vestibular neuronitis, and benign positional vertigo include meclizine, dimenhydrinate, antiemetics and benzodiazepines. These medications may help in alleviating symptoms but may cause drowsiness as their primary side effect. Acoustic neuroma is managed surgically and requires referral to an otolaryngologist.

Meniere's disease is a chronic disease that may potentially lead to permanent hearing loss. These patients require chronic therapy directed at the underlying disease, and not just symptomatic therapy. Diuretics, in particular acetazolamide or hydrochlorothiazide have been found to be helpful in managing Meniere's disease. Salt restriction is also considered an important adjunct to the use of diuretics. Vertigo associated with central vestibular disease is also often chronic in nature. Vestibular exercises and gait training may be beneficial to these patients along with therapy directed at the underlying disease. For example, in patients with vertebrobasilar disease blood pressure should be controlled, lipid levels should be lowered and aspirin or coumadin should be prescribed to help prevent additional events.

◆ KEY POINTS ◆

1. True vertigo occurs due to disease in the central or peripheral vestibular system.

2. Benign positional vertigo generally occurs as an isolated symptom and the vertigo is short-lived, recurrent and associated with particular head movements.

3. Vertigo, tinnitus and hearing loss are the cardinal features of Meniere's disease. The vertigo and hearing loss are initially fluctuating in nature.

4. In assessing for central versus peripheral causes for vertigo, important distinguishing features are the presence of isolated vertigo with or without hearing loss, which suggests peripheral disease, and associated brainstem or other neurological symptoms, which suggest a central disease.

5. Peripheral causes for vertigo are usually acute in nature and self-limited.

6. Medications used to treat labyrinthitis, vestibular neuronitis, and benign positional vertigo include meclizine, dimenhydrinate, antiemetics and benzodiazepines.

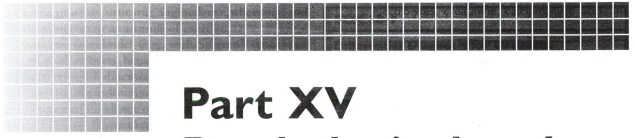

Part XV
Psychological and
Behavioral Disorders

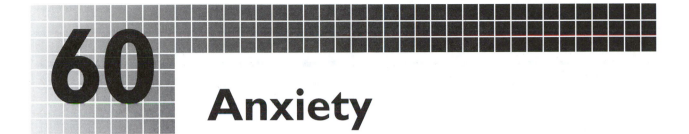

60 Anxiety

Anxiety is the experience of dread, foreboding, or panic, accompanied by a variety of physical symptoms. The distress can be both physical and psychological. It is a very common complaint and accounts for approximately 11% of all visits to a primary care physician. Box 60–1 lists brief definitions for the different types of anxiety disorders. Anxiety may also be a symptom of other psychological diseases, intoxication or withdrawal, or a symptom of a medical illness.

PATHOPHYSIOLOGY

Anxiety is a normal response to many situations. Pathological anxiety results when the anxiety occurs in the absence of appropriate stimulus or is of excessive duration and intensity. Both behavioral and biological theories exist for anxiety disorders. Biological theories implicate the involvement of several different monoamine and neuropeptide neurotransmitters. The locus caeruleus, which is the main central nervous system nucleus responsible for distributing norepinephrine throughout the brain, exhibits increased activity and is implicated in the pathology of some anxiety disorders. The inhibitory neurotransmitter, gamma-aminobutyric acid, may serve as an anxiolytic function in the nervous system.

CLINICAL MANIFESTATIONS

History

The history is an essential element of the evaluation. Inquiring about stresses, fears, substance use, and precipitating factors is important. Psychological complaints include apprehension, agitation, poor concentration, feeling on edge, difficulty sleeping, and heightened arousal. Physical symptoms are usually related to increased automatic activity. Typically, symptoms involve the cardiopulmonary system, gastrointestinal system, urinary system, and neurological system. Dyspnea, dizziness, palpitations, sweating, nausea, abdominal pain, diarrhea, frequent urination, sweaty palms, and difficulty swallowing are common symptoms. Anxiety may also cause heightened motor tension with trembling, twitching, muscle spasms, and easy fatigability.

Physical Examination

A physical examination is helpful to detect medical illness that may present as anxiety. For example, an enlarged thyroid or irregular heart rhythm may suggest an underlying organic etiology.

BOX 60–1

Glossary of Terms

Generalized Anxiety:
Excessive or unrealistic worry over at least two issues for more than six months.

Panic Disorder:
Episodic periods of intense fear or apprehension accompanied by at least four somatic complaints: (e.g., diaphoresis, dyspnea, dizziness, or flushing), accompanied by behavior changes because of unrealistic and persistent worry.

Phobia:
Persistent or irrational fear of a specific object, activity, or situation.

Obsessive-Compulsive Disorder:
Intrusive, unwanted thoughts (obsession); and repetitive behaviors performed in a ritualistic manner (compulsion).

Post-traumatic Syndrome:
Anxiety symptoms lasting at least one month that develop after an individual experiences a distressing event outside the normal human response (e.g., combat, natural catastrophe). There may be delayed onset and the patient may experience flashbacks.

Adjustment Disorder with Anxious Mood:
Anxiety develops as a maladaptive response to an identifiable stressor.

BOX 60–2

Medical Conditions That May Mimic Anxiety

Cardiopulmonary:
  Arrhythmias
  Hypoxia
  Ischemic Heart Disease
  Mitral Valve Prolapse
  Pulmonary Edema
  Pulmonary Embolus
  Asthma
  Congestive Heart Failure

Neurological Diseases:
  Encephalopathies
  Temporal Lobe Epilepsy
  Primary Sleep Disorders
  Post-Concussion Syndrome

Endocrine:
  Hyperthyroidism
  Pheochromocytoma
  Hypoglycemia
  Hypocalcemia
  Hypercalcemia
  Cushing's Disease
  Carcinoid Syndrome

Stimulant Toxicity:
  Withdrawal Syndrome

Hematological Disorders:
  Anemia

DIFFERENTIAL DIAGNOSIS

In addition to anxiety disorders, similar symptoms can be seen in a wide variety of psychological and medical illnesses. Medications such as sympathomimetics (pseudoephedrine), antihistamines, bromocriptine, bronchodilators, and excessive caffeine may all cause anxiety-like symptoms. Neuroleptics (e.g., phenothiazines) may cause akathisia and anxiety while some antidepressants (e.g., SSRIs) may cause anxiety-like reactions. Drug or alcohol withdrawal is an important differential consideration. Stimulant abuse (e.g., cocaine, amphetamines) can cause agitation, irritability, and anxiety. Other psychiatric disorders that may have anxiety as a prominent component include depression, manic-depressive disease, alcoholism, psychosis, or grief reaction. Medical illnesses may present with signs and symptoms of anxiety. Box 60–2 lists some of the conditions that may present as anxiety.

DIAGNOSTIC APPROACH

The diagnostic goal for the anxious patient is to assess for medical causes and psychiatric illnesses. The focus should be first to consider any clinical conditions the patient currently has and to review all medications. Attention should be given to those disorders such as hyperthyroidism, arrhythmia, and drug withdrawal that are more common and often have anxiety as a prominent feature. Laboratory testing may not be necessary and should be focused by clinical findings. For example, pulmonary function testing may be indicated in patients with wheezing or a CBC in patients with pallor and dizziness.

MANAGEMENT

Treatment strategies for anxiety include psychotherapeutic and pharmacological interventions. The primary care provider can provide supportive counseling consisting of empathetic listening, meaningful reassurance, education, guidance, and encouragement. Understanding that a patient may not be able to identify the cause of their anxiety coupled with an empathetic willingness to listen may help alleviate symptoms. Education begins with informing the patient of the diagnosis and discussing the underlying problems and potential treatment. Discussing the patient's fears of serious illness and of "going crazy" may have a cathartic effect.

An important element of treatment is assessing the degree of anxiety. Severely affected patients merit referral to a psychiatrist or psychologist. Non-pharmacological treatment that has been found beneficial includes psychotherapy, behavioral therapy, relaxation techniques, reconditioning, and cognitive-behavior therapy. These therapies are often augmented and enhanced by use of anxiolytic medicines. The goal of medication is to help the patient resume function and to alleviate anxiety symptoms that interfere with the patient's life. Medications should generally be of limited duration and administered using a scheduled dose, rather than on a "PRN" basis. Fixed goals should be set, for example improved sleep or reduction of intrusive symptoms.

Benzodiazepines (BZD) are the most frequently used medications and are regarded as the anxiolytic medication of choice. Side effects include physical dependency, tolerance, sedation, and impaired memory. To avoid dependence, physicians should prescribe a fixed amount and remain aware of signs of misuse, such as lost prescriptions. The patient should be seen regularly and if symptoms are under control, chronic therapy should be discontinued by tapering doses over several weeks. Abrupt cessation can result in withdrawal symptoms or even seizures. Antidepressants, beta-blockers, buspirone, and neuroleptics are also used.

Serotonin selective reuptake inhibitors (SSRIs) are another first line therapeutic agent. They can benefit patients with panic disorder, general anxiety disorder, post-traumatic stress disorder, and OCD. SSRIs may take a few weeks to become effective, so a BZD may be prescribed concomitantly for immediate relief and then tapered as the SSRI takes effect. Tricyclic antidepressants and monoamine oxidase inhibitors are also effective. Buspirone is a non-benzodiazepine medication that has mild anxiolytic effects. It is non-addictive and has no withdrawal, thus making it a good choice for patients at risk of abuse.

Beta-blockers blunt some of the adrenergic symptoms such as palpitations, tremors, and tachycardia. They can help patients with panic attacks who suffer from cardiovascular symptoms and are useful for treating stage fright on an as-needed basis.

◆ KEY POINTS ◆

1. Anxiety is the experience of dread, foreboding, or panic, accompanied by a variety of body symptoms.

2. Pathological anxiety results when the anxiety occurs in the absence of appropriate stimulus or is of excessive duration and intensity.

3. Medications such as sympathomimetics (pseudoephedrine), antihistamines, bromocriptine, bronchodilators, and excessive caffeine may all cause anxiety-like symptoms.

4. Treatment strategies for anxiety include psychotherapeutic and pharmacological interventions.

5. Benzodiazepines (BZD) are the most frequently used medications and are regarded as the anxiolytic medication of choice. Side effects include physical dependency, tolerance, sedation, and impaired memory.

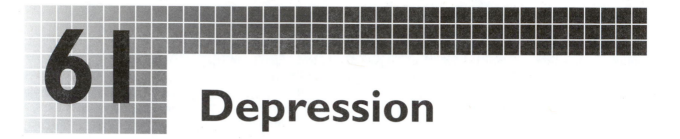

61 Depression

Feeling blue or sad is an appropriate response to a difficult situation. Clinical depression occurs if the reaction is more severe or prolonged than expected. Major depression is a mood disorder characterized by at least two weeks of depressed mood, a loss of interest or pleasure in usual activities, and a feeling of hopelessness associated with other findings such as sleep disturbances, or loss of energy. Major depression is a chronic debilitating disease with a lifetime prevalence of 7% to 12% in men and 20% to 25% in women. It often accompanies chronic medical illnesses and substance abuse.

Another form of less severe depression is dysthymia. It lasts at least two years and is described by some as a depressive type of personality. Although symptoms are not as severe as seen in major depression, they persist too long to be considered an adjustment reaction. Most patients with depression seek help from a family physician or general internist rather than a psychiatrist, making it important for the primary care physician to feel comfortable managing this illness.

PATHOPHYSIOLOGY

Most theories explaining depression emphasize a biological model. Depression is thought to be related to dysregulation of the brain's neurotransmitters. Although an imbalance in neurotransmitters provides an explanation for symptoms, it is still unclear why the imbalance develops. Research suggests genetic factors play a role

and that some individuals appear to be predisposed to developing depression in response to stressors. Potential stressors include medical illness, stressful life events, unresolved losses, poor support systems, and life changes impacting lifestyle such as divorce or financial loss. The process by which environmental factors interact with biological factors to cause depression is still poorly understood.

CLINICAL MANIFESTATIONS

History

Depression can cause a wide range of psychological and somatic complaints. Box 61–1 lists a summary of the criteria used for diagnosing depression. The average age of onset of depression is in the 20s. Identifiable stressors often play a role in the first episode of depression, but may play a limited role or have no role in subsequent episodes. Concerns expressed by a family member or friend about crying spells and depressed mood should trigger a physician to ask questions about depression. The patient's past medical history should be reviewed. Illnesses such as stroke, chronic fatigue syndrome, dementia, diabetes, cancer, rheumatoid arthritis, and HIV are frequently associated with depression. A family history of depression may be present. A careful review of medications is indicated since some medications can precipitate depression. Box 61–2 lists medications that have depressive symptoms as a side effect.

BOX 61–1

Diagnostic Criteria of Major Depression

The diagnosis requires two weeks of a depressed mood and/or disinterest with an impairment of function accompanied by four of the following:

- Weight changes
- Sleep disturbance
- Loss of energy
- Feelings of worthlessness or guilt
- Poor concentration
- Psychomotor retardation or agitation
- Thoughts of death
- Recurrent suicidal ideations

BOX 61–2

Common Medications Causing Depression

- Alpha-methyldopa
- Amphetamine withdrawal
- Beta blockers
- Digitalis
- Cimetidine
- Clonidine
- Indomethacin
- Isotretinoin
- Levodopa
- Oral contraceptives
- Phenothiazines
- Reserpine
- Steroids

Depression should be considered in patients with somatic complaints such as headache, backache, fatigue, chronic abdominal or pelvic pain, and a positive review of systems. An old adage states that if there are more than four complaints, consider depression.

Eliciting the patient's social history, particularly alcohol and other substance use, is important. Since some individuals presenting with depression have manic-depressive illness, it is important to ask about episodes of mania. Assessing the severity of depression by asking about suicidal thoughts and about psychotic symptoms is important. Risk factors for suicide include social isolation (e.g., divorce, widowed, living alone), substance use, elderly male, persons with terminal or chronic illnesses, and those who have developed a specific plan. Although women attempt suicide more often, men are successful more often.

Physical Examination

A physical examination is recommended to screen for medical disorders. Assessing mental status, for such things as appearance, mood, affect, speech, thought, content, perceptual disturbances, and cognition is important. Psychomotor retardation, poor eye contact, tearfulness, poor grooming, somber affect, and impaired memory are characteristics of depression.

DIFFERENTIAL DIAGNOSIS

Several conditions besides depression can cause a depressed mood. An adjustment disorder with a depressed mood occurs when an identifiable stressor causes more symptoms than expected, but does not last more than six months. Grief reactions may also present with symptoms mimicking depression; however, symptoms begin to improve after a period of a few months. An anxiety disorder can mimic depression, but is not usually accompanied by depressive symptoms such as loss of appetite and fatigue. A bipolar disorder or substance abuse may also present with symptoms similar to depression. In addition to psychological diseases, certain medications (see Box 61–2) and medical illnesses such as chronic infections (e.g., HIV, TB), endocrine disorders (e.g., hypothyroidism, hyperthyroidism, Cushing's disease, and Addison's disease), connective tissue diseases, neurological disorders, and cancers are associated with depression.

DIAGNOSTIC EVALUATION

The clinical interview is the most effective means of diagnosing depression. Laboratory testing should be limited to ruling out a medical disorder such as a TSH for suspected hypothyroidism. A baseline EKG should be performed in patients with a history of cardiac disease or over age 40 if tricyclic antidepressants are going to be prescribed. Neuroimaging and EEG should be considered with patients with new onset psychotic depression.

MANAGEMENT

Common treatments include supportive counseling and pharmacotherapy. Examples of supportive counseling include providing education, empathizing with the patient, challenging a patient's exaggerated negative or self-critical thoughts, and encouraging patients to be more active and to schedule enjoyable activities. Sometimes encouraging a patient to break down their problems into smaller components is helpful. Often a willingness to explore issues is therapeutic and the physician should not be expected to address and solve all problems. Patients with family or marital issues may benefit from therapy. Patients with persistent symptoms or major depression should be treated pharmacologically.

The different classes of antidepressant medications are equally effective. The choice of medication depends on the patient's symptoms, current medications, and side effect profile. If the patient has insomnia, a more sedating medication such as a tricyclic antidepressant, trazodone, or mirtazapine are good choices. If somnolence is a problem, a more energizing antidepressant such as an SSRI or bupropion is a good choice.

Although SSRIs are typically energizing, about 15% of patients experience sedation as a side effect. If anxiety or agitation is a complaint, SSRIs should be avoided as a first choice. Sedative antidepressants should be given in this situation. Although TCAs have been available for years, they have many unpleasant side effects. Their anticholinergic properties can precipitate an attack of acute angle glaucoma or bladder outlet obstruction. They can also cause constipation, dry mouth, orthostatic hypotension, tachycardia, cardiac arrhythmias, tremor, and weight gain. SSRIs appear to be safe in patients with cardiac disease and cause less orthostatic hypotension in elderly patients. Common side effects include gastrointestinal disturbances, headache, agitation, insomnia, sexual dysfunction, tremor, and somnolence. Trazodone has minimal anticholinergic side effects, but is very sedating and on rare occasion causes priapism in males. Venlafaxine combines SSRI properties with neuroadrenergic effects. It is often used for refractory depression, but its side effects limit its use as a first line agent. MAO inhibitors are effective but are less commonly used because of their potential for drug and food interactions.

For a first episode of depression, antidepressants should be continued for six to twelve months after symptoms improve. The highest risk for recurrence is within the first few months of tapering. Patients suffering relapses should promptly be restarted on medications and continued for at least another three months of therapy. Patients at high risk of relapse should be considered for long-term therapy. Patients who fail to respond to therapy should be referred to a psychiatrist. Patients who are suicidal, have accompanying psychosis, or symptoms of mania also should be referred to a psychiatrist.

◆ KEY POINTS ◆

1. Major depression is a mood disorder characterized by at least two weeks of depressed mood, a loss of interest or pleasure in usual activities, and a feeling of hopelessness associated with other findings such as sleep disturbances or loss of energy.

2. Major depression is a chronic debilitating disease with a lifetime prevalence of 7% to 12% in men and 20% to 25% in women.

3. Conditions such as stroke, pregnancy, chronic fatigue syndrome, dementia, diabetes, cancer, rheumatoid arthritis, and HIV are frequently associated with depression.

4. The different classes of antidepressant medications are equally effective. The choice of medication depends on the patient's symptoms, current medications, and side effect profile.

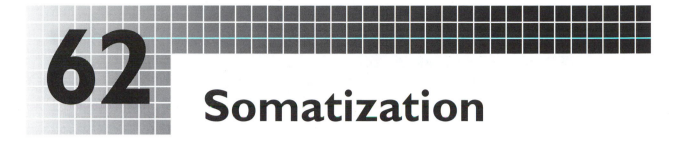

62 Somatization

Somatization is broadly defined as emotional or psychological distress that is experienced and expressed as physical complaints. Somatization can occur in the presence of physical illness, with symptoms either unrelated to the illness or out of proportion to objective findings. Somatization is an important problem in family medicine. Approximately one-third of all primary care patients have ill-defined symptoms not attributable to physical disease, and 70% of those patients with emotional disorders present with a somatic complaint as the reason for their office visit. Patients often view these physical symptoms as a more acceptable entry into the medical care system than an emotional complaint.

PATHOPHYSIOLOGY

The pathophysiology of somatization is not well understood. Multiple theories have been proposed, but no single underlying theory explains somatization. Common risk factors include sociocultural characteristics, biological characteristics, and individual risk factors such as being unmarried, female, lower educational level, and coming from a lower socioeconomic group. One theory is that the central nervous system regulates sensory information abnormally, resulting in symptoms. Behavioral theories suggest that somatization is a learned behavior in which the environment reinforces the illness behavior. Somatization is also thought by some to be a defense mechanism.

Precipitating factors include stressful life events, which can either be positive (such as marriage), or negative (such as a death in the family). Interpersonal conflict either at work or home is a common risk factor. Somatization can lead to symptoms in several ways. Patients may amplify symptoms of an acute or chronic problem or alternatively give several physical complaints while de-emphasizing psychological problems such as depression. Some patients experience physiological disturbances, such as palpitations or irritable bowel that may be mediated through the autonomic nervous system. In rare occasions, patients can experience conversion symptoms that may serve a symbolic function such as "hysterical blindness." Conversion symptoms typically do not conform to any known physiologic mechanisms.

CLINICAL MANIFESTATIONS

History

Symptoms for somatic patients range from occasional functional complaints to a full-blown syndrome that meets the DSM-IV criteria for a somatiform disorder. The most common of these entities is somatization disorder, which is characterized by multiple unexplained symptoms in multiple organs beginning before age 30. DSM-IV criteria require the presence of 4 pain symptoms, 2 gastrointestinal symptoms, one sexual symptom and one pseudoneurologic symptom drawn from an extended list of symptoms. Other somatiform disorders include hypochondriasis and conversion disorders. The prevalence of somatization disorder is about 2% in the general population, 6% in the general medical clinical population, and 9% among tertiary hospital inpatients.

A thorough history is helpful for determining the possibility of somatization. Unfortunately, the presence of a physical illness or abnormalities discovered on physical examination does not eliminate somatization. Clues that should raise suspicion for somatization disorder are listed in Box 62–1. Pain is the most frequent complaint. Symptoms often cluster around the cardiovascular system, such as atypical chest pain, palpitations, racing heart, and shortness of breath, neurological symptoms such as headache, dizziness, lightheadedness, and paresthesias, or the gastrointestinal system with complaints such as heartburn, gas, and indigestion.

Physical Examination

A careful and thorough physical examination is useful for eliminating organic disease. Several diseases, such as hyperparathyroidism and lupus erythematosis, can present with what appears to be somatization complaints.

DIFFERENTIAL DIAGNOSIS

The differential diagnosis includes anxiety, depression, post-concussion syndrome, hypochondriasis, schizophrenia, and malingering.

Medical disorders that affect multiple systems or produce non-specific symptoms that are either transient or recurring can be confused with somatization. Box 62–2 lists some illnesses that masquerade as somatization.

DIAGNOSTIC EVALUATION

A thorough history and physical examination are essential. Not only may an unsuspected illness be diagnosed, but a normal examination is also critical for providing effective reassurance and avoiding unnecessary testing. Unless there is evidence suggesting a specific disorder, extensive testing should be avoided.

BOX 62–1

Clues to Somatization

- Multiple and vague symptoms: Description of symptoms can be inconsistent or bizarre.
- Symptoms persist despite adequate medical treatment
- Illness begins with a stressful event
- The patient "doctor shops."
- History of numerous work-ups with insignificant findings.
- The patient refuses to consider psychological factors or discuss issues other than medical concepts.
- There is evidence of an associated psychiatric disorder
- The patient has a hysterical personality
- Demanding yet disparaging of the physician
- Unreasonable demands for a treatment and drugs
- Dwelling on symptoms and proud of suffering
- Complaints that are inconsistent with known pathophysiology

---

BOX 62–2

Differential Diagnosis of Somatization

- Chronic fatigue syndrome
- Dementia
- Fibromyalgia
- HIV
- Hyperparathyroidism
- Hyperthyroidism
- Lyme disease
- Systemic Lupus Erythematosus
- Substance abuse

MANAGEMENT

An important step is to legitimize and acknowledge the complaints, share the patient's frustrations, and express continued interest and hope. The treatment should focus mainly on restoring and maintaining function. An explanation of symptoms should be presented in functional or physiological terms if possible. If you cannot explain a symptom, share this with the patient.

A well-defined program should be initiated and presented to the patient. Even if treatment consists of reassurance and symptom control, definitive information about what to expect, and instructions for follow-up can help reduce anxiety. Treatments should be time-limited and expectations set. For example, a physician might say, "we will try this medicine for four weeks. Although it may not relieve your symptoms entirely, you should improve enough to participate in your weekly book club meeting. We will know how this is working by whether you miss any meeting dates. I will see you in four weeks so we can see how you are managing." Often engaging the patient in behavioral methods, such as keeping a diary, helps. Consultation with a psychologist or a mental health counselor can help by confirming the diagnosis and recommending effective treatments. Pharmaceuticals can benefit patients with major depres-

sion or an anxiety disorder that presents with somatic symptoms. Medication should be used sparingly and in low doses. Patients with somatization often have poor tolerance for side effects. There is rarely an indication for using narcotics in this population.

◆ KEY POINTS ◆

1. Somatization is defined as emotional or psychological distress that is experienced and expressed as physical complaints.

2. A thorough history and physical examination are essential in order to eliminate the possibility of organic disease.

3. Unless there is evidence suggesting a specific disorder, extensive testing should be avoided.

4. An important step in management is to legitimize and acknowledge the complaints, share the patient's frustrations, and express continued interest and hope.

5. Pharmaceuticals can benefit patients with major depression or an anxiety disorder that presents with somatic symptoms.

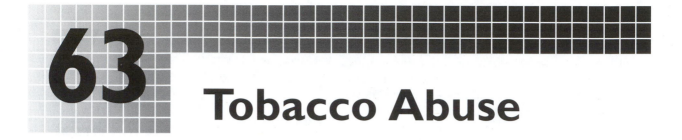

63

Tobacco Abuse

Tobacco abuse is the leading preventable cause of death and disability in the United States. Each year in the United States approximately 400,000 deaths can be attributed to tobacco use. Although the percent of smokers has declined to about 25%, millions of Americans continue to smoke and the incidence of adolescent smoking has fallen very little since its peak in the 1970s. Smoking among teenage girls has even increased.

PATHOPHYSIOLOGY

Smoking is a complex behavior that is still not completely understood. Pharmacological and psychological models have been proposed. The psychological and behavioral models propose that smoking is a learned behavior that continues because the individual receives gratification from smoking. Smoking also becomes a habit, triggered by certain situations such as stress or alcohol. There also appears to be a link between depression and smoking.

The pharmacological model emphasizes the physical addiction to smoking. There is abundant evidence that nicotine is an addictive drug capable of creating tolerance, physical dependence, and causing withdrawal symptoms. According to this model, smokers use tobacco to maintain their nicotine levels and avoid withdrawal. Withdrawal symptoms include craving for cigarettes, restlessness, irritability, poor concentration, headache, and nausea. Withdrawal varies greatly among smokers. Clinically, those individuals that need to smoke shortly after rising, smoke at least one pack per day, or have difficulty abstaining for even a few hours are at greatest risk for withdrawal symptoms. Although withdrawal symptoms explain why many smokers fail to quit during the first week, it does not explain why many smokers have trouble abstaining for long periods of time.

Epidemiological data clearly identifies multiple benefits for smoking cessation. Box 63–1 lists some health consequences of smoking. Even older individuals benefit from stopping tobacco use after years of smoking or quitting after a smoking-related illness. Lung cancer risks drop significantly ten years after abstaining. Coronary risk reduction occurs much more rapidly; the excess risk of a second MI is cut in half within one to two years after quitting.

CLINICAL MANIFESTATIONS

History

Smokers may present with symptoms of one of the smoking-related illnesses listed in Box 63–1. More commonly, smokers complain of cough, sore throat, shortness of breath, and frequent infections. The history should focus on when and why the patient began to smoke. Smoking can be quantified by multiplying the average number of packs smoked per day by the number of years of smoking to calculate the number of smoking

BOX 63–1
Health Consequences Associated with Smoking

Cancers:
   Lung cancer
   Oral cancers
   Larynx cancers
   Pharyngeal cancers
   Esophageal cancers
   GU cancers—kidney, bladder, cervical
   GI cancers—pancreas, stomach

Cardiovascular:
   Myocardial infarction
   Cerebral vascular disease
   Peripheral vascular disease

Pulmonary:
   Chronic obstructive pulmonary disease
   Recurring respiratory infections

Secondary-Hand Smoke-Related Problems:
   Higher incidence of respiratory tract infections
   Asthma in children of smokers
   High risk of lung cancer in household members

Pregnancy:
   Lower birth weight babies
   Higher incidence of SIDS

Others:
   Osteoporosis
   Peptic Ulcer Disease
   Skin wrinkling

pack years. Asking whether the patient has thought about quitting, tried to quit, or intends to quit helps assess readiness and motivation to quit. Understanding past failures or fears about quitting may help address barriers to smoking cessation.

Physical Examination

Physical examination may show signs of underlying smoking-related disease. The mouth and oral cavity should be examined for lesions that may represent cancer. The tongue in smokers often has a brownish dis-

coloration due to exposure to the tar in smoke. Wheezing and diminished breath sounds may indicate chronic obstructive lung disease. Peripheral pulses may be diminished suggesting vascular disease.

DIFFERENTIAL DIAGNOSIS

In general, laboratory tests are not helpful for the diagnosis, but may be indicated to evaluate consequences of smoking. Pulmonary function tests may help quantify pulmonary damage and provide evidence of the importance of smoking cessation. If the tests are normal, it is important to stress the importance of stopping smoking now to prevent further damage.

EVALUATION

Providing all smokers seen in the office with even brief advice increases the proportion of smokers who quit. The National Cancer Institution lists four "A"s for office-based intervention.

1. **Ask**—about smoking at every opportunity. Ask those who smoke if they are interested in stopping.

2. **Advise**—every smoker with a clear, unambiguous direct message. Tailor the advice to the patient's individual situation.

3. **Assist**—patients in their efforts to stop. For smokers ready to quit, ask the smoker to set a quit date. Provide self-help material and offer pharmacological therapy, such as nicotine replacement. Consider a referral to a formal smoking cessation program. If the individual is not ready to quit, discuss the benefits and barriers to smoking cessation. Make the information as relevant to the individual as possible. Advise the smoker to avoid exposing family members to second-hand smoke. Indicate a willingness to help in the future when the smoker is ready and continue to ask about it in future follow-up visits.

4. **Arrange**—Negotiate a follow-up appointment, generally within one to two weeks after the quit date. For those who have quit, make sure you congratulate and reinforce the benefits of giving up smoking. Discuss high-risk situations for relapse and review coping mechanisms. For those who fail to quit, provide positive reinforcement in taking the

first steps toward quitting. Ask about what obstacles were encountered and discuss strategies to overcome these problems in the future. Encourage the smoker to set another quit date.

TREATMENT

The most effective approaches address nicotine addiction and behavioral dependence. Nicotine replacement mitigates some of the symptoms of withdrawal by continuing nicotine exposure, although at reduced and tapered doses. Nicotine delivery can be achieved with transdermal patches, nicotine-containing chewing gum, or nicotine inhalers. All are ideally used for two to three months in patients and then discontinued.

Nicotine replacement is not a panacea, but does improve the quit rate. For example, nicotine patches double quit rates. They should be offered to smokers willing to set a quit date, who will not smoke while on the patch, and who ideally will follow a behavioral program either individually or in a group setting. The side effects of the patch are mild, generally limited to skin irritation. Nicotine gum was the original form of nicotine replacement. Side effects of the gum are mostly related to vigorous chewing and the release of excess nicotine. These symptoms include sore jaw, mouth irritation, nausea, dizziness, and headache.

Bupropion originally marketed as an antidepressant, also enhances quit rates. It is contraindicated with seizures. It is useful for people who do not want nicotine replacement or have been unable to quit with nicotine replacement. Generally, it is started one week before the target quit date. Bupropion has been used in conjunction with nicotine replacement, and some evidence suggests the combination of the two is more effective than either approach alone.

The behavioral model has also stimulated a host of strategies to help manipulate the environment. The physician can work with the patient to develop strategies like spending time in places where smoking is not permitted or rewarding oneself with money saved by not smoking. Organized group programs such as those sponsored by the American Cancer Society or the American Lung Association may also be of benefit. These societies sponsor telephone services that provide education, encouragement, advice, and referral.

◆ KEY POINTS ◆

1. Tobacco abuse is the leading preventable cause of death and disability in the United States.

2. Even older individuals who stop smoking after many years or quit after a smoking-related illness benefit.

3. Providing all smokers seen in the office with even brief advice increases the proportion of smokers who quit.

4. Bupropion has been used in conjunction with nicotine replacement, and some evidence suggests the combination of the two is more effective than either approach alone.

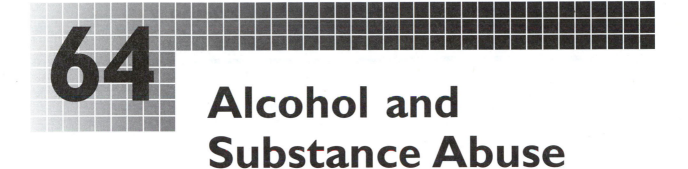

Alcohol and Substance Abuse

Alcohol and substance abuse are among the most serious social and medical problems in the United States. The estimated prevalence of substance abuse disorders ranges from 10% to 20%, with an estimated 5% of the adult population using illicit substances. The estimated societal cost of alcohol is in excess of 165 billion dollars per year due to the associated health problems, lost productivity, crime, deaths, and fires. Each year there are approximately 100,000 deaths resulting from alcohol abuse and another 20,000 deaths from the use of illicit substances.

PATHOPHYSIOLOGY

Substance problems encompass a wide range of severity. Abuse is defined as continued use of a psychoactive substance despite repeated adverse consequences of such use. These consequences can include legal problems, health problems or continued use in the face of recurrent social, work-related, or interpersonal problems.

Physical dependence is a physiological phenomenon of either tolerance or withdrawal. Withdrawal is the development of a typical set of symptoms after stopping a substance. Tolerance is when a drug that is used repeatedly begins to have less effect. Tolerance can lead to an escalation of use. Some individuals, such as those who take chronic narcotics, may have physical dependence without substance abuse. The pneumonic CPR, standing for compulsivity, preoccupation, and relapse, is useful for remembering the essential features of dependence.

The cause of substance abuse is not completely understood, but is most likely multifactorial. Genetic factors appear to play a role. Individuals with an alcoholic parent have a 3–4 times greater risk of becoming dependent on alcohol and identical twins have a greater concordance of alcoholism than fraternal twins.

Environmental factors also appear to play a role. Emotional stress or interpersonal stress may serve as an initiator and maintainer of alcohol abuse. Parental and peer values can contribute to substance abuse. Adults who grew up in a dysfunctional family and/or are in a dysfunctional family situation are at increased risk for alcohol abuse. Changes in societal perception may account for the increasing use of alcohol among women and adolescents.

Another model to explain substance abuse is the psychodynamic model. In this model, the individual's substance abuse is related to underlying psychopathology such as depression or anxiety. In this situation, patients use substances to self-medicate and the substance abuse is the symptom of the underlying pathology.

CLINICAL MANIFESTATIONS

History

Symptoms of substance abuse vary greatly. Early diagnosis and treatment, before irreversible health problems or major psychosocial consequences, should be the goal of the primary care physician. A commonly used screening tool for alcohol abuse is the Cage Test (Box 64–1).

BOX 64–1

Cage Questions

- Have you ever felt the need to **C**ut down on your drinking?
- Are you **A**nnoyed by people criticizing your drinking?
- Have you ever felt **G**uilty about your drinking?
- Do you ever need a drink in the morning to steady your nerves or help a hangover? (**E**ye-opener)

TABLE 64–1

Alcohol-Related Symptoms

Psychosocial complaints:	Physical complaints:
Absenteeism from work	Blackouts
Antisocial behavior	Falls
Anxiety	Gastrointestinal problems
Child abuse	Gout
Depression	Headache
Domestic violence	History of trauma
Financial problems	Motor vehicle accident injuries
Interpersonal relationship problems	Muscle cramps
Irritability	Nasal congestion
Job-related problems	Nocturia
Legal problems	Palpitations or chest pains
School-related problems	Peripheral neuropathy
Suicidal ideation	Poor memory
	Recurrent infections
	Sleep disturbances
	Weight changes

In the primary care setting, two "yes" answers have a sensitivity that ranges from 70% to 85% and specificity from 85% to 95%. The other screen, the Two-Item Conjoint Screen, has nearly an 80% sensitivity and specificity. This involves asking two questions:

- In the past year, have you ever drank or used drugs more than you meant to?
- Have you ever felt a need to cut down on your drinking or drug use?

Other clues that patients abuse alcohol and other substances include anxiety, insomnia, depression, legal problems, and a family history of alcoholism. Table 64–1 lists concerns or complaints that may be presenting symptoms of alcoholism or illicit drug use.

Inquiring into a patient's use of substances is best approached by using a non-judgmental, supportive manner. A detailed social history is important since many early symptoms are psychosocial. It is important to elicit the type of substance used, the frequency, the quantity, and pattern of use. Examining the setting for abuse, time, place, pattern, and social relationships of the patient is also helpful. Denial is a common defense mechanism, and it may be necessary to interview family members to obtain accurate information.

PHYSICAL EXAMINATION

The physical examination should be thorough and detailed. However, physical complications of substance abuse may not be evident early in the disease. High blood pressure may be a sign of withdrawal or cocaine abuse. Cirrhosis, ascites, edema, palmar erythema, tes-

ticular atrophy, rosacea, cardiomegaly, and peripheral neuropathy characterize end-stage alcoholism and are usually associated with heavy drinking for at least ten years. Binge drinking can sometimes precipitate cardiac arrhythmias or the "holiday heart" syndrome. Nasal irritation, septal perforation, tachycardia, chest pain, and paranoia are associated with cocaine. Smoking marijuana can cause cough and dark-colored or bloody sputum. Dilated pupils can be a sign of stimulant abuse, while constricted pupils in combination with sedation suggest opioid use.

DIFFERENTIAL DIAGNOSIS

The psychosocial and physical problems outlined in Tables 64–1 and 64–2 also form the differential diagnosis for substance abuse. In evaluating patients present-

TABLE 64–2

Alcohol-Related Health Problems

Cardiovascular	**Hemopoietic System**
Hypertension	Anemia
Cardiomyopathy	Thrombocytopenia
Arrhythmias	**Neurological System**
Endocrine	Cognitive impairment
Testicular atrophy	Dementia
Feminization	Korsakoff's psychosis
Amenorrhea	Wernicke's encephalopathy
Gastrointestinal	Peripheral neuropathy
Hepatitis	**Musculoskeletal**
Cirrhosis	Cramps
Esophagitis	Osteoporosis
Gastritis	**Skin**
Diarrhea	Rosacea
Pancreatitis	Telangiectasia
Gastrointestinal	Palmar erythema
bleeding	
Pregnancy	
Low birth weight	
Fetal Alcohol	
Syndrome	

ing with these various complaints, consideration of underlying substance abuse is very important. Clinical and lab evidence of substance abuse may be not be evident in early stages, and the diagnosis depends on a constellation of medical, social, and psychological clues. Substance abuse may be preceded or complicated by anxiety, depression, chronic pain, or marital distress, and these need to be considered when evaluating the patient.

DIAGNOSTIC EVALUATION

Although laboratory tests are not diagnostic of substance abuse, they are occasionally helpful. Liver enzyme abnormalities can provide objective evidence of problem drinking. Serum gamma-glutamyl transferase (GGT) is the most sensitive indicator of alcohol-induced liver damage; however, it is not specific. Elevation of the liver enzyme aspartate amino-transferase (AST) to alanine amino-transferase (ALT) in a ratio greater than 1 is typical of alcohol-related hepatitis. In cases of alcoholism, a CBC may reveal an elevated MCV or anemia. Hyperlipidemia and elevated uric acid levels are also often present.

MANAGEMENT

The goal of treatment is to reduce the consequences of the patient's substance abuse and prevent further substance abuse. For at-risk individuals or for those with a short history of abusing alcohol, evidence suggests that even brief interactions may be of benefit. This may consist of a brief counseling session when the physician educates the patient about the consequences of continued use and recommends quitting or cutting down. Setting specific goals and making a follow-up appointment to review progress are also an important part of a brief intervention.

Self-help groups, such as Alcoholics Anonymous, are a mainstay of treatment for patients willing to participate. Similar groups exist for other substances such as Narcotics Anonymous. Programs are also available for relatives and friends of individuals with substance abuse problems. A referral to an outpatient treatment center or to an addiction specialist is another treatment option. Counseling sessions may be individual, group, or family. Inpatient programs are usually reserved for those who fail outpatient therapy.

Pharmacological therapy can augment behavioral programs. Alcohol withdrawal can range from minor symptoms such as tachycardia, elevated blood pressure, shakiness, and irritability to life-threatening manifestations such as seizures, delirium tremors (DTs), and coma. Treating withdrawal is aimed at reducing the patient's discomfort and preventing symptoms from progressing. Normalization of vital signs and moderate sedation are two of the end-points for managing withdrawal. Long-acting benzodiazepines (BZD) such as diazepam or chlordiazepoxide either given as a loading dose until the patient is sedated or using symptom-adjusted dosing is effective. Short-acting BZD, such as lorazepam, are preferred in patients with severe liver disease. Beta-blockers, such as atenolol, can help reduce adrenergic symptoms and control blood pressure and tachycardia. Although they may reduce benzodiazepine requirements, they should not be used as monotherapy because they do not prevent seizures, hallucinations, or DTs. Clonidine, a central acting antihypertensive medicine, can also be used to help control blood pressure and withdrawal symptoms. Thiamine and magnesium should be given to patients at risk for alcohol withdrawal.

Outpatient therapy is appropriate for patients with mild withdrawal symptoms and a supportive social structure. Inpatient care is needed for those with more severe symptoms, a history of severe withdrawal, or a poor social support network. Withdrawal from BZD is best accomplished with a long-acting BZD or phenobarbital over a period of 8 to 12 weeks. Withdrawal of other sedative hypnotic drugs is usually managed using phenobarbital. Opiate withdrawal can be treated either with propoxyphene or methadone. Clonidine is useful as an adjunctive therapy. No drug is currently indicated for managing cocaine withdrawal, although tricyclic antidepressants, serotonin reuptake inhibitors, and dopamine agonists such as bromocriptine may reduce cravings.

Some patients seeking total abstinence from alcohol may request disulfiram. Disulfiram therapy sensitizes patients to alcohol and causes reactions such as flushing, palpitations, headache, nausea, and vomiting if a patient consumes alcohol. Nalexone, an opioid antagonist, is also useful in alcohol abuse. It appears to inhibit the pleasurable effects of alcohol and reduce cravings. Contraindications include opiate use and hepatocellular disease.

◆ KEY POINTS ◆

1. The estimated prevalence of substance abuse disorders ranges from 10% to 20%, with an estimated 5% of the adult population using illicit substances.

2. Liver enzyme abnormalities can provide objective evidence of problem drinking. Serum gamma-glutamyl transferase (GGT) is the most sensitive indicator of alcohol-induced liver damage; however, it is not specific.

3. The goal of treatment is to reduce the consequences of the patient's substance abuse and prevent further substance abuse.

4. Outpatient therapy is appropriate for patients with mild withdrawal symptoms and a supportive social structure. Inpatient care is needed for those with more severe symptoms, a history of severe withdrawal, or a poor social support network.

5. Disulfiram therapy sensitizes patients to alcohol and causes reactions such as flushing, palpitations, headache, nausea, and vomiting if a patient consumes alcohol.

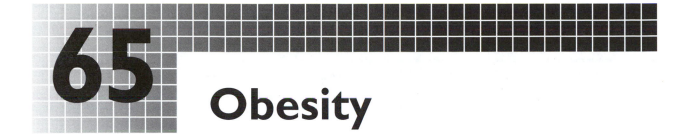

65 Obesity

Obesity is the presence of an abnormally large amount of adipose tissue. The preferred method to measure obesity is to use a measure known as the body mass index (BMI). The BMI is calculated by dividing the weight in kilograms by the height in meters squared. The BMI has the advantage of being gender and frame size independent and serves as a surrogate measure of body fat. Using the BMI, overweight is defined as BMI of 25–29.9 kilograms per meter squared and obesity as a BMI greater than 30 kilograms/meters squared. Morbid obesity is defined as a BMI greater than 40.0. In the United States, approximately 20% of men and 25% of women meet the criteria for obesity. Unfortunately, the percentage of obese Americans is increasing, particularly among children and adolescents. Minority populations are disproportionately affected. About one-third of Mexican-American and African-American women are obese.

Several studies suggest that central obesity may be associated with more adverse health conditions than lower body obesity. Central obesity can be determined by calculating a waist-hip ratio. Central obesity is present if the waist-hip ratio is greater than 0.85 in women and 1.0 in men.

PATHOPHYSIOLOGY

People gain weight when the caloric intake exceeds the body's energy expenditure. The reasons why an individual's caloric intake may exceed demand is complex and probably represents a heterogeneous disorder reflecting genetic, socioeconomic, and environmental influences. Clinically, physicians should view obesity as a chronic metabolic disease with health consequences rather than solely as a cosmetic or behavioral problem.

The current American social environment facilitates obesity. Many individuals have sedentary lifestyles that reduce or eliminate calorie-burning activities and eat at restaurants, where large portions of high-calorie foods contribute to added weight. In addition to environmental and social influences, some individuals overeat in response to emotional stress.

Studies of identical twins indicate that energy expenditure and fat distribution appear to be influenced by heredity. Recent studies have also explored the role of an appetite-controlling hormone, leptin. This hormone is secreted by fat cells and may signal the hypothalamus with a measure of the level of stored fat. There have been case reports of obese individuals having mutations of the leptin gene. In a few cases, genetic syndromes such as Prader-Willi cause obesity. These syndromes are usually identified in childhood.

There is some evidence that the body regulates its weight around a certain weight or set point. The body defends the set point by adjusting the metabolic rate and one theory proposes that obese patients regulate their weight around a higher set point. Some experts believe that physical activity and the amount of dietary fat may help modify this set point. Despite advances in understanding the pathophysiology of obesity, it is unlikely that these advances will lead to significant improvements in treatment in the near future.

CLINICAL MANIFESTATIONS

History

Obese patients generally have symptoms related to decreased exercise tolerance or to illnesses associated with obesity. Box 65–1 lists some health conditions associated with obesity. In addition, obese individuals may suffer from psychological impairment such as poor self-image or social isolation.

The history should also include information about current diet, previous diets attempted and their outcome, motivation to lose weight, and knowledge about health and diet. A complete review of medical problems and screening for symptoms of neuroendocrine disorders and co-morbid conditions listed in Box 65–1 is important.

Physical Examination

The physical examination should include the patient's blood pressure, height, weight, and the BMI. Although anthropomorphic measures are important, visual assessment of the patient generally is accurate—that is, if the patient looks overweight, then they are overweight. In addition, signs of obesity-influenced conditions should be sought and an assessment made of the patient's mobility.

BOX 65–1	
Conditions Associated with Obesity	
Cancer of the uterus, breast, prostate, and colon	Coronary disease
Degenerative arthritis	Diabetes
Fatty Liver	Gallbladder disease
Gout	Hyperlipidemia
Hypertension	Increased operative risk
Low back pain	Reflux esophagitis
Sleep apnea	Low self-esteem
Thromboembolic disease	Intertrigo

DIFFERENTIAL DIAGNOSIS

Obesity can either be primary or secondary. Secondary causes of obesity account for less than 1% of cases. Medicines associated with weight gain include tricyclic antidepressants, beta-blockers, phenothiazines, glucocorticoids, oral contraceptives, sulfonylureas, and insulin.

Neuroendocrine problems such as hypothyroidism, Cushing syndrome, and hypothalamic disease can also cause obesity. Genetic disorders causing obesity are usually clinically evident in childhood.

DIAGNOSTIC EVALUATION

Few tests are routinely indicated in the obese patient. Laboratory evaluation will depend on the individual and age, but should usually include a fasting blood glucose and lipid profile. A TSH is helpful in cases of suspected of hypothyroidism.

MANAGEMENT

Obesity is a chronic problem that can be frustrating for both the patient and the physician. Individuals need to be motivated to lose weight and to make lifestyle changes in diet and exercise. Poorly motivated patients are unlikely to adhere to a weight loss program.

Treatment options include diet, exercise, drugs, and surgery. The degree of obesity and the presence of associated illness should influence management strategies. Conservative therapy relying on diet and exercise form the basis of most weight loss programs. High cost programs or hazardous procedures such as surgery should be reserved for patients at greatest risk from obesity.

Most obese people would like to achieve an "ideal body weight." Unfortunately, short of surgery, most diet, exercise, or drug programs result in about a 10% weight loss. For many individuals, the goal might be to achieve a healthful weight rather than an ideal weight. Even modest weight reduction (5–10%) can be clinically significant, especially in obese individuals with diabetes or hypertension. Emphasizing realistic goals and then reinforcing them help prevent failure and contributing further to poor self-esteem. Sometimes prevention of further weight gain may be the most appropriate goal for someone who is unwilling or unable to lose weight.

Ideally, the patient and physician should work together to create a nutritionally sound diet that incorporates the patient's food preferences. A dietitian is also helpful in planning a diet. The loss of 1 pound of fat requires a 3500 calorie deficit. Therefore, a calorie deficit of 500 to 1000 calories per day will result in a weight loss of 1 to 2 pounds per week, which is appropriate for most patients. Gradual dietary changes tend to produce better long-lasting results. Simple suggestions include eating three meals per day, eating only during mealtime and limiting portions to one serving. Reducing dietary fat to 20% to 30% of total calories also enhances weight loss and is consistent with recommendations to reduce the risk of cardiac disease. Very low calorie, medically supervised diets have a limited role in management and are usually reserved for morbidly obese or very high-risk individuals, such as those with sleep apnea. A minimum of 800 calories per day is recommended. Risks for very low calorie diets include cardiac arrhythmias and gallstones. Exercise alone without calorie restriction is not an efficient weight loss program. However, exercise enhances overall health, improves weight to hip ratio, and helps to keep an individual's metabolic rate from resetting during periods of caloric restriction. Studies show that people who exercise regularly are more likely to maintain weight loss.

Exercise is most likely to be sustained if the exercise is something that the patient enjoys and can fit into their lifestyle. Opportunities should be explored to integrate exercise into daily activities whenever possible, such as climbing stairs instead of taking the elevator.

Drug therapy should be considered for morbidly obese individuals or those with significant co-morbidities. Medications include appetite suppressants, such as phentermine. Side effects include insomnia, hypertension, tachycardia, nausea, diarrhea, and anxiety.

Amphetamines and amphetamine-like products are rarely used because of their side effects and addiction.

Sibutramine is a serotonin-norepinephrine reuptake inhibitor, which is approved for long-term use in obesity management. Side effects include insomnia, dry mouth, headache, constipation, and small increases in pulse and blood pressure in some patients.

Orlistat is a gastrointestinal lipase inhibitor that interferes with fat absorption. Side effects are primarily gastrointestinal and include oily stools, diarrhea, and leakage of stool. Symptoms usually improve with time and adhering to a low-fat diet. Surgery for obesity, such as gastric stapling, should be reserved for patients with morbid refractory obesity. Liposuction can remove localized deposits of fat by a suction probe. However, serious complications, including fat embolus, hemorrhage, and even death have been reported.

Childhood obesity is increasing, and children who are overweight by age 6 are at much greater risk for being obese as adults than other children. Involvement of the parents in managing the diet and activity of younger children is essential. Often slowing weight gain is the goal so the child can grow out of his obesity. In adolescents, the degree of parent involvement should be individualized.

◆ KEY POINTS ◆

1. The BMI is the weight in kilograms divided by the height in meters squared. The BMI is independent of gender and frame size.
2. Obesity is defined as a BMI greater than 30.
3. Obesity is a heterogeneous disorder reflecting genetic, socioeconomic, behavioral and environmental influences.
4. The loss of one pound of fat requires a 3500-calorie deficit.

Part XVI
Dermatology
Problems

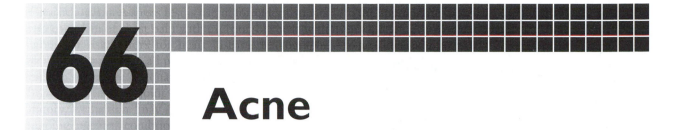

66 Acne

Acne is the most common chronic skin condition treated by physicians. It affects about 17 million people in the United States, including more than 85% of adolescents and young adults. Although most commonly seen in teenagers, acne may occur transiently in neonates and may persist beyond puberty into the third and fourth decades of life.

PATHOPHYSIOLOGY

Acne is caused by hyperkeratosis and the blockage of the pilosebaceous canal, increased growth of *Propionibacterium acnes*, overproduction of sebum, and inflammation. Androgen production stimulates the sebaceous gland, causing an increase in cell turnover, an increase in sebum production, and cohesivity of keratinocytes at the pilosebaceous canal. This alteration in keratinization, referred to as *cohesive hyperkeratosis*, causes the keratinous material in the follicle, which is normally loosely organized, to become more "sticky" causing a blockage of the canal. The blocked pilosebaceous gland produces a small cystic swelling (raised area) of the follicular duct just below the epidermis, referred to as a microcomedone. If the duct dilates with stratum corneum cells causing an opening of the follicular mouth it is referred to as an *open comedone* or "blackhead," if the mouth remains closed it is referred to as a *closed comedone* or "whitehead."

The combination of sebum, desquamated cells, and obstruction of the follicular opening creates an environment conducive to the overgrowth of the gram negative anaerobic diphtheroid bacteria, *Propionibacterium acnes*, which normally resides there. *P. acnes* secretes a low molecular weight chemotactic factor and lipase enzymes that break down the triglycerides of sebum into free fatty acids, which irritate the follicular wall and lead to formation of an erythematous *papule* on the skin. Neutrophils release hydrolases that may further disrupt the integrity of the follicular wall causing rupture and leakage into the underlying dermis, leading to the formation of a *pustule*. If this inflammatory process continues, it will eventually lead to formation of a *nodule* and subsequently a *cyst*.

Androgens are a primary stimulus of sebaceous gland proliferation and increased sebum production, which explains why acne often develops during puberty. Since girls reach puberty at an earlier age than boys, the peak of acne in girls is reached between 14 and 17 years of age, compared to ages 16 to 19 in boys. *Neonatal acne* is caused by maternal androgens that stimulate the sebaceous glands that have not yet involuted to their childhood state of immaturity. Neonatal acne is usually mild and can be observed during the second to fifth month of life, after which time the pilosebaceous units involute, only to reemerge again near puberty.

CLINICAL MANIFESTATIONS

History

The history should include onset and distribution of skin lesions and any associated aggravating or alleviating factors. The patient should be asked about aggravating foods, whether temperature affects their skin, and if there are seasons of the year during which the lesions are worse. Cosmetics, topical skin preparations, or exposure to heavy oils or greases may contribute to follicular plugging. Medications, such as corticosteroids, androgens, anticonvulsants, and lithium may contribute to acne. Patients should be asked about other symptoms of androgen excess, such as voice change and change in hair growth and distribution. The sudden onset of widely distributed severe acne may be associated with androgen excess, either from an androgen secreting tumor or from exogenous androgen ingestion.

Physical Examination

Physical examination focuses on characterizing the skin lesions. Acne lesions usually develop in areas with the greatest density and size of sebaceous glands. The face is almost always involved. Other common areas of involvement are the chest, shoulders, and upper back. There are no sebaceous glands in the palms or soles. Additional note should be made of hair pattern, and in cases of suspected virilization, a genital examination should be performed to assess for pelvic masses or clitoromegaly.

The prime focus of the exam in patients with acne is to characterize and classify the acne. Acne lesions can be classified into either *comedonal* (whiteheads, blackheads) or *inflammatory* (papules/pustules, nodules/cysts). Most cases of acne are pleomorphic and include comedones, papules, pustules, and nodules. Patients with mild acne usually have whiteheads and blackheads, a few papules, and some pustules. Moderate acne consists of many papules, pustules, and a few nodules. Severe acne, also referred to as nodulocystic acne, consists of many papules, pustules, and nodules or cysts.

DIFFERENTIAL DIAGNOSIS

Common conditions that mimic the lesions of acne vulgaris include acne rosacea, folliculitis and perioral dermatitis. Acne rosacea is a chronic vascular inflammatory disorder affecting mainly adults between the ages of 30 and 50. It is characterized by a vascular component (redness, telangiectasia, flushing, blushing) and an eruptive component (papules and pustules) affecting only the face. Patients are extremely sensitive to facial vasodilatory factors such as exposure to extreme heat or cold, excessive sunlight, and ingestion of alcohol, spicy foods, hot liquids, and highly seasoned food. Folliculitis is the infection of hair follicles from the epidermal surface by *Staph. aureus* bacteria, often from shaving. Perioral dermatitis is an eruption around the mouth, nose, and eyes affecting young women and thought to have a bacterial etiology. Patients have papules and pustules resembling folliculitis, there are no whiteheads or blackheads, and there is a clear zone around the vermilion border. Androgen excess and medications can be causes of acne. Drug acne is mainly seen in patients who take oral corticosteroids, potent topical corticosteroid preparations, isoniazid, anticonvulsants (phenytoin and trimethadione) or lithium containing medications.

DIAGNOSTIC APPROACH

There are no special tests required in evaluation of acne other than skin examination. In those women with suspected androgen excess, serum testosterone and dehydroepiandrosterone sulfate levels may help in guiding further evaluation and therapy.

MANAGEMENT

Topical agents such as tretinoin (Retin A) are often the first lines of therapy. Tretinoin increases cell turnover and reduces the cohesion between keratinocytes helping to unplug the follicle. The medication usually causes some redness, burning, and peeling of the skin within the first 3 to 4 weeks of treatment, and comedones may be more visible causing many patients to prematurely stop using their medication. However, with continued use, most patients improve after the sixth week, with best results seen at 9 to 12 weeks of treatment. Retin-A also causes the skin to become much more sensitive to irritants such as sun exposure, wind, dryness and cold temperatures. Other, milder comedolytics include Salicylic acid, Sulfur preparations and azelaic acid. Azelaic acid has antibacterial and keratolytic properties and is useful in patients with mild to moderate acne who cannot tolerate tretinoin.

The goal of treatment for mild to moderate acne is to reduce the follicular bacterial population using topical antibiotics (Erythromycin or Clindamycin) and keratolytics. Benzoyl Peroxide has bacteriostatic properties, which makes it an effective treatment for mild inflammatory acne. Patients should be advised that this medication can dry the skin and can bleach clothes and pillowcases. There are topical preparations that combine benzoyl peroxide with a topical antibiotic (Benzaclin, Benzomycin), which should be applied to the affected areas once or twice a day. If topical retinoids are used in conjunction with topical antibacterials, they should be applied at different times (i.e., antibacterial in a.m. and retinoid in p.m.). If lesions do not improve after 6 weeks of treatment, an oral antibiotic is usually added to the regimen. The antibiotics that have proven most efficacious are tetracycline, doxycycline, minocycline, and erythromycin. In adolescent females oral contraceptives can be an effective second line medication. The main effect of oral contraceptives is to suppress ovarian androgen production and thus reduce sebum production.

Severe acne, also referred to as nodulocystic acne, consists of many papules, pustules and nodules or cysts.

If the combination of oral and topical antibiotics is insufficient, prescribing Isotrenitoin (Accutane) is often helpful. Accutane is associated with significant toxicity and requires close monitoring under the direction of an experienced dermatologist.

◆ KEY POINTS ◆

1. Acne vulgaris affects approximately 85% of adolescents.
2. Overproduction of sebum and *Propionibacterium acnes* are etiologic agents leading to development of acne.
3. Comedonal acne is treated with topical Keratolytics (Retinoids) and/or Benzoyl peroxide.
4. Inflammatory acne is treated with either topical or oral antibiotics.
5. Isotretinoin (Accutane) is reserved for severe acne or moderate acne that is unresponsive to treatment.

67

Infections of the Skin

Skin serves as a barrier to fluid loss and protects internal organs against mechanical injury, infections, temperature changes, noxious agents, and trauma. When the skin defenses are altered or destroyed, bacteria, viruses, fungi, and parasitic organisms can infect or infest the skin.

PATHOPHYSIOLOGY

Clinical infection results from breaks in the skin (i.e., abrasions, needle punctures, catheters), loss of local immunity, and changes in the skin flora. Although more than 100 bacteria have been identified as causing cellulitis, two gram positive cocci, *Staphylococcus aureus* and group A beta-hemolytic streptococcus account for the majority of skin and soft tissue infections. *S. aureus* can cause folliculitis, cellulitis, and furuncles (abscess/boil). Toxins elaborated by *S. aureus* can result in bullous impetigo and staphylococcal scalded skin syndrome. Streptococci are usually secondary invaders of traumatic skin lesions and can cause impetigo, erysipelas, cellulitis, and lymphangitis.

Viruses damage host cells by entering the cell and replicating at the host's expense. Herpes simplex virus (HSV) infections can occur anywhere on the skin, and are caused by two types of the virus: HSV-1 and HSV-2. HSV-1 is usually seen in oral infections while HSV-2 is associated with genital infections. HSV infections have two phases, the primary infection transmitted by

respiratory droplets or by direct contact with an active lesion or infected secretions, and the secondary phase, representing a reactivation of latent virus from the dorsal root ganglion.

The varicella virus, which causes chickenpox, is a highly contagious viral infection transmitted by airborne droplets or vesicular fluid. Patients are contagious from 2 days before onset of the rash until all lesions have crusted. Herpes zoster is a cutaneous reactivation of varicella typically involving the skin of a single dermatome.

Warts are benign skin tumors confined to the epidermis resulting from human papilloma virus (HPV), which is transferred by touch and commonly occurs at sites of trauma. Molluscum contagiosum is caused by a poxvirus and produces an umbilicated skin lesion that is spread by autoinoculation, scratching or touching a lesion.

The dermatophytes, or ringworm fungi, infect and survive only on dead keratin, namely the top layer of the skin (stratum corneum), the hair and nails. Dermatophyte infections are clinically classified by body region with varying disease responses. "Tinea" means fungus infection, so the term "tinea capitis" refers to a fungal infection of the scalp.

The yeast-like fungus Candida albicans and other Candida species live normally in the mouth, vaginal tract and gut and may become pathogenic and produce budding spores, pseudohyphae (elongated cells) or true hyphae with altered cell mediated immunity, pregnancy, oral contraceptives, antibiotics, diabetes, skin maceration, topical steroid therapy and some endocrinopathies. The yeast infects the stratum corneum of mucous membranes (mouth, anogenital tract) and warm, moist intertriginous skin areas (axillae, groin, breast folds, digit spaces).

Scabies infestation begins when a fertilized female mite burrows through the stratum corneum to begin a 30-day life cycle of egg laying and fecal deposition (scybala). After eggs have hatched and the mites have increased and migrated to other areas like the finger webs, wrists, extensor surfaces of the elbows and knees, axillae, breasts, waist, sides of hands and feet, ankles, penis, buttocks, scrotum, and palms and soles of infants, symptoms intensify. The disease is transmitted by direct skin contact with an infected patient.

Three kinds of lice infest humans: Pediculosis humanus var. capitis (head louse), var. corporis (body louse) and Pthirus pubis (pubic or crab louse). Pediculosis capitis is most common in children. Live nits fluoresce and can be detected by Wood's light. Pediculosis corporis is a disease of poor hygiene where the lice live and lay their nits in the seams of clothing and return to the skin surface only to feed. Pediculosis pubis is an extremely contagious sexually transmitted disease, and may involve not only the groin but also other hairy areas of the body. Eyelash infestation in a child may be a sign of sexual abuse by an infested adult.

CLINICAL MANIFESTATIONS

History

The onset of the skin lesions and associated symptoms, such as fever, warmth or pruritus, should be part of the history. Tenderness, pain, mild paresthesias or burning may occur at the site of inoculation with herpes virus infections. A prodrome of localized pain, tender lymphadenopathy, headache, generalized aching and fever may occur. Shingles may also present prior to the eruption with a prodrome of itching, pain and burning in the affected dermatome. Associated underlying skin conditions or trauma should be noted. Local trauma or systemic changes like menses, fatigue, or fever may trigger a recurrence of herpes simplex infections. Known contact with cases of scabies, lice, viral, or fungal infections may suggest transmission has occurred.

Medications and medication allergies may be important in determining other potential causes for the rash and in determining therapy. An attack of chickenpox usually confers lifelong immunity, but a previous infection with varicella can be reactivated and cause shingles. Unlike chickenpox, an episode of shingles does not confer lifelong immunity.

Physical Examination

The lesions of impetigo are superficial and are characterized by honey colored crusts. Erythema, warmth, edema, pain, and sometimes fever characterize cellulitis. Folliculitis is characterized by a pustule in association with a hair follicle. Furuncles are larger fluctuant erythematous lesions also in association with hairy regions. Nikolsky's sign aids in the diagnosis of Staphylococcal scalded skin syndrome and is elicited when local skin separation occurs after minor pressure.

Herpes simplex appears as grouped vesicles on an erythematous base appear, and are uniform in size, unlike the vesicles seen in herpes zoster. The chickenpox rash has a centripetal distribution, starting at the trunk and spreading to the face and extremities. Lesions appear as a "dew drop on a rose petal" with a thin walled vesicle with clear fluid on a red base, and appear as a constellation of different stages at the same time. In the eruptive phase, vesicles appear in different sizes, unlike in herpes simplex where the vesicles are uniformly shaped. Warts are small tumors of the skin that obscure normal skin lines, have a mosaic surface pattern, and may have thrombosed vessels appearing as black dots on the surface. The lesions of molluscum contagiosum are discrete, 2 to 5 mm, slightly umbilicated, flesh-colored, dome shaped papules occurring on the face, trunk, axillae and extremities in children, and the pubic and genital areas in adults.

Fungal infections are characterized by erythematous as well as hypo or hyperpigmented lesions associated with scaling. They occur on various parts of the body. The classic ringworm lesion has central clearing of the lesion.

Lice are suspected when a patient itches without an apparent rash. Lice and nits may be identified on close visual examination. Scabies are associated with linear burrows on the distal extremities and scattered pruritic papules on the rest of the body.

DIFFERENTIAL DIAGNOSIS

The differential diagnosis for bacterial infections includes other forms of dermatitis such as eczema and contact or stasis dermatitis. Herpes viral infections including shingles, chickenpox and herpes simplex may also initially be confused with eczema, impetigo or contact dermatitis. The lesions of molluscum may be confused with warts or herpes simplex. Both warts and molluscum contagiosum may be confused with skin tags, dermatofibromas or nevi. The differential diagnosis for fungal infections includes pityriasis alba, pityriasis rosea, eczema, or in some instances psoriasis or seborrheic dermatitis. Scabies lesions may form vesicles leading to consideration of diagnoses such as herpes and contact dermatitis.

DIAGNOSTIC APPROACH

Skin infections are commonly diagnosed clinically. Additional diagnostic measures that are obtained to assist with diagnosis include blood cultures, wound cultures, viral cultures of suspicious lesions, and microscopic exam of skin scrapings or suspected organisms (Table 67–1). Blood cultures are often negative, but occasionally bacteremia can occur. Wound cultures are in general not helpful, though some advocate obtaining "leading edge" cultures obtained by injecting and aspirating from the edge of the infection. More helpful is a

TABLE 67–I

Diagnostic Testing and Treatment of Common Skin Infections

Infection	Diagnostic test	Treatment
Impetigo	Clinical exam	Topical mupirocin, oral dicloxacillin, cephalexin
Cellulitis	Clinical exam, blood or wound cultures	Oral or intravenous dicloxacillin, cefazolin, cephalexin
Furuncles	Clinical exam, culture of drainage	Incision and drainage, antibiotics
Herpes simplex	Clinical exam, Tzanck smear, culture	Antivirals: acyclovir, famcyclovir, valacyclovir
Chickenpox, herpes zoster	Clinical exam, culture, serology	Antivirals as for herpes above
Warts	Clinical exam, biopsy	Electrocautery, cryotherapy, topical salicylic acid or imiquimod
Molluscum contagiosum	Clinical exam, biopsy	Curettage, cryotherapy, Retinoin, salicylic acid
Fungal infections	Clinical exam, Wood's light, KOH microscopy, culture (fungal media)	Topical or oral antifungals; Nails and hair require oral therapy
Scabies	Clinical exam, microscopy	Topical lindane, permethrins, crotamiton, sulfur; clothing and bedding washed in hot water; treat close contacts
Lice	Clinical exam, microscopy	Topical lindane, permethrins, pyrethrins, malathion; must treat twice and remove nits

sterilely obtained culture from a purulent infection such as an abscess or furuncle. Viral culture is the most definitive method for diagnosis of herpes infections. Diagnosis of fungal infections is by potassium hydroxide wet mount preparation, which allows direct visualization under the microscope of the branching hyphae of dermatophytes in keratinized material. Culture is necessary for scalp, hair and nail fungal infections to identify the true source of infection for proper treatment. Mycosel agar, Dermatophyte Test Medium and Sabouraud's dextrose agar are the most common fungal culture media.

with Lindane (gamma benzene hexachloride) must be used exactly as directed to avoid potential neurotoxicity. Persistent itching may be treated with topical steroids if inflammation is present, or with oral antihistamines. Nit removal is an important component of lice treatment because they may hatch and reinfest. Cream rinse with formic acid (Step 2 Cream Rinse), vinegar compresses, and a metal nit comb are effective. Petrolatum jelly, baby shampoo, manual plucking of lice, and fluorescein drops are methods of treating eye infestations (see Table 67–1).

MANAGEMENT

Treatment generally involves use of a topical or oral medication directed at the offending organism. More extensive bacterial infections may require hospitalization and intravenous antibiotics. Furuncles are self-limited and usually respond to frequent moist, warm compresses followed by incision, drainage, and packing. Antibiotics are often prescribed, but may not be necessary for furuncles that have been properly drained.

Treatment for herpes simplex and varicella infections consists of measures to relieve discomfort, promote healing and prevent recurrence. Antiviral agents decrease the duration of viral excretion, new lesion formation and vesicles. Antipruritic lotions, antihistamines and antibiotics for secondary bacterial infections are also recommended. Antiviral agents started within the first 48 to 72 hours may shorten the course of illness and in the case of herpes zoster may decrease the likelihood of developing postherpetic neuralgia. Acyclovir and varicella-zoster immune globulin (VZIG) are also indicated in immunocompromised patients.

In addition to topical or systemic antifungal agents, treatment of candidal infection should include keeping the infected skin area clean and dry. Scabies treatment

◆ KEY POINTS ◆

1. Clinical infection results from breaks in the skin (i.e., abrasions, needle punctures, catheters), loss of local immunity, and changes in the skin flora.

2. Although more than 100 bacteria have been identified as causing cellulitis, two gram positive cocci, *Staphylococcus aureus* and group A beta-hemolytic streptococcus, account for the majority of skin and soft tissue infections.

3. HSV-1 is usually seen in oral infections while HSV-2 is associated with genital infections.

4. Wart treatment depends on the site and severity of the wart, and options include electrocautery, blunt dissection, topical salicylic acid, liquid nitrogen, or tape occlusion.

5. Oral antibiotics are usually effective for treating most cases of cellulitis and because of staphylococcal penicillin resistance, penicillinase-resistant antibiotics (cloxacillin or dicloxacillin) or cephalosporins (e.g., cephalexin) should be selected.

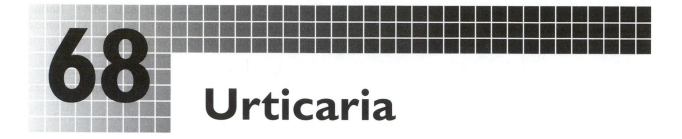

Urticaria

Urticaria, known as hives or wheals, is a pruritic, immune-mediated skin eruption that consists of well circumscribed lesions on an erythematous base affecting any part of the body. Angioedema is a related condition that affects deeper layers of the skin and often involves the face, tongue, extremities, or genitalia. Urticaria and angioedema can occur together. Urticaria affects 10% to 20% of the population and is classified as acute (less than 6 weeks' duration) or chronic (more than 6 weeks). Urticaria and angioedema can be a manifestation of many conditions and determining the underlying cause can be very challenging.

PATHOPHYSIOLOGY

A number of stimuli, such as medications or foods, may serve as antigens that bond to IgE receptors on mast cells causing them to degranulate. In other cases, physical or chemical stimuli may directly cause mast cell degranulation. Hypersensitivity to acetylcholine triggers mast cell degranulation in the physical urticarias. Autoimmune diseases associated with immune complex formation are additional causes of urticaria. These various stimuli trigger release of chemical mediators that increase blood flow and capillary permeability, causing leakage of protein-rich plasma from the local postcapillary venules resulting in hive formation.

Angioedema occurs with massive transudation of fluid into the dermis and subcutaneous tissues. Pruritus is usually present but to a milder degree in angioedema because there are fewer mast cells and sensory nerve endings in the deeper tissues.

CLINICAL MANIFESTATIONS

History

The history is a critical element in trying to establish the cause for urticaria. Having the patient keep a log of activities may be helpful for identifying triggers in chronic cases. All medications taken within 2 weeks of onset should be considered as a potential cause of urticaria or angioedema. Foods and food dyes may also cause urticaria. Occasionally a patient may have urticaria or angioedema with a seasonal pattern due to a seasonal allergen that is inhaled, ingested, or contacted. Such patients may have other manifestations of atopy such as allergic rhinitis or asthma to the same allergens.

Viral infections, such as infectious hepatitis and infectious mononucleosis, and parasitic infections may cause urticaria. The physical urticarias occur due to environmental factors such as a change in temperature or by direct stimulation of the skin from pressure, stroking, vibration, or light. In exercise induced urticaria, pruritus, urticaria, angioedema, wheezing, and hypotension occur as a result of exercise.

Systemic vasculitides (e.g., with Sjögren's syndrome, rheumatoid arthritis, hepatitis, and SLE either with or without cryoglobulinemia) are associated with lesions that are visually indistinguishable from urticaria. There is an increased incidence of urticaria in association with thyroid disease (hyperthyroidism and hypothyroidism) that may resolve with control of the thyroid disease. Urticaria with carcinoma of the colon, rectum, or lung and with lymphoid malignancies such as Hodgkin's disease and B cell lymphomas has been reported. Hereditary complement deficiencies may also result in severe angioedema with symptoms including laryngeal edema and abdominal pain.

Physical Examination

At the time of the office visit, the patient may be free of lesions. Skin lesions that are present should be examined and their characteristics and distribution may help identify possible causes. For example, typical urticarial lesions will be erythematous plaques that blanch with pressure. Non-blanching purpuric lesions raise the possibility of an underlying vasculitis. Swelling that involves the face, lips and periorbital region suggests angioedema.

A thorough examination looking for other associated or underlying diseases is warranted. The exam should include examination of the ears, pharynx, sinuses, teeth and lungs for signs of underlying infection. The abdomen should note presence of hepatosplenomegaly or tenderness. Lymphadenopathy and joint swelling, effusion or warmth should be documented.

DIFFERENTIAL DIAGNOSIS

In addition to idiopathic urticaria, the differential diagnosis includes underlying systemic diseases such as the connective tissue diseases, infections, neoplasm, and thyroid disease. Studies examining the frequency of the different forms of urticaria and underlying causes vary depending upon the study population. However, food and medications are thought to account for a significant percentage of cases, with physical and contact urticarias occurring less often. Underlying thyroid disease was found in 12% of one study population and sinus disease was present in 17% in another study. In up to 90% of cases of chronic urticaria, no cause is identified. The

---

BOX 68–1
Differential Diagnosis for Urticaria

Idiopathic

Food and food additives

Medications

Infections (e.g., sinusitis, vaginitis, hepatitis, infectious mononucleosis)

Environmental allergens

Insect stings

Physical urticarias (heat, cold, pressure, exercise, vibration, sunshine)

Connective tissue disease

Malignancy

Hereditary C1 inhibitor deficiency

Hyperthyroidism

---

differential diagnoses for urticaria are outlined in Box 68–1.

DIAGNOSTIC EVALUATION

For patients with acute urticaria, the history and physical examination will direct any further evaluation. Once patients have chronic urticaria, diagnostic testing may include a complete blood count, liver and renal function tests, urinalysis and sedimentation rate. Further work-up is directed by clinical history and physical examination keeping in mind the differential diagnosis listed in Box 68–1. In patients with chronic urticaria and no apparent cause, referral to an allergist for allergy testing is warranted. In addition to testing for the standard allergens, evaluation of patients with urticaria or angioedema may include those procedures outlined in Table 68–1. Despite evaluation, many patients remain undiagnosed.

MANAGEMENT

Underlying diseases, such as connective tissue diseases, thyroid disease and infections should be treated and any identified triggers should be avoided. Medications that

TABLE 68–1

Testing Procedures for Urticaria and Angioedema

Food and drug reactions	Elimination of offending agent, challenge with suspected foods, lamb and rice diet, special diets eliminating natural salicylates and food additives
Inhalant allergens	Skin tests, in vitro histamine release from human basophils, radioallergosorbent test (RAST)
Collagen vascular diseases and cutaneous vasculitis	Skin biopsy, CH_{50}, C4, C3, factor B, immunofluorescence of tissue
Malignancy with angioedema	CH_{50}, C1q, C4, C INH determinations
Cold urticaria	Ice cube test
Solar urticaria	Exposure to defined wavelengths of light, red cell protoporphyrin, fecal protoporphyrin, and coproporphyrin
Dermographism	Stroking with narrow object (e.g., tongue blade, fingernail)
Pressure urticaria	Application of pressure for defined time and intensity
Vibratory angioedema	Vibration with laboratory vortex for 4 minutes
Aquagenic urticaria	Challenge with tap water at various temperatures
Urticaria pigmentosa	Skin biopsy, test for dermographism
Hereditary angioedema	C4, C2, C INH by protein and function
Familial cold urticaria	Challenge by cold exposure, measurement of temperature, white blood cell count, sedimentation rate, and skin biopsy
C3b inactivator deficiency	C3, factor B, C3b inactivator determinations
Idiopathic	Skin biopsy, immunofluorescence (negative), autologous skin test

may be causing urticaria or angioedema, such as an ACE inhibitor, should be switched to an alternative medication. For those patients with an acute attack, the severity of the attack and the presence or absence of respiratory or mucosal involvement dictate treatment measures. Those with mild symptoms are treated with histamine-1 receptor blockers. These medications include the classic antihistamines such as diphenhydramine and the newer non-sedating antihistamines such as loratadine. Those with severe symptoms should receive subcutaneous epinephrine, antihistamines and a tapering course of corticosteroids. Many patients with severe reactions are hospitalized for observation and therapy.

Therapy for chronic urticaria is often empiric since only a fraction of cases have any identifiable cause. Therapy includes antihistamines. In refractory cases H2 blockers, such as cimetidine, to block the H2 receptors present in the skin can be used in combination with antihistamines. Steroids in 7 to 14 day tapering courses are sometimes used for acute control of exacerbations; patients with hereditary angioedema who have frequent, recurrent or severe disease may benefit from use of anabolic steroids, such as danazol, which is thought to increase levels of C1 esterase inhibitor and thus lessen severity of the disease. Most cases of chronic urticaria or angioedema resolve within one year and only 10% to 20% will have long-term symptoms.

◆ **KEY POINTS** ◆

1. Urticaria is extremely common, affecting up to 10% to 20% of the population.

2. In addition to allergens as triggers of urticaria, the differential diagnosis should include consideration of the presence of systemic disease, most notably the connective tissue diseases, infections, neoplasm and thyroid disease.

3. Despite evaluation, many patients remain undiagnosed.

4. For those patients with an acute attack, the severity of the attack and the presence of absence of respiratory or mucosal involvement dictate treatment measures. Therapy for chronic urticaria is often empiric since only a fraction of cases have any identifiable cause.

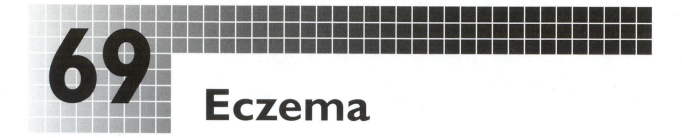

Eczema

69

Atopic Dermatitis (AD) is a clinical term, which describes one of the most common skin diseases and the most common form of eczematous dermatitis. The term *atopy* refers to a group of patients who have a personal or family history of hay fever, asthma, dry skin (xerosis), or eczema. AD is an eczematous eruption that is itchy, recurrent, symmetric and commonly involves the skin in the flexural creases (e.g., popliteal and antecubital regions). It begins early in life, followed by periods of remission and exacerbation and usually resolves by the age of 30. The highest incidence is among children with 60% of cases presenting within the first 12 months of life.

PATHOPHYSIOLOGY

The precise pathogenesis of atopic dermatitis is unclear. Genetic factors, altered immune function and abnormalities within the epidermis are thought to play a role in development of AD. Individuals with AD appear to inherit cellular changes that lead to mast cell and basophil hyperactivity in association with IgE mediated cross-linking and activation of these cells. With activation, histamine, leukotrienes and other factors are released leading to vascular leakage, which is manifest as erythema, edema and pruritus. During the late phase response and with chronic disease, inflammatory cells are present in the skin. These abnormalities in mast cell and basophil reactivity are not specific to the skin, and patients with AD frequently have other manifestations of atopic disease, such as asthma or allergic rhinitis.

CLINICAL MANIFESTATIONS

History

Atopic dermatitis may present in slightly different patterns at different ages. The age of the patient and any past history of skin disease are helpful in narrowing the differential diagnosis. In addition, it is important to ask about family history of atopic disease and to get detailed information about potential triggers for the patient's AD. Infants may present around 3 months of age with inflammation occurring initially on the cheeks, and later involving the forehead, extensor surfaces of arms and legs while sparing the diaper area. AD will resolve in approximately 50% of infants by 18 months of age, and the rest will progress into childhood.

During childhood, there may be lichenification and inflammation of flexural areas including the antecubital and popliteal fossae, neck, wrists and ankles. Exudative lesions, which are more typical of the infant phase, are less common. Other areas, such as the hands, eyelids, and anogenital regions are more commonly involved in adolescents and adults.

AD tends to remit and exacerbate. Factors that cause dryness of the skin or increase the desire to scratch will worsen and often trigger AD. These include: excessive washing (especially with hot water), decreased humidity, occlusive clothing, sweating, contact with irritating substances (wool, cosmetics, some soaps, fabric softeners, household chemicals, etc.), contact allergy, and aeroallergens (dust mites, pollen, animal dander, molds, etc.). Stress and foods such as eggs, milk, seafood, nuts, wheat or soy can also provoke exacerbations of AD.

Physical Examination

The location and nature of any skin lesions should be noted. During an acute eruption of AD, the skin may have papules and vesicles with eventual crusting of the vesicles. Chronic skin lesions suggesting possible AD include scaling plaques and lichenification of the skin, particularly in the flexural creases. Dry skin and keratosis pilaris are other common associated skin findings. Signs of secondary bacterial infection should be noted, as the skin of patients with AD is more susceptible to infections with Staphylococcus or streptococcal bacteria. The examination should also include a search for other manifestations of atopic disease, such as asthma, allergic rhinitis, and allergic conjunctivitis.

DIFFERENTIAL DIAGNOSIS

Eczema can also include diseases other than AD such as dyshidrotic eczema and lichen simplex chronicus. In addition to these, the differential diagnosis for eczema includes other skin and systemic diseases as outlined in Box 69–1.

BOX 69–1

Differential Diagnosis of Atopic Dermatitis

- Hand dermatitis
- Dyshidrotic eczema
- Lichen simplex chronicus
- Stasis dermatitis
- Seborrheic dermatitis
- Contact dermatitis
- Psoriasis
- Scabies
- Fungal infections
- Immunodeficiency diseases

DIAGNOSTIC APPROACH

The diagnosis of AD can be made clinically by the presence of three essential criteria: personal or family history (first degree relative) of atopy, pruritus, and the specific patterns of eruption.

AD is an itch that when scratched will erupt leading to the phrase "it is not the eruption that itches, but the itchiness that erupts." The skin lesions generally do not appear before rubbing or scratching traumatizes the skin. Patients with AD often have abnormally dry skin and a lowered threshold for itching. The findings of papules, vesicles, and plaques located in the flexural creases are supportive of the diagnosis of eczema. In addition, lichenification and dry scaly skin should raise the suspicion for eczema even in the absence of active lesions. Allergy testing should be considered to identify triggers of the patient's eczema, particularly in those who are refractory to therapy and with no triggers identified by history.

MANAGEMENT

The goal of therapy is to decrease inflammation, promptly treat secondary infections, and to preserve and restore the stratum corneum barrier. In general, steroids are used to suppress the inflammation and antibiotics are used to treat any secondary infection. Trigger avoidance, emollients, and antihistamines are used to try and maintain the integrity of the skin.

During an acute exacerbation, weeping and vesiculated lesions may be dried with domeboro compresses and Aveeno baths may aid dry lesions. Both types of skin lesions are then treated most commonly using topical steroid ointments or creams. Many physicians prefer to use ointments in patients with AD due to the added moisturizing effects of the ointment. Antihistamines are useful in helping to control the pruritus.

Chronically, trigger avoidance and keeping the skin moist are important aspects of treatment. Chemical irritants should be avoided. The hands should be protected from prolonged water exposure. Cotton clothing should be worn and mild soaps, such as Dove or Basis, should be recommended. Bathing should be in warm, but not hot water and daily moisturizing creams, oils or petroleum jelly should be applied. Scratching should be kept

TABLE 69–1

Treatment of Atopic Dermatitis

Topical	Topical Steroids
	Tar
	Moisturizers—should be applied after showers and handwashing
	Lipid-free lotion cleansers
Antibiotics (suppress S. aureus)	Erythromycin (250 mg QID)
	Dicloxacillin (250 mg QID)
	Cephaloxin (250 mg QID) or Cefadroxil (500 mg BID)
Antihistamines (sedation & controlling pruritus)	Hydroxyzine
	Doxepin, Hyphenhydranol
Severe Cases	Oral Prednisone
	IM triamcinolone
	PUVA
	Tar plus UVB
	Topical Steroids

to a minimum through use of antihistamines and topical steroids. Other medications that have been used for treating AD include tars, oral steroids and UV light. Patients do not usually tolerate topical tar medications due to the inconvenience and staining associated with their use. Patients not controlled with topical steroids, antihistamines, use of emollients and trigger avoidance merit referral to a dermatologist or allergist. Treatment for eczema is summarized in Table 69–1.

◆ **KEY POINTS** ◆

1. The highest incidence of atopic dermatitis is among children with 60% of cases presenting within the first 12 months of life.

2. Lichenification and inflammation of flexural areas (antecubital/popliteal fossae, neck, wrists and ankles) are common findings in atopic dermatitis.

3. The mainstays of therapy are steroids, trigger avoidance, emollients, and antihistamines.

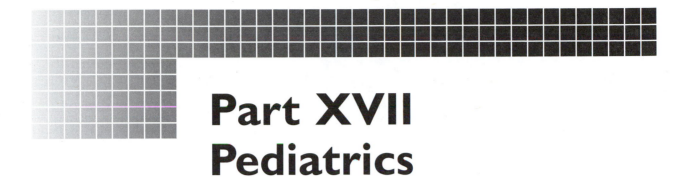

Part XVII
Pediatrics

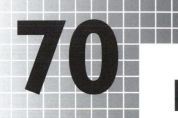

70 Newborns

Birth is a time of joy but it is also accompanied by significant parental anxiety. Most families, especially first time parents, need education, reassurance, and encouragement. Ideally education should begin during the prenatal period and continue during and after the hospital stay. Topics should include nutrition, sleeping, infant behavior, bathing, and elimination habits. The newborn examination and lab screening are also important in infant assessment and parental reassurance.

NUTRITION

Either infant formula or breast milk can meet infant nutritional needs for at least 4 to 6 months. However, authorities encourage breast-feeding because there are numerous advantages to breast-feeding including promoting maternal infant bonding, convenience, and low cost. In addition, breast milk contains all the nutrients required for good growth with the possible exception of vitamin D. Supplementation with vitamin D (400 units) is usually recommended if there are questions regarding adequate sun exposure. Breast milk is easily digestible, non-allergenic, and breast-fed babies produce softer stools. Breast milk contains immunoglobulins such as IgA, which result in fewer enteric and respiratory infections in breast-fed infants. The disadvantages of breast-feeding include the need to feed more frequently and the difficulty posed by mothers returning to work. However, working mothers can either pump their breasts and refrigerate or freeze the breast milk or breast-feed part time and formula feed part time. Contraindications to breast-feeding are rare and include metabolic diseases that require special formulas, maternal ingestion of medications secreted in breast milk and harmful to the infant, or maternal infectious disease such as AIDS. The best way to determine if breast-feeding is adequate is to monitor weights. A method that parents may use to gauge adequate intake is monitoring the number of wet diapers per day (>6).

Complications of breast-feeding include mastitis, cracked nipples, breast milk jaundice, and poor infant weight gain due to inadequate milk supply or letdown. Jaundice from breast-feeding peaks at 10 to 14 days of age. If jaundice is from breast-feeding, holding breast-feeding for 12 to 24 hours often results in a significant drop in the bilirubin. In external cases, phototherapy or exchange transfusion may be necessary.

Formula provides adequate infant nutrition and mothers who choose not to breast-feed should not be pressured and made to feel guilty. Iron fortified formulas are recommended. Most formulas have 20 cal/oz. Initially feeding the infant 1 to 2 ounces of formula every 3 to 4 hours and on demand is appropriate. Fluoride supplementation is recommended for infants living in areas that do not have fluoride in the water.

SLEEP

Although sleep patterns vary among infants, a newborn sleeps up to 20 hours per day. Infants should sleep on their backs since the prone position has been associated with an increased risk for Sudden Infant Death Syndrome (SIDS).

INFANT BEHAVIOR

All babies cry. Crying may be a sign of hunger, discomfort, a wet diaper, frustration, or a desire for attention. The average infant cries for 1 to 3 hours per day, and daily periods of crying can occur. These periods of fussiness often occur in the afternoon and evening. Rhythm rockers, pacifiers, swaddling, and cuddling are common methods to reduce crying. Uncontrollable crying can be a sign of illness and merits medical evaluation. Infant colic is characterized by paroxysmal crying or irritability in the evening hours in an otherwise healthy infant. The crying episodes last for more than 3 hours per day and occur more than 3 days per week. Infants with colic generally have the onset by 3 weeks of age and resolution occurs by 4 months of age in almost 90% of cases.

In addition to inconsolable crying, the infant who feeds poorly, shows signs of respiratory difficulty, or exhibits skin color changes (e.g., cyanosis, jaundice) should be evaluated by a physician. Though infants may not mount a fever with infection, the presence of fever mandates physician evaluation. The parents should be instructed with proper methods for obtaining a rectal temperature on their infant.

BATHING

Sponge baths are recommended until the umbilical cord falls off (10–14 days of age). After this, the child can be immersed in a tub and baby soap used. Baths should be limited to every other day to avoid dry skin. The scalp should be washed once or twice a week. A mild shampoo can be used in children with cradle cap.

STOOLS

Breast-fed babies have between 3 to 8 stools a day. Formula-fed infants generally have fewer. Many parents have concerns regarding infant constipation because of the grunting and facial redness associated with passage of bowel movements or due to lack of daily bowel movements. Infants and toddlers usually have visible straining for passage of normal bowel movements. After 2 weeks of age, infants may have less frequent bowel movements. Some babies may have bowel movements every 3 or 4 days. As long as the infant is passing soft stools, having bowel movements every 3 to 7 days, and is feeding and otherwise well, then the parents can be reassured.

Diaper rashes are common and usually respond to keeping the diaper area clean and dry. Harsh soaps should be avoided and leaving the diaper area open to air is helpful for almost all types of diaper rashes. Satellite lesions and involvement of the inguinal folds often identify a secondary infection with yeast. A yeast infection usually improves with topical antifungal preparations and frequent diaper changes.

EXAMINATION AND SCREENING

All infants require a careful physical examination. The first examination is a screening procedure aimed at discovering disorders open to early treatment. The examination should be systematic. It is important to identify congenital heart disease, orthopedic problems such as congenital hip dysplasia, cataracts, and dysmorphic features suggestive of a congenital syndrome (e.g., low set ears and a palmar crease in Down's syndrome). Many abnormalities occur in the midline and it is important to examine these areas (e.g., palate, anus, and genitalia) carefully. Respiratory disorders may be more easily seen than heard. Checking pulses and auscultation of the heart are important. The examination should also assess the baby's behavior and responsiveness. Box 70–1 lists common minor cutaneous abnormalities often identified on the first exam.

Routine neonatal screening differs from state to state but usually includes hypothyroidism, phenylketonuria, and galactosemia. Early recognition and treatment of these metabolic disorders can prevent irreversible damage. Neonates also receive prophylactic antibiotic eye ointment to prevent infections with gonorrhea or chlamydia that may be acquired as the infant passes through the birth canal. Vitamin K is administered to prevent hemorrhagic disease of the newborn. Infants exposed in utero to HIV, syphilis, or hepatitis B need testing and appropriate treatment. Many doctors recommend giving the first hepatitis B immunization prior to discharge from the hospital.

BOX 70–1

Common Cutaneous Abnormalities Seen on Newborn Exam

- Caput succedaneum
- Macular hemangiomas (e.g., "stork bites")
- Blue-black pigmented areas in sacral region (Mongolian spots)
- Erythema toxicum
- Dermal sinuses
- Breast enlargement
- White pimples on nose/cheek (milia)
- Skin tags
- Extra digits
- Sacral dimples

◆ KEY POINTS ◆

1. Breast milk contains immunoglobulins such as IgA, which result in fewer enteric and respiratory infections in breast-fed infants.

2. Contraindications to breast-feeding are rare and include metabolic diseases that require special formulas, if the mother takes a medication that is passed in the breast milk and is harmful to the infant, or if the mother has a contagious illness such as AIDS.

3. Infant colic is characterized by paroxysmal crying or irritability in the evening hours in an otherwise healthy infant. The crying episodes last for more than 3 hours per day and occur more than 3 days per week.

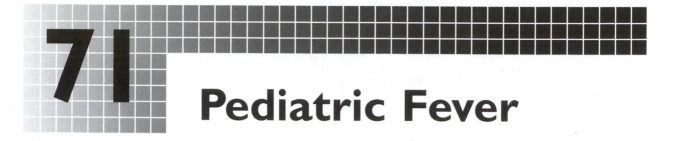

71

Pediatric Fever

Normal body temperature is 98.6 degrees Fahrenheit (F) or 37 degrees Celsius (C). Fever is defined as a temperature greater or equal to 100.4 degrees F or 38.0 degrees C using rectal temperature measurements. The majority of pediatric patients presenting with fever will have an obvious source for the temperature elevation, such as a viral upper respiratory infection, otitis media, or gastroenteritis. However, the source of infection is not always obvious and fever is not always due to infection. For example, fever can also occur with malignancies and connective tissue diseases. A thorough history and physical examination is necessary in evaluating children with fever. In children without an apparent source for fever after completion of the history and physical examination, further evaluation is needed, and in performing this evaluation, an age-dependent approach is often employed. The sources of fever, organisms causing infections, and the host immune response to infection can vary by age. Thus, the clinical approach will also vary by age with the most common age categories being: birth to 3 months, 3 months to 3 years, and 3 years and older. A fever that persists for longer than 14 days in a child without an identifiable cause is defined as a fever of unknown origin.

PATHOPHYSIOLOGY

Fever is caused by the release of endogenous pyrogenic cytokines (e.g., interleukins, tumor necrosis factor and interferons), in response to exotoxins from gram-positive organisms, endotoxins from gram-negative organisms, endogenous immunologic stimuli (e.g., malignancy), or medications. Monocytes, macrophages and endothelial cells are the major cell types responsible for releasing these cytokines, which are also known as pyrogens. These pyrogens stimulate release of prostaglandins from the central hypothalamus, which then act on the preoptic and anterior hypothalamus to increase the thermoregulatory set point. Increase of this set point increases heat production and conservation, thus elevating the body temperature. Medications used to treat fever are active in either inhibiting prostaglandin production (nonsteroidal anti-inflammatory medications) or blunting the hypothalamic response to altering the thermoregulatory set point (acetaminophen).

CLINICAL MANIFESTATIONS

History

Parents should be questioned regarding the onset of the fever, how the temperature was taken, and the height of the fever. In addition, associated symptoms, such as vomiting, diarrhea, rhinorrhea, respiratory difficulty, cough and presence of rash should be elicited. Inquiry into the child's behavior is an important part of the history. For example, pulling on an ear may indicate an ear infection, decrease in oral intake and number of wet diapers may indicate early dehydration, and refusal to walk may indicate a joint or extremity as the source of pain or infection. Activity level and oral intake by the child are important in helping to assess the severity of illness. History of travel or exposure to illness and a thorough past medical history, birth history, immunization history and review of systems should be included.

Physical Examination

Physical examination often will direct the intensity and direction of further work-up of the febrile child. Temperature, vital signs and weight should be recorded. Temperature in infants and toddlers should be obtained rectally using either a glass or electronic thermometer. Older children may have their temperature taken orally. Tachycardia or tachypnea out of proportion to the temperature elevation suggest presence of sepsis, dehydration, or a primary cardiac (e.g., myocarditis, pericarditis) or respiratory (e.g., pneumonia, brochiolitis) condition.

Examination of the child should include an assessment of the general appearance, including alertness, irritability, and respiratory effort. Auscultation is often one of the initial parts of the exam and can be performed while the parent is holding the child. Examination of the abdomen, skin and extremities, including range of motion should be included. Testing for meningimus and palpation of the fontanelles should be performed. Finally, inspection of the ears and oropharynx can be performed, usually after other parts of the exam that require the patient to be quieter or more cooperative.

DIFFERENTIAL DIAGNOSIS

The first and foremost consideration in the initial evaluation of the child with fever is an infectious etiology. The history and physical examination may help to determine the specific cause. For example, the parents may report a history of vomiting and diarrhea, suggesting gastroenteritis as the cause. The patient may have rhinorrhea or an erythematous bulging tympanic membrane on physical examination, establishing the diagnosis of an upper respiratory tract infection or otitis media. However, it is not uncommon for a child to present without localizing symptoms and a broader differential diagnosis must be entertained. The most common causes for fever in children are presented in Box 71–1. When the fever persists and is classified as fever of unknown origin (>14 days), then additional diseases need to be considered (Box 71–2).

BOX 71–1

Common Causes for Pediatric Fever

Systemic viral infections
—fifth disease
—roseola
—mumps
—measles
—rubella
—infectious mononucleosis

Occult bacteremia

Respiratory infections
—upper respiratory infections
—pharyngitis
—otitis media
—sinusitis
—bronchiolitis
—croup
—pneumonia

Gastrointestinal
—viral gastroenteritis
—bacterial gastroenteritis
—viral hepatitis

Nervous system
—viral meningitis
—bacterial meningitis
—encephalitis

Genitourinary
—pyelonephritis
—pelvic inflammatory disease

Musculoskeletal/Skin
—osteomyelitis
—septic joints
—cellulitis

BOX 71–2

Causes for Fever of Unknown Origin

Infectious
—endocarditis
—sinusitis
—abscess
—tuberculosis
—infectious mononucleosis
—viral hepatitis
—cytomegalovirus
—malaria
—rheumatic fever
—AIDS

Collagen Vascular
—juvenile rheumatoid arthritis
—lupus erythematosus
—vasculitis

Gastrointestinal
—ulcerative colitis
—Crohn's disease

Malignancy
—lymphoma
—leukemia
—neuroblastoma
—Wilms' tumor

Other
—drug-induced fever
—Kawasaki syndrome
—hyperthyroidism
—environmental
—factitious

DIAGNOSTIC APPROACH AND MANAGEMENT

The approach to the child with fever varies depending upon the age of the child. For example, clinical assessment of infants between birth and 3 months of age cannot reliably distinguish those with serious infections from those with less serious causes for fever. The approach to infants in this age group often involves a full septic work-up that entails a complete blood count (CBC), blood cultures, chest x-ray, urinalysis, urine culture, and lumbar puncture. For neonates (age birth to 1 month) and ill-appearing infants 1 to 3 months of age, hospitalization and empiric antibiotic coverage is indicated to cover the most common bacterial pathogens until culture results are available. Infants 1 to 3 months of age who appear well, have normal laboratory studies, and have a white blood cell count between 5000 and 15,000 may be discharged with a follow-up visit in 24 hours. Empiric antibiotic coverage (e.g., ceftriaxone IM) is commonly provided pending follow-up and culture results.

Children between the ages of 3 months and 3 years of age are more likely to have an identifiable source of fever and the clinical assessment is more reliable in establishing the severity of illness. Children without a source for their fever can be divided based upon their clinical appearance and height of the temperature. Toxic appearing children should be admitted to the hospital for evaluation and blood cultures, urinalysis, urine culture, and a chest x-ray. If the child has clinical signs of meningitis or appears seriously ill, then lumbar puncture may be warranted. Empiric antibiotic coverage is usually provided pending culture results. Well appearing children without a source for fever and a temperature less than 102 degrees Fahrenheit (39 degrees Celsius) may be followed clinically. Children with temperatures above 102 degrees F (39 degrees C) are at increased risk for occult bacteremia and an underlying bacterial illness. One approach to these children is to first obtain a CBC. In those individuals with WBC counts greater than 15,000, urine and blood cultures should be ordered. A chest x-ray is indicated in those with respiratory symptoms. Children in whom cultures are obtained should generally receive empiric antibiotic coverage until the culture results are available. Children between 3 months and 3 years of age with temperatures above 102 degrees F should have follow-up the next day.

In children older than age 3, occult bacteremia is significantly less common and clinical evaluation including a thorough history and physical examination can usually identify the source for fever. Laboratory evaluation in these older children is dictated by the clinical findings.

◆ KEY POINTS ◆

1. Fever is defined as rectal temperature of 100.4 degrees Fahrenheit (38 degrees Celsius).

2. The majority of children with fever will have a common identifiable source, such as upper respiratory infection, otitis media, or gastroenteritis.

3. Important factors in evaluating febrile children without an apparent source includes age of the child, height of the fever, and appearance of the child.

4. Febrile children from birth to age 3 months warrant a laboratory evaluation including CBC, cultures, chest x-ray, and often lumbar puncture.

5. Clinical appearance of the child and height of the fever dictate the work-up of febrile children from age 3 months to 3 years.

6. Clinical assessment will usually identify the source of fever in children over 3 years of age.

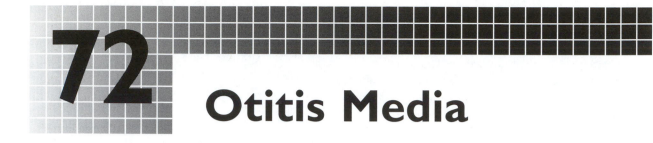

Otitis Media

The term otitis media encompasses four conditions: acute otitis media (AOM), recurrent otitis media (ROM), otitis media with effusion (OME) and chronic suppurative otitis media (CSOM). Acute otitis media is defined as a purulent infection involving the middle ear and is characterized by fever and ear pain. These ear infections are more common in the winter months, often occurring in association with upper respiratory infections. The highest incidence of ear infections is seen in children who are between 6 and 36 months of age. Other risk factors include bottle feeding, prematurity, age less than 2 years, Native American ethnicity, exposure to passive smoke, and day care attendance. Recurrent otitis media is defined as 3 to 4 episodes of acute otitis media within 6 months or 6 episodes within one year. Otitis media with effusion is diagnosed when there are no signs and symptoms of infection but on the physical exam there is fluid behind the tympanic membrane (TM). This condition is often preceded by acute otitis media. It is generally asymptomatic, but may manifest as hearing loss. Chronic suppurative otitis media is characterized by foul smelling otorrhea.

PATHOPHYSIOLOGY

For anatomic reasons, children less than 2 years of age are more likely to develop otitis media. In children, the eustachian tube is shorter and is more horizontal than in adults, allowing easier passage of bacteria from the nasopharynx into the middle ear. Furthermore, the canal of the eustachian tube is very narrow and is subject to occlusion by the surrounding adenoids and lymphoid follicles. Even mild upper respiratory tract infections can cause these lymphoid tissues to enlarge and obstruct the drainage of fluid from the middle ear. Upper respiratory infections also cause a loss of the ciliated epithelium of the eustachian tube that increase the likelihood of bacteria adhering to the wall, predisposing the individual to a superimposed bacterial infection. The cause of ear pain is secondary to the increasing pressure due to fluid accumulation and inflammation.

The most common bacteria associated with otitis media are *Streptococcus pneumoniae* followed by *Hemophilus influenzae* and *Moraxella catarrhalis*. About 30% of cases of acute otitis media are due to viruses such as respiratory syncytial virus (RSV), parainfluenza, and rhinovirus. Acute otitis media is often followed by otitis media with effusion that usually resolves over 4 to 12 weeks. OME that is persistent or interferes with normal hearing requires evaluation and treatment.

CLINICAL MANIFESTATIONS

History

The presenting complaint of acute otitis media can vary depending on the age of the child. Ear pain is the most common complaint in children able to complain of pain. However, younger children may present with irritability, sleep disturbances, fever, or history of pulling on the affected ear. Otitis media may also cause nausea, vomiting, and diarrhea. Older children may also complain of hearing loss, whereas in younger children this may manifest as inattention, loss of balance, dizziness or tinnitus.

Physical Examination

Acute otitis media is usually associated with an upper respiratory infection. Some children may be totally asymptomatic thus making the diagnosis difficult. The examination of the ear should focus on the color and appearance of the tympanic membrane (TM) and the presence of pus or air bubbles behind the TM. The affected TM may be dull or erythematous. Patients with AOM will also often have a bulging or retracted TM. Mobility of the TM, assessed using the pneumatic otoscope, is decreased in both AOM and OME. In otitis media with effusion, there is no fever or other signs of infection and the TM may appear dull or normal, but is not erythematous. Children with chronic suppurative otitis media will have otorrhea that may be foul smelling. They are also likely to have hearing loss and examination of the TM will usually demonstrate a perforation.

DIFFERENTIAL DIAGNOSIS

Vigorous crying may cause a reddened TM and be the cause of an abnormal examination. Infectious causes of a hyperemic tympanic membrane include acute otitis media, recurrent otitis media, or chronic suppurative otitis media. Other causes of ear pain may include otitis externa, TMJ, and pain referred from a dental source.

DIAGNOSTIC APPROACH

The diagnosis of otitis media is based on the history and physical exam and rarely requires laboratory studies. However, if the child is less than 6 weeks old, and has a fever, a full sepsis work-up is indicated. If symptoms persist despite the use of different antibiotics, tympanostomy to obtain fluid for culture and sensitivity may be needed to direct antibiotic therapy.

It is also important to differentiate otitis externa from otitis media. In otitis externa, the ear canal may appear red with purulent material in the canal and is very tender to touch. The ear canal is not erythematous or tender to the touch with acute otitis media. Otitis media with effusion is diagnosed when there are no signs of infection but pneumatic otoscopy shows TM immobility indicating fluid behind the TM. Tympanometry can be a helpful diagnostic tool in confirming the presence of fluid in the middle ear. In addition, in children with OME, hearing evaluation may be warranted to document the impact of the fluid on the child's hearing. A chronic history of ear discharge along with the physical finding of perforated TM with visible discharge suggests the presence of chronic suppurative otitis media.

TREATMENT

Many infections of the middle ear resolve spontaneously. However, most experts agree that there is an advantage to using antibiotics. The goals of treatment are to prevent recurrent infections that can lead to chronic otitis media and persistent otitis media with effusion. Persistent OME may affect a child's hearing and thus language development.

Children who are less than 6 weeks are at a higher risk of developing sepsis and meningitis. As a result, a full sepsis work-up is recommended before starting any antibiotics. If the child has a fever, parental antibiotics such as ampicillin and gentamycin may be used.

Children older than 6 weeks may be treated in a more conservative way. For most patients the drug of choice is amoxicillin for 10 days. If there is no response within 48 to 72 hrs, high dose amoxicillin (80 mg/kg/day) or a different antibiotic should be prescribed. High dose amoxicillin or a second-line drug is also used initially for patients at risk for a resistant organism. Markers of high risk include a history of multiple infections, day care attendance, and recent therapy with amoxicillin. Secondary choices of antibiotics include amoxicillin with clavulanic acid, second or third generation cephalosporins (e.g., cefixime, cefuroxime), erythromycin with sulfasoxazole, and sulfonamides. Children who have persistent symptoms despite multiple courses of antibiotics should have tympanocentesis with culture and sensitivity testing. Also immunocompromised children may require a tympanocentesis before starting antibiotics.

Supportive therapy including antipyretics and local heat may be helpful for relieving symptoms. Parents should be advised not to expose children to passive smoking. Follow-up in 7 to 10 days is recommended to ensure symptom resolution and subsequent follow-up should monitor for persistent otitis media with effusion.

Patients who have recurrent otitis media may be started on prophylactic antibiotics. Amoxicillin 20 mg/kg at bedtime for 6 months is recommended. Sulfasoxazole may also be used in penicillin-allergic patients. If this fails, the child should be referred to an otolaryngologist for possible tympanostomy tube placement. Children who have OME that persists for more than 4 to 6 months in spite of antibiotics may be candidates for myringotomy and tympanostomy tube placement. If there is significant hearing loss, tympanostomy may be performed earlier.

◆ KEY POINTS ◆

1. Acute otitis media is diagnosed when there is a hyperemic tympanic membrane with decreased mobility.

2. Recurrent otitis media is more than 3 to 4 episodes within 6 months or more than 6 episodes within a year.

3. Most common bacterial pathogens are *Streptococcus pneumoniae*, *Hemophilus influenzae*, and *Morexalla catarrhalis*.

4. The drug of choice is amoxicillin, unless infection with a resistant organism is suspected.

5. Myringotomy and tympanostomy tube placement is indicated for recurrent infections despite antibiotic prophylaxis or for persistent effusion associated with hearing loss.

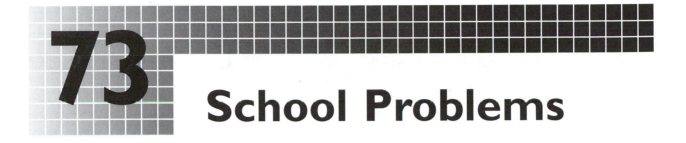

73 School Problems

The primary care physician is often asked to evaluate a child performing poorly in school. The primary care physician should be aware of the multiple factors that can contribute to school failure. These can be grouped into four major categories: 1) neurological, 2) cognitive disorders, 3) environmental interference, and 4) emotional disorders.

NEUROLOGICAL

Most children develop the social and mental skills necessary for school participation by the age of 5. Not all children develop at the same pace and, hence, not all children are ready for school at 5 years of age. Thus, one cause for school problems may be that the child enters school at too early an age. In assessing a child for school readiness and making a recommendation, one must balance the potential of holding the child back versus forcing them to compete with a more mature group.

Sensory impairments can cause poor school performance and may be correctable. One potentially reversible problem is hearing impairment. Although the child with congenital deafness is usually identified well before entering school, some children have diminished hearing that may have escaped detection, but impairs performance. Similarly, visual impairment can be missed and form the basis for a child's poor scholastic performance.

COGNITIVE DISORDERS

Generally, the presence of delayed milestones will identify children with severe retardation well before school age. Mild mental retardation may first become noticeable in school when there is a lag or dysfunction in fine motor skills and more complex speech development. Mild mental retardation also may be difficult to distinguish from a learning disability or an emotional disability. An evaluation by a psychologist and testing may be needed to differentiate among these conditions. Specific learning disabilities severe enough to cause problems at school affect an estimated 5% to 10% of people. Learning disabilities affect specific areas such as reading, writing, spelling, communication, memory, and listening. They are not due to sensory or motor impairment, mental retardation, or a poor environment, although these problems often occur concomitantly with a learning disability. Evaluation of a suspected learning disability requires a multidisciplinary approach involving teachers, psychologists, pediatric neurologists, speech pathologists, and psychiatrists. The family physician can serve as an advocate for the child and be aware of the community resources that can evaluate and manage a child with learning disabilities. Attention deficit disorder (ADD) can also contribute to a child's problems in school. Poor attention span, impulsivity, inability to finish tasks, inability to sit still, and easy distractibility are signs of ADD. Psychoactive drugs, such as Ritalin, have helped children with ADD focus their attention and control their behavior. The decision to start these drugs should not be taken lightly. If these medications are used, close follow-up and discussion with parents and teachers to evaluate the effects of these medications is imperative.

ENVIRONMENTAL

Several issues may play a role in creating a poor learning environment. A school may lack appropriate resources or a conflict between a child and teacher may result in school failure. If a child is bullied, this may also create an uncomfortable learning environment. Language barriers may create problems for a child who speaks another language at home. In this case, bringing the problem to the attention of the school can allow them to make the appropriate accommodations.

Absenteeism from illness may create problems that can potentially be addressed by tutoring or a home program. Other causes of absenteeism include a home crisis or family dysfunction that draws a child away from school. Dysfunction in the family may result from illness in a parent, alcoholism, divorce or separation, or substance abuse and may cause poor school performance independent of absenteeism. Truancy is another cause for absenteeism. Truancy can result from many potential reasons, including harassment, embarrassment about a learning disability, drug use, poor self-esteem, or becoming involved with "a bad crowd." Involving a social worker can help with these issues.

EMOTIONAL DISORDERS

Poor school performance is often a red flag for depression or other psychiatric disease. Thus, children who are struggling with poor school performance should be asked about their moods, fears, and involvement with activities and relationships with others.

Poor motivation may account for poor performance. This may stem from a lack of role models or undue influence from peers who are doing poorly in school. A lack of motivation may also be a protective mechanism to avoid failure or hide a learning disorder.

◆ KEY POINTS ◆

1. Addressing a child's failure at school often involves a team effort with the family physician coordinating the efforts and facilitating communication among multiple disciplines.

2. Use of school and community resources, such as school counselors, teachers, social workers, and a psychiatrist or psychologist may help to find the underlying cause for poor school performance.

3. Referral for neuropsychiatric testing may lead to discovery of a learning disorder.

4. Once the factors contributing to these school problems are identified, resources can be provided to help the child improve his or her performance.

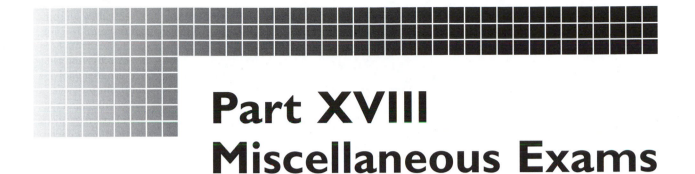

Part XVIII
Miscellaneous Exams

74 Preparticipation Evaluation

Over thirty million children participate in organized sports, and many more adults and children participate in unorganized sporting activities. Sports participation promotes physical fitness, provides opportunities for psychosocial growth, promotes self-confidence, and fosters healthful lifetime habits and hobbies. The physician's role in sporting activities is to provide preparticipation health examinations, counseling regarding appropriate participation, and care for injuries and illnesses. The purpose of the preparticipation evaluation is to identify medical conditions that may interfere with athletic performance and to identify possible life-threatening conditions that may prevent an athlete from safely participating in his or her sport. The preparticipation examination also creates an opportunity to evaluate healthy individuals who may not otherwise seek medical care, thus providing an opportunity to assess an athlete's general health and counsel about preventive issues such as tobacco avoidance and safe-sex practices. Recently, an emphasis has been placed on the PPE as a way of identifying those athletes at risk for sudden cardiac death. Sudden cardiac death is defined as a non-traumatic, non-violent, unexpected event resulting from sudden cardiac arrest within 6 hours of a previously witnessed state of normal health. The incidence of sudden cardiac death among high school and college athletes is thought to be roughly 1 in 200,000, with about 50 deaths occurring annually. Although sudden cardiac death has a very low frequency, it can devastate the community, family, and medical personnel associated with it.

Consequently, it is recommended that all athletes in high school and beyond participate in some form of sports preparticipation evaluation.

PATHOPHYSIOLOGY

Physicians generally suggest that individuals participate in some form of physical exercise. However, physical exertion places the body in a stressful state that may exacerbate an underlying medical condition and place the participating individual at risk for harm. For example, risk of injury to a solitary kidney or enlarged spleen may preclude such an individual from participation in contact sports. The presence of coronary artery disease or asymmetric hypertrophic cardiomyopathy may preclude any sports participation until evaluation and therapy have been initiated. When determining an individual's risk for sports participation, the physician will need to determine the type of activity involved with participation.

Dynamic activity is highly aerobic and includes activities such as running, cross country skiing, and swimming. These athletes need to maintain elevated cardiac output for an extended period of time that leads to an increase in wall thickness and volume of the left ventricle. Athletes who regularly engage in dynamic activity often have an increase in baseline vagal tone and may have resting pulses as low as 30 beats per minute.

Static or isometric exercise includes activities such as weight lifting. This type of exercise involves a tremendous brief increase in cardiac output against elevated peripheral resistance. Athletes who frequently engage in isometric exercise develop symmetric left ventricular thickening, in contrast to asymmetric thickening, which indicates possible pathology. Activities are then sorted by level of dynamic and static activity (e.g., billiards is low dynamic and low static; football is high dynamic and high static).

In addition, activities may also be categorized according to type of interaction with other athletes. For example, football, lacrosse, and rugby are examples of collision sports whereas contact sports include sports such as soccer, basketball, and wrestling. Non-contact sports typically include tennis, track, golf, and swimming.

In adults over the age of 40 and in those with a family history of heart disease, coronary artery disease is the most common cause of sudden cardiac death. Individuals with coronary artery disease are prone to myocardial infarction or ischemia resulting from atherosclerotic plaque rupture occurring in association with physical exertion. Hypertrophic cardiomyopathy is the most common cause of sudden death in athletes younger than 35 years of age, accounting for roughly 40% of cases. Hypertrophic cardiomyopathy is an autosomal dominant trait with variable expression, thus not everyone with the gene expresses the trait. Mutations of the beta cardiac heavy myosin chain result in asymmetric left ventricular wall thickening, which, with significant physical exertion, predisposes individuals to arrhythmias.

CLINICAL MANIFESTATIONS

History

The history can identify many athletes at risk for sudden cardiac death as well as those with medical conditions that might place them at an increased risk when participating in athletics. The patient's age, complete past medical history, including previous surgeries and injuries, medications, heart murmurs, rheumatic fever, and previous athletic experience should be documented. Patients should be asked specifically about episodes of chest tightness, chest pain, palpitations, shortness of breath with little or no exertion, lightheadedness, head trauma, and syncope. Family history of sudden cardiac death before the age of 40, cardiomyopathy, Marfan's syndrome, and prolonged QT syndrome should be assessed. In women, menstrual history is important. Use of illicit drugs such as cocaine and anabolic steroids should also be asked about.

Physical Examination

The patient's vital signs, height, and weight should be reviewed. General inspection should observe for body habitus consistent with Marfan's syndrome (unusually tall, arm span greater than height, pectus excavatum, myopia, displaced lenses). Cardiovascular assessment includes femoral and radial pulses to evaluate for coarctation of the aorta. Careful cardiac auscultation to determine the presence of any murmurs and noting how they change with deep inspirations, during standing and sitting positions, and with valsalva is also important. Benign flow murmurs typically diminish or do not change with valsalva while the murmur associated with asymmetric hypertrophic cardiomyopathy will increase with valsalva. Any extra heart sounds or clicks should be documented. Abdominal exam should note any surgical scars and the presence of hepato- or splenomegaly. The male genital exam should note developmental state and the presence of an inguinal hernia.

Another important area for focus, in addition to the cardiovascular exam, is the musculoskeletal exam. Assessment of the neck, spine, shoulders, elbows, wrists, fingers, hips, knees, ankles, and feet for range of motion and stability should be performed. Asymmetry should be noted and lead to a more focused exam. The spine should be examined for kyphoscoliosis. Upper extremity strength should be assessed by testing the different muscle groups and the duck walk can be performed to assess the lower extremities.

DIAGNOSTIC TESTING

The history and physical exam is sufficient evaluation for the vast majority of those who undergo sports preparticipation evaluations. Routine screening EKGs and echocardiograms are not cost-effective interventions due to the low incidence of cardiac abnormalities.

In patients with suspected hypertrophic cardiomyopathy, a CXR, EKG, and echocardiogram are indicated. In patients with a history of syncope and no murmurs on physical exam, an event monitor or 24-hour Holter may be helpful in addition to the EKG and echocardiogram. A stress test is useful for older patients who complain of chest pain with exertion or those with significant risk factors for heart disease. Radiographs should be obtained in all patients with history of recent fracture to ensure adequate healing and may be indicated in others with joint complaints or findings. Laboratory evaluation may be useful in patients with ongoing medical conditions such as hepatitis or diabetes, but is seldom indicated otherwise.

to the appropriate specialist (e.g., nephrologist with solitary kidney, neurologist with seizure disorder) may assist in providing additional counseling regarding all the risks associated with participating in athletics.

Finally, in those with a worrisome past medical history, significant family history, or an abnormality on cardiovascular exam or testing, cardiology consultation may be warranted to provide additional information regarding safe sports participation.

MANAGEMENT

The vast majority of athletes who participate in preparticipation evaluations are cleared to play. When deciding to not allow an athlete to participate, the rationale for exclusion needs to be thoroughly discussed with the athlete, family, coaching staff, and other medical staff, and emphasis should be placed on the activities in which they can participate.

Athletes with active contagious infections should be excluded from all sports until their infection resolves. Participants with skin lesions such as tinea corporis, impetigo, or herpes simplex should not participate in contact sports. Individuals with joint injuries should rehabilitate the joint prior to returning to participation. Individuals with medical conditions such as recent concussion or splenomegaly should avoid sports that may involve collision contact. In athletes with an active medical illness such as uncontrolled diabetes or asthma, appropriate tests and treatment are recommended before allowing the athlete to participate. In patients with certain congenital or acquired conditions, referral

◆ KEY POINTS ◆

1. The purpose of the preparticipation evaluation is to identify medical conditions that may interfere with athletic performance and to identify possible life-threatening conditions that may prevent an athlete from safely participating in his or her sport.

2. The history and physical exam is sufficient evaluation for the vast majority of those who undergo sports preparticipation evaluations.

3. In patients with suspected hypertrophic cardiomyopathy, a CXR, EKG, and echocardiogram are indicated.

4. When deciding to not allow an athlete to participate, the rationale for exclusion needs to be thoroughly discussed with the athlete, family, coaching staff, and other medical staff and emphasis should be placed on the activities in which they can participate.

75

Preoperative Evaluation

More than 25 million Americans undergo surgery every year. Primary care physicians are often asked to evaluate these patients preoperatively. This evaluation serves to identify and prepare higher-risk patients requiring surgical interventions. The physician must understand the risk factors associated with the surgical procedures and incorporate this information into the evaluation and treatment recommendations for the individual patient.

At least one surgical complication occurs in 17% of patients undergoing surgery. Surgical morbidity and mortality generally fall into one of three categories: cardiac, respiratory, or infectious complications. These complications are increased for certain populations of patients. Identification of at-risk patients along with preoperative assessment and preparation may help in reducing the risks of surgery.

RISK FACTORS

Certain patient factors increase the likelihood of complications. Patients with angina, recent myocardial infarction, arrhythmias, congestive heart failure, and diabetes are at significantly increased risk for cardiac complications of perioperative myocardial infarction, heart failure or arrhythmias. Some increased risk for cardiac complications is also present in elderly patients and those with abnormal EKGs, low functional capacity, history of stroke, and uncontrolled hypertension. Procedures that are considered high risk for cardiac complications include vascular surgeries, emergency surgeries, and those with increased blood loss.

Patients at risk for pulmonary complications include those with lung disease (e.g., asthma or chronic obstructive lung disease), obesity, smokers, and those with undiagnosed cough or dyspnea. Procedures that increase risk for pulmonary complications are primarily abdominal or thoracic surgeries, with the rule being that the closer the surgery is to the diaphragm, the higher the risk of complications.

Wound infections are the most common infectious complications following surgery, followed by pneumonia, urinary tract infections, and systemic sepsis. Diabetes and vascular disease are patient factors associated with increased risk for wound infections. Surgeries with potential spillage of infectious material, such as abscess drainage or gastrointestinal surgery, are at higher risk for wound infections or potentially even sepsis. Instrumentation of the urinary tract, as occurs during bladder catheterization or genitourinary surgery, can lead to development of urinary tract infections.

CLINICAL EVALUATION

Preoperative evaluation consists of a thorough history and physical and risk assessment, which then directs preoperative testing and perioperative medical management. The history should include information about the patient's current condition requiring surgery, any past surgical procedures, and the patient's experience with anesthesia. It is also important to assess the patient's exercise tolerance. In children, past medical history including birth history, perinatal complications, congenital chromosomal or anatomic malformations and recent infections, particularly upper respiratory infections or pneumonia are important elements of the preoperative evaluation. The physician must inquire about any chronic medical conditions, particularly those involving the heart and lungs. Medications, including over-the-counter medications must be noted. Medication dosing may need to be adjusted in the perioperative period. Aspirin and non-steroidal anti-inflammatory medications should generally be discontinued 1 week prior to surgery to avoid excessive bleeding.

During the evaluation, immunization status can be assessed and updated if necessary. A history of smoking, alcohol, and drug use should be elicited, and ideally, the patient should quit smoking 8 or more weeks preoperatively to minimize the risk of pulmonary complications. A functional assessment should be performed, and the physician should review the patient's social supports and potential need for assistance after hospital discharge. For example, a patient undergoing hip replacement with limited assistance available at home may require home services or temporary placement in a rehabilitation facility. Planning for these needs can occur prior to hospitalization.

The physician must pay particular attention during the physical examination to the bedside cardiopulmonary assessment. More than 20% of patients undergoing elective surgery have some form of cardiovascular disease. Key features that may warrant further evaluation include elevated blood pressure, heart murmurs, chest pain, signs of congestive heart failure, shortness of breath, and lung disease—most commonly obstructive lung disease. After assessment or therapy, patients with identified cardiopulmonary disease may warrant a second examination just prior to hospitalization. In children with upper respiratory infections, a second visit to assess the current state of the infection can allow consultation with the surgeon regarding cancellation of the procedure (persisting fever, wheezing or significant nasal discharge), or allowing the surgery to proceed.

DIAGNOSTIC TESTING

Preoperative laboratory studies once routinely included ordering CBC, chemistry profiles, urine analyses, PT, PTT, EKG, and chest x-rays. Subsequently, many studies have shown that many of these tests were ordered without a clear indication and only a very small percentage of these results were unexpectedly abnormal. Among this small percentage of patients with unexpected abnormal results, patient management was rarely affected. Current recommendations call for fewer routine tests and for selective ordering of laboratory tests based upon patient-specific indications.

Routine preoperative testing includes hemoglobin, urinalysis, and in patients over age 40, a serum glucose and EKG. Urine pregnancy tests should be considered in women of childbearing age. All other testing should be dictated by specific indications found through the history and physical examination.

Patients with risk factors for cardiac complications undergoing elective or semi-elective surgeries may require preoperative cardiac evaluation. Those requiring emergency surgery will have to have postoperative cardiac assessment and management. In addition to an EKG, an echocardiogram may be used to evaluate murmurs, left ventricular function, check for hypertrophy, and assess wall motion abnormalities. Patients with major clinical predictors (decompensated CHF, unstable angina, recent MI, severe valvular disease, arrhythmias) warrant cardiology consultation and possibly angiography. For the remainder of patients, assessment of functional capacity can assist with decision-making. Patients with good functional capacity can climb two flights of stairs, walk up a hill effortlessly, or walk four or more blocks easily. Patients with poor functional capacity are limited to activities such as personal care, walking indoors around the house, or walking slowly on level ground. Patients with intermediate predictors (history of MI, angina, compensated CHF, diabetes) and poor functional capacity should have stress testing performed, as should patients with intermediate predictors undergoing high-risk procedures, such as vascular surgery. For patients with minor clinical predictors, only those patients with poor functional capacity *and* undergoing high-risk procedures require stress testing. Those patients with positive stress test results warrant cardiologic consultation prior to proceeding with surgery.

A baseline chest x-ray may be helpful in patients at risk for pulmonary complications. Guidelines for ordering pulmonary function tests have been published, but have not been shown to be predictive of complications. Pulmonary function testing may be helpful in diagnosing and assessing disease severity. Other than for lung resection surgery, there are currently no preoperative guidelines that absolutely define prohibitive lung function.

PROPHYLACTIC THERAPIES

Prophylaxis against postoperative infections, namely wound or surgical site infections, includes using antibiotics 30 minutes before the start of surgery and for prolonged procedures may include additional doses of antibiotics during the procedure. Administering postoperative antibiotics is controversial, although many surgeons give one additional postoperative dose of antibiotic. Additional doses should generally only be used for those with suspected or documented infection. Antibiotic selection depends on the type of surgery. For most surgeries, cefazolin or vancomycin is used to cover skin flora, namely *Staphylococcal aureus*, responsible for wound infections. Gram-negative coverage is recommended for gastrointestinal, oral, head and neck, and genitourinary surgeries and anaerobic coverage should be provided for gastrointestinal and oral surgeries. Cefoxitin is commonly used for gastrointestinal surgeries, ciprofloxacin for genitourinary, and the combination of gentamicin and clindamycin are commonly recommended for head and neck surgeries.

Endocarditis prophylaxis should be provided for patients with valvular heart disease and prosthetic heart valves who undergo oral, upper respiratory, gastrointestinal or genitourinary procedures. Not all procedures require antibiotic prophylaxis. For example, cystoscopy with sterile urine and gastrointestinal endoscopic procedures without biopsy do not require antibiotics. Generally, amoxicillin is used for oral and upper respiratory procedures and amoxicillin, ampicillin, or vancomycin with or without gentamicin are used for gastrointestinal or genitourinary procedures. For penicillin allergic patients undergoing oral procedures, clindamycin or azithromycin are suitable alternatives.

Planning for surgery should also include deep vein thrombosis prophylaxis and efforts to maximize the patient's pulmonary function. Prophylaxis to prevent venous thromboembolism should be provided to most surgical patients. Risk for developing deep venous thrombosis (DVT) with resultant pulmonary embolism is approximately 15% to 30% in the general surgical patient and increases to 50% to 60% for patients undergoing hip surgery. Risk factors for developing DVT include age over 40, obesity, orthopedic surgery, CHF, prior or family history of DVT, stroke, malignancy, immobilization, trauma, and estrogen use. Accepted prophylactic therapies for lower risk patients include early ambulation, gradient compression stockings, pneumatic compression stockings and low-dose subcutaneous heparin. For high-risk patients, either low molecular weight heparin or coumadin should be considered. In cases where bleeding risk may be too high for use of anticoagulants (e.g., certain neurosurgical procedures), pneumatic compression stockings are generally used. Maximizing preoperative pulmonary function in at-risk patients (e.g., COPD) may include treatment of any apparent infections and use of bronchodilators in those with reversible airway disease. High-risk patients should be trained in use of an incentive spirometer before surgery.

◆ KEY POINTS ◆

1. Routine preoperative evaluation includes a thorough history and physical, with additional testing based upon patient characteristics.

2. Risk factors for cardiac disease, in concert with the surgical procedure and the patient's functional status, drive the need for cardiac evaluation.

3. Incentive spirometry and smoking cessation can help to limit pulmonary complications.

4. Laboratory testing for the otherwise healthy patient includes a hemoglobin and urine analysis, and in those over age 40, a serum glucose and EKG.

5. Antibiotic prophylaxis is warranted for those procedures with high infection rates, those involving implantation of prosthetic devices, and those in which the consequence of infections are particularly serious.

6. DVT prophylaxis is warranted for most surgical patients.

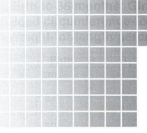

Questions

1. A 25-year-old female comes to the office complaining of vaginal itching and burning. The pH of the vaginal discharge is 4. The most likely diagnosis is:

   a. Atrophic vaginitis

   b. Candida vaginitis

   c. Trichomonas

   d. Bacterial vaginosis

2. A 40-year-old male presents to the office with a painful, swollen right knee and a low-grade temperature. The most useful test for this individual is:

   a. CBC

   b. Uric acid level

   c. ESR

   d. Joint fluid analysis

3. A previously healthy 26-year-old male presents to the office with abdominal cramping and fever for 2 days. He has had 10 stools in the last 24 hours. A stool specimen reveals the presence of blood and white blood cells. The most likely diagnosis is:

   a. Staphylococcal food poisoning

   b. Rotavirus

   c. Crohn's disease

   d. Shigella

   e. Irritable bowel disease

4. A 30-year-old obese female presents to the clinic with complaints of right upper quadrant pain and low grade fever. Her symptoms started 2 weeks ago with myalgias, fatigue, and anorexia. The symptoms are progressively worsening and now she has nausea and vomiting. Her physical exam reveals mild jaundice and right upper quadrant pain. Complete blood count shows mild elevation of the white blood cell count. Hemoglobin, hematocrit and platelet levels are within normal limits. The liver function test shows elevated AST, ALT, and total bilirubin with a high conjugated fraction.
Which of the following is the best management option?

   a. Since the patient has abdominal pain with nausea and · vomiting, admit the patient for possible appendicitis.

   b. Since she has three risk factors for gallstone disease and right upper quadrant pain, she needs a cholecystectomy.

   c. Her jaundice is secondary to hemolysis and should be evaluated and treated accordingly.

   d. Advise the patient to continue oral fluids, bed rest, and order a hepatitis profile to determine the type of hepatitis.

5. A 30-year-old obese female presents with acute onset of sharp intermittent right upper quadrant pain associated with eating. She denies any fever or

chills. On examination there are no abdominal masses or tenderness. Complete blood count is normal. Liver function tests show elevated total and conjugated bilirubin levels as well as alkaline phosphatase. The next step in management is:

a.   Ultrasound of right upper quadrant

b.   Magnetic resonance imaging of abdomen

c.   Esophagogastroduodenoscopy (EGD)

d.   Empiric proton pump inhibitor therapy

6.   A 76-year-old male comes in with complaints of progressively worsening fatigue over the past 6 months. He has difficulty walking 2 blocks because of the fatigue. He also has a poor appetite and has lost 15 pounds. Physical exam reveals pale conjuctiva. Lungs are clear to auscultation bilaterally. Heart rhythm is regular and the rate is 96 beats per minute. There are no heart murmurs. Complete blood count shows hemoglobin of 7 with decreased mean corpuscular volume (MCV). Total iron binding capacity is increased and the ferritin level is low. This patient's anemia is most likely secondary to:

a.   Thalassemia

b.   Anemia of chronic disease

c.   Iron deficiency anemia

d.   B12 or folate deficiency

7.   A 70-year-old male presents with complaints of fatigue for the past 6 months. His condition has been progressively worsening. Now he is beginning to notice weakness and unsteadiness in his gait. Physical exam shows pale conjunctiva. His lung and heart exams are unremarkable but the neurologic exam shows a decreased vibration sense. The hemoglobin level is 8 and the mean corpuscular volume (MCV) is high. The most common cause of his condition is:

a.   Iron deficiency anemia

b.   Folate deficiency

c.   Pernicious anemia

d.   Anemia of chronic disease

8.   A 32-year-old Gravida 3 Para 2, 0, 0, 2 presents for her prenatal visit. Based on her last menstrual period, the current gestational age is 10 weeks and

4 days. Patient states that she is sure of her dates. She denies any problems. Her blood pressure is 125/80. On physical exam, the uterus is barely palpable above the pubis. Fetal heart sounds are heard at a rate of 140 beats per minute. Management of this patient should include:

a.   Laboratory evaluation for preeclampsia

b.   Routine care with follow-up in 4 weeks

c.   Ultrasound to confirm gestational age

d.   Abdominal x-ray to rule out any pelvic masses

9.   A 30-year-old G1 P1 female at 16 weeks gestation comes in for her second trimester prenatal visit. She has had prenatal care since her pregnancy diagnosis at 8 weeks and has had all routine prenatal testing performed according to schedule. In continuing to provide routine care, which one of the following tests should be offered at this time?

a.   Complete blood count to rule out anemia

b.   Atypical antibody screen

c.   Hepatitis B surface antigen

d.   Triple marker screen

10.   A 20-year-old male with no past medical problems comes in with complaints of a runny nose for several months. The nasal discharge is watery and clear. He also has a nonproductive chronic cough for which he has tried several over-the-counter medications with no relief. His symptoms are worse at night. On physical exam, the patient has a pale nasal mucosa. The bridge of the nose also has a nasal crease. The most likely diagnosis is:

a.   Vasomotor rhinitis

b.   Allergic rhinitis

c.   Sinusitis

d.   Rhinitis medicamentosa

11.   A 40-year-old male with no past medical problems comes in with complaints of left sided chest pain with no radiation. He denies any nausea or diaphoresis. His pain is located at midclavicular line at the fourth intercostal space. The pain is worsened with inspiration. His vital signs are stable. Physical exam shows a tender spot at the fourth intercostal space. The remainder of the physical

exam is unremarkable. ECG shows a normal sinus rhythm at 70 beats per minute. The most likely diagnosis is:

a. Myocardial infarction

b. Pneumonia

c. Costochondritis

d. Esophageal spasm

12. A 50-year-old male comes in with complaints of recurrent chest pain that radiates down his left arm and has been occurring over the past 9 months. The pain is described as a retrosternal pressure. It is brought on by walking or other strenuous exercise and is relieved by 2 minutes of rest. His vital signs are stable and the physical exam is unremarkable. The most likely diagnosis is:

a. Myocardial infarction

b. Stable angina

c. Unstable angina

d. Pericarditis

13. A 55-year-old male with history of hemorrhoids presents with complaints of weakness and dizziness. Over the last 2 days, he has had several episodes of painless rectal bleeding. He denies any fever or chills. Vital signs are: BP 100/60; temperature 98.4°F; respiratory rate 22; heart rate 98. The conjunctiva are pale. His lungs and heart exam are unremarkable. The abdomen is not distended. The bowel sounds are active. There is no abdominal tenderness. Rectal exam shows bright red blood per rectum (BRBPR). His hemoglobin level is 7 and the white blood cell count is 8000. Diagnostic considerations include all of the following except:

a. Diverticulosis

b. Colon cancer

c. Colon polyps

d. Irritable bowel syndrome

14. A 55-year-old male comes in with complaints of left lower quadrant abdominal pain, fever, and chills for the past 2 days. His appetite is poor and he feels nauseous. Vital signs are: BP 140/90; temperature 101°F; respiratory rate 22; and heart rate 90. The patient looks sick and appears to be in pain. The

lung and heart exam are unremarkable. His abdomen is distended with decreased bowel sounds. The left lower quadrant is tender to palpation. The rectal exam is normal. Complete blood count shows a leukocytosis of 15,000 and hemoglobin of 12. The test of choice to diagnose this patient's condition is:

a. Ultrasound

b. CT scan of abdomen

c. Barium enema

d. Bleeding scan

15. A 20-year-old male with no prior medical problems presents with a complaint of a dry cough for the past month. He denies any fever, chills, or night sweats. The cough started with a runny nose and a low-grade fever. All the other symptoms resolved within a week but the cough has been persistent. His vital signs are stable and the physical exam is unremarkable. The most likely diagnosis is:

a. Sinusitis

b. Post-viral syndrome

c. Pneumonia

d. Psychogenic cough

16. A 20-year-old female waitress comes in to the office with complaints of cough and a low-grade fever. She feels tired and has shortness of breath on exertion. She denies any pleuritic pain or night sweats. Her temperature is 100.6°F, heart rate is 100, and her respiratory rate is 22. Exam of the ears, nose, and throat are normal. Auscultation of the lungs reveals few fine crackles at the right lung base. Heart rate is regular with no murmurs. The next step in the management of this patient is:

a. Treat with antibiotics for sinusitis

b. Treat with a cough suppressant for post-viral syndrome

c. Order a chest x-ray for suspected pneumonia

d. Obtain sputum for gram stain and culture

17. A 9-month-old Native American male child is brought in by his mother with a fever of 101°F since yesterday. She denies any diarrhea, nausea, or vomiting. Lately he has been pulling on his right ear. All

his symptoms started after a cold, which started a couple of days ago. He has had four other similar episodes in the past 6 months. Mom is very concerned and states that antibiotics usually take care of the problem. His vitals show a temperature of 100°F. The child is irritable but consolable. Examination of the ear shows erythematous tympanic membrane with decreased mobility. The remainder of the physical exam is unremarkable. Best management option for this child should include:

a. Observation—this is most likely a viral URI

b. Treat for acute otitis media with antibiotics

c. Antibiotics for acute otitis and then prophylaxis for 6 months

d. Refer to ENT specialist for myringotomy and tympanostomy tube placement

18. A 5-year-old child is brought by mom for follow-up. The child was diagnosed with acute otitis media 2 weeks ago and was given an antibiotic. The child's fever and ear pains have resolved. On exam you note that the effusion behind the ear is still present. The tympanic membrane is normal. Management of this child should include:

a. Antibiotics

b. Tympanostomy tube

c. Observation

d. Refer to ENT specialist

19. A 68-year-old male presents for routine physical examination. In addition to obtaining a complete history and exam, which of the following would you routinely recommend?

a. Chest x-ray

b. Hepatitis B vaccine

c. Dual beam x-ray absorptiometry (DEXA) scan

d. Pneumococcal vaccine

e. Electrocardiogram

20. A 42-year-old woman returns from a business trip and notes sudden onset of dyspnea along with a pleuritic right sided chest pain. Her past medical history is unremarkable. She is currently on birth control pills. Her vital signs are: blood pressure 120/70, heart rate 100, and regular, respiratory rate 24, and temperature 98.6°F. Cardiac and lung exams are unremarkable. There is no chest wall tenderness. Examination of her extremities reveals no cyanosis or clubbing, but there is pitting edema in her right leg. Testing should be done promptly to exclude which of the following diagnoses:

a. Fibromyalgia

b. Costochondritis

c. Pulmonary embolus

d. Lymphedema

e. Varicose veins

21. A 52-year-old male presents with complaints of dyspnea for the preceding 8 months. He has had minimal prior medical care, notes no prior medical problems and denies any medication use. He admits to smoking one pack of cigarettes daily for the past 30 years. He is currently stable and his physical examination is remarkable for prolonged expiratory phase and diminished breath sounds bilaterally. In evaluating this patient, causes of chronic dyspnea that are part of the differential diagnosis include all of the following except:

a. Congestive heart failure

b. Chronic obstructive pulmonary disease

c. Anemia

d. Myocardial infarction

e. Pleural effusion

22. A 60-year-old female presents with chronic dyspnea and a long history of smoking. Based upon the history and physical examination findings, you diagnose chronic obstructive pulmonary disease and initiate treatment to help the patient's symptoms. In addition to this therapy, additional recommendations should include:

a. Spiral computed tomography scan of the chest

b. Exercise avoidance

c. Smoking cessation

d. Hemophilus influenza B vaccination

23. A 40-year-old woman with complaints of intermittent palpitations presents for evaluation. The palpitations began 3 weeks ago and occur daily. The symptoms are not associated with any medication use, activity, or other associated symptoms. The physical examination, including heart rate, is within normal limits. Testing may be useful in diagnosing all of the following except:

    a. Menopause

    b. Cardiac arrhythmias

    c. Anemia

    d. Panic attacks

    e. Hyperthyroidism

24. A 70-year-old male has been treated with therapy for an *H. pylori*-positive gastric ulcer diagnosed 6 weeks ago. He presents for follow-up and is asymptomatic. Current recommendations should include which of the following:

    a. Lifetime proton pump inhibitor use

    b. Rotating antibiotic use every 6 weeks

    c. Esophagogastroduodenoscopy (EGD)

    d. Observation for recurrence of symptoms

25. A 23-year-old female comes into your office with a complaint of dizziness. On questioning she relates that she feels the room spinning at times. She has no significant past medical history, is on no medications, and has not been ill recently. On physical examination, she is noted to have vertical nystagmus unaffected by position. Her physical examination, including vital signs and orthostatic blood pressure and pulse readings are normal. Hearing evaluation is performed and is within normal limits. Which of the following diagnoses should be considered in further evaluation of this patient?

    a. Multiple sclerosis

    b. Meniere's disease

    c. Benign positional vertigo

    d. Vestibular neuronitis

    e. Psychiatric disease

26. A 65-year-old male presents for preoperative medical evaluation for a planned carotid endarterectomy following a transient ischemic attack (TIA) 2 weeks ago. He has a past medical history of hypertension that has been well controlled the past 2 years with ACE inhibitor therapy. He is on no other medications other than one aspirin per day. He has had two prior uncomplicated surgeries for an inguinal hernia and a herniated lumbar disk. He quit smoking 10 years ago. Other than a carotid bruit, his physical examination is within normal limits. The surgeon has requested that he have a complete blood count, basic metabolic profile, EKG, and chest x-ray performed. What other testing is indicated in this patient before proceeding with surgery?

    a. Prothrombin time

    b. Cardiac stress test

    c. Pulmonary function tests

    d. Echocardiogram

27. The parents of a 4-year-old and a newborn child present for wellness care and are seeking counseling with regards to vaccinations for their children. Which of the following is a true statement that may be part of the counseling you provide to encourage appropriate vaccination?

    a. Hepatitis A vaccine is recommended for all children

    b. Inactivated poliovirus vaccine (IPV) has been associated with vaccine related polio infection

    c. Pneumococcal vaccine is recommended only for high-risk adults

    d. Chronic hepatitis B infection develops in up to 90% of infected infants

    e. Children receiving aspirin therapy should not receive influenza or varicella vaccines

28. A mother brings in her 12-year-old son for a routine health care visit. She expresses concerns about their family's history of elevated cholesterol and heart disease. She would like her son to have his cholesterol evaluated. A true statement regarding cholesterol and cholesterol screening in children is:

a. Normal cholesterol in children is ≤240 mg/dl

b. Childhood cholesterol levels are predictive of adult levels

c. Screening is recommended for children with a parental history of hypercholesterolemia

d. Cholesterol values in children are unaffected by diet and physical activity

e. Screening is recommended for children beginning at 12 months of age

29. A 35-year-old male presents for an initial physical examination. He has had no significant past medical history and reports that both of his parents are alive and well, as are his siblings. He does not smoke or drink and exercises regularly. His last tetanus shot was 5 years ago. His physical examination, including vital signs and weight, is normal. You now recommend which of the following:

a. Electrocardiogram

b. Chest x-ray

c. Lipid profile

d. Exercise stress test

e. Occult blood testing of stool

30. You are seeing a 15-month-old male in the office for follow-up on a pruritic skin rash that you have diagnosed as atopic dermatitis. The child has erythema, scaling, and lichenification of the flexural creases of the arms and legs. There is a family history of eczema and allergies. No identifiable triggers have been identified for the child's atopic dermatitis and he is otherwise well. The mother is concerned about the long-term implications of this condition. You advise her that:

a. Over 20% of children are affected by this condition

b. Resolution of the atopic dermatitis by age 2 is common

c. Over half of affected children will go on to develop allergic rhinitis or asthma

d. All of the above

31. A 15-year-old adolescent female presents with recurrent episodes of wheezing that occur three or four times per year in association with upper respiratory infections. During the episodes, medical evaluation has documented a peak expiratory flow of 70% predicted. She has no nocturnal symptoms and no other significant past medical history. You diagnose asthma and now recommend which of the following therapies:

a. Oral steroids daily

b. Short acting B-agonists as needed

c. Inhaled steroids daily

d. Inhaled nedocromil daily

e. Antibiotics to be used with exacerbations

32. A 10-year-old male presents for evaluation of his asthma. He reports daily symptoms and awakening once per week from sleep with symptoms. He is currently using albuterol as needed for his symptoms, which occur daily. Current therapeutic recommendations should include:

a. Oral steroids daily

b. Antibiotics for 10 days

c. Nedocromil daily

d. Inhaled steroids and long acting B-agonists

e. No change in therapy

33. A 45-year-old previously healthy male presents for a physical examination. His last physical examination was performed 10 years ago and was normal. He has no significant past medical history and is on no medications. He does not smoke and consumes 2 to 3 alcoholic drinks weekly. His family history is significant for hypertension in his mother. He denies any physical complaints. His physical examination is normal with the exception of a blood pressure of 148/98. You recommend a recheck on his blood pressure in 1 month and the repeat measurement is 150/100. Further evaluation of this patient should include which of the following:

a. Serum and urine catecholamines

b. Cardiac stress testing

c. Electrocardiogram

d. No testing

e. Renal scan

34. An 18-year-old male presents for a preparticipation sports examination. He has no significant past medical or family history and a normal physical examination. His mother asks whether or not he should have any cardiac screening performed. Which of the following statements are true and helpful in addressing her concerns?

   a. Routine screening with EKGs or echocardiogram has not been shown to be cost effective.

   b. History taking is used to identify those at risk for sudden cardiac death.

   c. In those over the age of 40, coronary artery disease is the most common cause of sudden cardiac death.

   d. All of the above.

35. An asymptomatic 15-year-old male presents for a preparticipation sports examination and is found to have a systolic ejection murmur at the left sternal border that decreases with squatting and increases upon standing. With regards to hypertrophic cardiomyopathy, which of the following is NOT true?

   a. Most with hypertrophic cardiomyopathy are without symptoms.

   b. It is the most common cause of sudden cardiac death in those under the age of 35.

   c. It is an autosomal recessive trait.

   d. Diagnosis is made via echocardiogram.

36. A 20-year-old female presents with concerns that her thyroid gland is "overactive" because her mother had a similar condition and she has not been feeling well. When evaluating this patient, which of the following is NOT a sign or symptom of hyperthyroidism?

   a. Palpitations

   b. Weight loss

   c. Constipation

   d. Exophthalmos

37. A 32-year-old female presents with palpitations, tachycardia, and exophthalmos. You are concerned she may have Grave's disease. With regard to Grave's disease, which of the following statements is true?

   a. Serum TSH is decreased while Free T4 is elevated.

   b. Thyroid scan shows a "hot" nodule.

   c. Tests for thyroid antibodies are negative.

   d. Both serum TSH and Free T4 are elevated.

38. A 31-year-old female presents to your office with complaints of fatigue, cold intolerance, and dry skin. She has no other medical problems and takes birth control pills. Physical exam is normal. Laboratory evaluation reveals TSH to be elevated at 8.9. The next step to evaluate her thyroid function would be:

   a. Thyroid scan

   b. Free T4

   c. TRH

   d. Start her on thyroxine and recheck TSH in 3 months

39. A 26-year-old male presents to the emergency department with complaints of acute onset of the "worst headache of my life." Appropriate diagnostic evaluation includes which of the following?

   a. Sumatriptan 6 mg SC

   b. CT scan of the head which, if negative, should be followed by lumbar puncture

   c. CT scan of the head

   d. Ibuprofen 600 mg po q 6 hours

40. A 22-year-old female presents to her physician's office complaining of a severe, unilateral, throbbing headache accompanied by emesis and photophobia. The patient has a history of "bad headaches" and states that her mother and sister also have "headache problems." The patient takes no medications, is afebrile, and other than being moderately uncomfortable, has a normal physical exam. The most likely diagnosis is:

   a. Tension headache

   b. Migraine headache

   c. Meningitis

   d. Temporal arteritis

Answers

1. b (chapter 39)

Atrophic vaginitis is usually seen in postmenopausal women. In menstruating women, trichomonas, bacterial vaginosis (BV), and candida cause 90% of vaginitis symptoms. All three may cause itching, but the discharge seen in BV and trichomonas usually has a pH > 4.5. The diagnosis can be confirmed by examining a wet mount and then adding KOH to the slide, which will dissolve epithelial cells but not the spores and hyphae seen in candida infections.

2. d (chapter 56)

Although a CBC, uric acid level, and an ESR are useful tests, a joint fluid analysis is critical to determine if this patient has a septic joint and to detect uric acid crystals (gout) or calcium pyrophosphate crystals (pseudogout).

3. d (chapter 26)

The presence of white blood cells, and blood in the stool is consistent with an inflammatory process. Food poisoning, rotavirus and irritable bowel are non-inflammatory processes. Although Crohn's disease can cause bloody stools with white blood cells, there is no previous history of gastrointestinal complaints. The most likely cause is diarrhea from a bacterial infection, such as Shigella.

4. d (chapter 30)

The subacute course, myalgias, fatigue and elevated liver function tests are suggestive of hepatitis. Patients with appendicitis have nausea and vomiting along with right lower quadrant pain, but do not have elevated liver enzymes. Although she does have risk factors for gallstones, patients with cholelithiasis typically present more acutely and have intermittent pain that is aggravated with food. Although hemolysis can cause jaundice, it is unlikely to be the cause of her problems as the complete blood count is normal, and in hemolytic disease, the unconjugated fraction of bilirubin is elevated. Supportive care is generally recommended for patients with hepatitis. Determining the specific viral cause may help in determining follow-up testing, likelihood of developing chronic hepatitis and in counseling family members regarding testing.

5. a (chapter 30)

This patient most likely has cholelithiasis. She has risk factors for gallstone disease and her total and conjugated bilirubin levels are elevated, indicating that the stone may be obstructing the common bile duct. She may ultimately need endoscopy and Endoscopic Retrograde Cholangiopancreatography (ERCP), but an ultrasound or CT scan is generally done prior to the ERCP to confirm the diagnosis. MRI is not indicated in this situation. Peptic ulcers can sometimes present with right quadrant pain, however do not cause liver enzyme abnormalities.

---

6. c (chapter 50)

This patient has iron deficiency anemia as indicated by low ferritin levels and increased total iron binding capacity. The most probable cause of his anemia is a chronic gastrointestinal bleed, possibly from a colon cancer. Patients with thalassemia can have microcytic anemia, however the iron binding capacity and the ferritin levels would be normal. Similarly the serum ferritin levels are normal or increased in anemia of chronic disease. B12 or folate deficiency cause megaloblastic anemias.

---

7. c (chapter 50)

The patient has macrocytic anemia as indicated by the high MCV. Iron deficiency and anemia of chronic disease typically cause microcytic anemia. Both vitamin B12 and folate deficiencies may cause megaloblastic anemia, however, only B12 deficiency causes neurologic symptoms. The most common cause of B12 deficiency is pernicious anemia.

---

8. c (chapter 43)

Although this patient is sure of her last menstrual period (LMP), the physical findings do not correlate with the gestational age by LMP. At 10 weeks the uterus is not palpable about pubis and it is unlikely that fetal heart tones would be detected by Doppler. As a result, an ultrasound is needed to confirm the gestational age as well as to document a single fetus and normal uterus. Preeclampsia does not occur before 20 weeks of gestation. Abdominal x-rays should be avoided in pregnancy as the radiation may affect the fetus.

---

9. d (chapter 43)

Triple marker screen should be offered to the patient in the second trimester. It includes the maternal serum AFP, estriol, and hCG. This is a screening test for neural tube defects and Down's syndrome. High levels of MSAFP are associated with neural tube defects. Low levels of MSAFP are associated with trisomy 21. However, dating errors

and multiple fetuses should be ruled out before ordering further testing for neural tube defects or trisomy 21. Not all women choose to have the triple screen performed. Counseling about the tests, possible test results, additional testing for abnormal results, and options available to the woman faced with an abnormal fetus should be provided to assist in her making the decision to be tested. All other listed tests are done in the first trimester.

---

10. b (chapter 15)

This patient has the typical symptoms and signs of allergic rhinitis. The nasal crease is a sign of chronic nasal itching, a common symptom associated with allergic rhinitis. Vasomotor rhinitis is characterized by chronic nasal congestion with pink nasal mucosa that is brought on by sudden changes in temperature, humidity, or odor. Although rhinitis occurs with sinusitis, it's unlikely that the patient has sinusitis. The nasal discharge in sinusitis is purulent rather than watery. Rhinitis medicamentosa is a condition caused by chronic use of cocaine or nasal decongestants. There is nothing in the history to suggest that the rhinorrhea may be secondary to rhinitis medicamentosa.

---

11. c (chapter 20)

This patient has the classic signs and symptoms of costochondritis. The history and the fact that his pain is reproducible indicates that it is not cardiac but rather musculoskeletal. In pneumonia, patients can have chest pain worsened with inspiration, but they also have other symptoms such as cough and fever, along with physical exam findings such as inspiratory rales. Esophageal spasm is often associated with eating or drinking but is not affected by breathing.

---

12. b (chapter 20)

This patient has the classic presentation for stable angina. Typical cardiac pain is a substernal pressure with radiation to left arm, shoulder, or jaw. A distinguishing feature in this case is the duration of the pain. In myocardial infarction the pain usually lasts longer than 20 minutes. The pain in stable angina lasts less than 10 minutes. Unstable angina by definition occurs at rest or with increasing frequency or less strenuous activity. The pain of pericarditis is sharp, persistent, and worsened with breathing.

---

13. d (chapter 29)

Patients with diverticular disease, colon cancer, or colon polyps can present with painless gastrointestinal bleeding as in this patient. Although hemorrhoids can cause bleeding from the rectum, the bleeding is generally not enough to cause a significant anemia or the symptoms mentioned above. Before assuming that the bleeding is due to the patient's hemorrhoids, the patient should undergo diagnostic testing to eliminate other causes for his anemia. Irritable bowel syndrome is a benign condition—where people feel cramping abdominal pain, relieved with a bowel movement—and is not associated with gastrointestinal bleeding.

---

14. b (chapter 29)

This patient has diverticulitis. Although a barium enema can help diagnose diverticular disease, it should not be done in acute diverticulitis because of the risk of perforation. In the acute setting, the test of choice is the CT scan. Ultrasound is useful in diagnosing appendicitis and other abdominal disorders, but has not been shown to be a useful test for diagnosing diverticulitis.

---

15. b (chapter 16)

This patient had a viral illness prior to the onset of the cough. Post-viral syndrome can cause cough for up to 8 weeks. It is unlikely that the patient has sinusitis without nasal congestion, headaches, or any other symptoms of sinusitis. Pneumonia is unlikely in the absence of fever, dyspnea, or sputum production. Psychogenic cough is a possibility but the viral prodrome and the short duration of symptoms make it unlikely.

---

16. c (chapter 16)

With symptoms of fever and dyspnea and abnormal findings on lung exam, this patient most likely has pneumonia and this may be documented by obtaining a chest x-ray. Sinusitis is not likely given the absence of nasal symptoms, headaches and a normal ear, nose, and throat exam. Symptomatic treatment with cough suppressants may be appropriate, however evaluation and treatment of the underlying condition is the first priority in a patient with these signs and symptoms. Sputum cultures are generally not very helpful in the outpatient setting. However, if the patient doesn't respond to antibiotics, then a sputum culture may be considered.

---

17. c (chapter 72)

This child has recurrent otitis media. Acute otitis media is often associated with a URI. Treatment should be initiated with antibiotics that cover *Streptococcus pneumoniae*, *Hemophilus influenzae*, and *Moraxella catarrhalis*. Children with recurrent otitis media should be started on prophylactic antibiotics for 6 months to suppress recurrent infections and allow fluid resolution. Otitis media tends to occur less frequently as children advance in age and the prophylactic antibiotics may allow the child to grow and develop further while also suppressing recurrent infections. Myringotomy and tympanostomy tube placement is an option for those who fail suppressive therapy and for children with persistent otitis media with effusion, particularly when associated with hearing loss.

---

18. c (chapter 72)

Middle ear effusions may persist for several weeks following an episode of acute otitis media. At 2 weeks, 60% of children will still have effusions. Further therapy may be indicated if the effusions persist *and* are associated with hearing loss. Though antibiotics and systemic corticosteroids have been studied and may be helpful as medical therapy, most effusions resolve spontaneously within 2 to 3 months. Bilateral effusions that persist for greater than 4 to 6 months and are associated with bilateral hearing deficits of 20 decibels or more are indications for tympanostomy tube placement.

---

19. d (chapter 10)

Of those tests and vaccines listed, only pneumococcal vaccine is part of the routine recommendations for health care in a 68-year-old male. The heptavalent pneumococcal vaccine is currently recommended for children. The 23-valent pneumococcal vaccine is recommended for all patients over age 65 and for high-risk individuals of other ages (e.g., asplenia, diabetes, asthma, COPD). Chest x-rays are not routinely recommended in any age group. Hepatitis vaccine is recommended for children and for adults who are at risk. DEXA scanning is not routinely suggested for men. Electrocardiograms, though often routinely performed during physical examinations, are not recommended for routine screening.

20. c (chapter 17)

Pulmonary embolus (PE) is high on the list of possible diagnoses in the patient presented. She has two significant risk factors for developing PE, namely history of recent travel and use of oral contraceptives. Fibromyalgia is a chronic non-life-threatening disease that may present with chest pains, but will be associated with pain elsewhere as well as trigger points on physical examination. In addition, peripheral edema is not a characteristic of fibromyalgia. Costochondritis may cause chest pain and on occasion may be associated with dyspnea. The chest pain is typically reproduced by palpation of the costochondral margin. Both costochondritis and fibromyalgia are clinical diagnoses and there are no diagnostic tests to diagnose either. Varicose veins may be associated with development of edema and are a risk factor for developing deep vein thrombosis and PE, however varicose veins themselves are not life-threatening and do not cause dyspnea or chest pain. Lymphedema can cause swelling in the lower extremity but would not typically cause dyspnea.

21. d (chapter 17)

The most common cause for chronic dyspnea in a smoker who presents like this patient with no significant prior medical problems is chronic obstructive pulmonary disease. When evaluating this patient, other causes for chronic dyspnea must also be considered. A chest x-ray and laboratory work can help to exclude other causes such as pleural effusion, congestive heart failure, and anemia. When the diagnosis is in doubt, additional testing, including pulmonary function testing, may help in arriving at the diagnosis. Patients with myocardial infarction present with acute dyspnea.

22. c (chapter 18)

Patients with chronic obstructive pulmonary disease are commonly treated with bronchodilators, anticholinergics and inhaled steroids. During acute exacerbations, antibiotics and oral steroids are commonly used for therapy. Non-medication recommendations include smoking cessation and pulmonary rehabilitation, which includes exercise. Spiral CT scanning is not recommended routinely in patients with chronic obstructive pulmonary disease, except to assist in diagnosis of suspected pulmonary embolus, lung cancer, or other structural lung lesions that may complicate or contribute to a patient's symptoms. Routine vaccinations that are recommended for patients with COPD include pneumococcal vaccine and an annual influenza vaccine. Hemophilus influenza B vaccine is not recommended for patients with COPD.

23. d (chapter 21)

All of these conditions are diagnoses with palpitations as significant symptoms. Diagnostic testing is often warranted to evaluate patients presenting with a complaint of palpitations. Cardiac evaluation may include an echocardiogram, 24-hour Holter monitor, or event monitor. The echocardiogram evaluates cardiac structure. A 24-hour Holter monitor may detect arrhythmias occurring on a daily basis, whereas an event monitor may detect those that occur more sporadically. A CBC, TSH, and FSH may help in diagnosing the other listed causes for palpitations. Panic disorder is diagnosed clinically, and thus diagnostic testing, though useful in excluding other potential causes, does not diagnose panic disorder.

24. c (chapter 28)

Following therapy for gastric ulcers, ulcer healing must be documented to help ensure that the ulcer did not represent a gastric carcinoma. Once ulcer healing is documented, then observation for recurrence of symptoms is appropriate. Repeated therapy with antibiotics or extended use of proton pump inhibitors is not necessary in an asymptomatic patient, provided the EGD results are normal. If the ulcer persists and remains *H. pylori*-positive, then a repeat course of antibiotics and proton pump inhibitors may be warranted.

25. a (chapter 59)

A central cause is likely in this patient with vertigo in light of the physical finding of vertical nystagmus. Vertical nystagmus does not occur with peripheral etiologies. The lack of association of the patient's symptoms with positional changes and the normal findings on hearing evaluation also help to localize the process to a central etiology. Evaluation for possible multiple sclerosis should be performed with MRI scanning of the brain and possibly use of Brainstem Auditory Evoked Responses. A psychiatric cause is unlikely and would not cause the finding of vertical nystagmus.

26. b (chapter 75)

The patient presented is undergoing vascular surgery, which is a high-risk surgery for concomitant coronary artery disease. Thus, a cardiac stress test should be ordered. A prothrombin time has been shown in several studies to not be warranted as a routine test, but is indicated for those requiring coumadin therapy and for those with suspected liver disease. Pulmonary function testing may help to define the severity of lung disease but is not recommended as a screening test and does not define a prohibitive level of lung function for surgeries other than lung resection. An echocardiogram may help in assessing patients with known or suspected congestive heart failure or valvular heart disease.

27. d (chapter 6)

Hepatitis A generally is a mild self-limited infection in children. Vaccination for hepatitis A is recommended for children living in or visiting endemic areas or for those who attend daycare. Hepatitis B, on the other hand, is associated with chronic infection and can cause lifelong liver disease. Oral poliovirus has been associated with vaccine related infection and has led to recommendations for universal use of IPV, which has not had this association. Pneumococcal is recommended for all children as well as high-risk adults, although the vaccine for

children is different than the one for adults. Individuals who require chronic aspirin therapy should receive influenza and varicella vaccines to limit the risk for developing Reye's syndrome.

28. c (chapter 5)

Some controversy surrounds the issue of cholesterol screening in children because childhood values are not predictive of future adult values. Cholesterol values tend to be variable and affected by diet and level of physical activity and thus if elevated need to be confirmed on one or more occasions. Elevated levels are those greater than 200 mg/dl, with values of 170–199 mg/dl considered borderline and those less than 170 mg/dl normal. Screening is currently recommended for children greater than 2 years of age with a family history of premature cardiovascular disease ($\leq$age 55) in the parents or grandparents, or a parental history of hypercholesterolemia.

29. c (chapter 9)

Routine health care of a healthy 35-year-old with no medical disease, no significant family or social history, and a normal physical examination including blood pressure will involve minimal lab work. The primary focus of the examination is review of risk factors, including those for accidents, injury and exposures to sexually transmitted diseases, cigarettes and drugs. Routine electrocardiogram, chest x-ray, and stress testing is not supported by the literature in any age group. Occult blood testing of the stool generally commences at age 50 and at age 40 in those with a family history of colon cancer. Lipid profile evaluation is recommended at age 35 in males and beginning at age 45 in females.

30. d (chapter 69)

Atopic dermatitis is a common disease affecting infants, with over 60% of cases diagnosed by 1 year of age and an additional 30% diagnosed by age 5. The lifetime incidence for atopic dermatitis is over 20%, however, many of these cases will spontaneously resolve by age 2, with most of the remaining cases resolving during the teen years. Atopic dermatitis is associated with other allergic diseases and children who develop atopic dermatitis may go on to develop allergic rhinitis or asthma.

lesterol, electrolytes, creatinine, calcium, uric acid, and urinalysis.

31. b (chapter 19)

The patient described has mild intermittent asthma for which short acting B-agonists are recommended as needed for the acute exacerbations. Oral steroids may be used for acute exacerbations, but are generally reserved for those with severe symptoms. Daily medication use is reserved for those with mild, moderate, or severe persistent asthma. Patients with persistent asthma have symptoms more than twice per week and/or nocturnal symptoms more than twice per month. Chronic oral steroids are reserved for those with chronic persistent asthma, refractory to other therapies. Antibiotic therapy is not recommended for treatment of uncomplicated asthma.

32. d (chapter 19)

The patient described has moderate persistent asthma for which daily therapy with inhaled steroids and long acting B-agonists are recommended. The presence of daily symptoms requires daily medications to suppress the inflammation and reactivity of the airways of asthmatic patients. Oral steroids are reserved for severe persistent asthma and those with severe acute exacerbations. Nedocromil is useful for mild persistent asthma and may be used in combination with other therapies for more severe disease.

33. c (chapter 22)

Ninety-five percent of patients with a diagnosis of hypertension have primary or essential hypertension. Evaluation for secondary causes is generally reserved for those refractory to medical therapy or for those presenting with hypertensive crisis. Though this patient may be at increased risk for cardiac disease in the future, screening cardiac stress testing is not routinely recommended for any patient. Testing is recommended to detect the secondary effects of hypertension, evaluate other cardiovascular risk factors, and to help in choosing medical therapy. Recommended testing includes electrocardiogram, chest x-ray, complete blood count, glucose, cho-

34. d (chapter 74)

An important part of the preparticipation evaluation (PPE) is to identify those at risk for sudden cardiac death. Although EKG and echocardiogram may be appropriate in those at risk for sudden cardiac death, these tests have not been shown to be effective in mass screening of those with a normal history and physical. Because the incidence of coronary artery disease increases with age, it is the most common cause of sudden cardiac death in athletes over the age of 40.

35. c (chapter 74)

Hypertrophic cardiomyopathy is an autosomal dominant trait with variable expression and is the most common cause of sudden death in those younger than 35 years. Most patients with this condition are asymptomatic and sudden cardiac death may be the initial presentation. Definitive diagnosis is made via echocardiogram, which shows asymmetric septal hypertrophy and left ventricular outflow obstruction.

36. c (chapter 49)

Constipation is most common in those with hypothyroidism and is uncommon in those with hyperthyroidism. Patients who complain of palpitations, unintended weight loss, loose stools, heat intolerance, nervousness, or have goiter, exophthalmos, or atrial fibrillation on physical exam should be evaluated for hyperthyroidism.

37. a (chapter 49)

Grave's disease is a common cause of hyperthyroidism and is the result of serum thyroid stimulating antibodies. These antibodies act on the TSH receptors of the thyroid, which causes excessive release of thyroid hormone. As a result, TSH is low and Free T4 levels are high. Thyroid scan shows diffuse uptake and thus helps differentiate between Grave's disease and a nodular disorder.

ANSWERS

38. b (chapter 38)

The most appropriate next step is to determine the levels of Free T4. TSH levels are useful to screen for thyroid dysfunction while Free T4 levels provide information about the amount of thyroid hormone being produced by the thyroid gland. If the Free T4 levels are normal, the patient most likely has subclinical hypothyroidism, while if the levels of Free T4 are low, she has overt hypothyroidism and requires medication.

39. b (chapter 57)

Sudden onset of a severe headache, especially the "worst headache of my life" should illicit concern about subarachnoid hemorrhage (SAH). Diagnostic steps include an emergent CT scan of the head. Because the CT scan will identify only 90% of all SAH, a negative scan should be followed up by a lumbar puncture to avoid missing 1 out of every 10 subarachnoid hemorrhages.

40. b (chapter 57)

Migraine headaches are characterized by severe unilateral, throbbing pain, which is often accompanied by photophobia, nausea, and emesis. Migraines that are preceded by auras (transient neurological abnormalities such as the sensation of flashing lights or strange odors) are called classical migraines while those not associated with auras are called common migraines. A family history of migraines occurs in the majority of cases and is an important diagnostic clue.

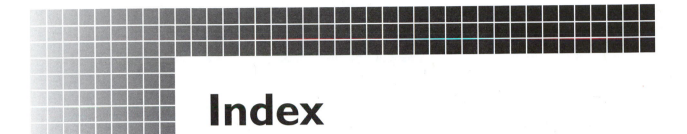

Index

A-V nicking, 87
Abdominal examination
  for diverticulitis, 115
  for weight loss, 47
Abdominal pain, 115t
Abdominal x-rays, 107
Abscess, breast, 158
Abusers, in family violence, 172
Acanthosis, 180
Accessibility, 3
Accidents
  from 5–18 years, 31, 32t
  from 13–18 years, 33
  from 18–40 years, 34
Accutane, 277
ACE inhibitors. *See* Angiotensin
    converting enzyme inhibitors
Acetaminophen
  for headache, 241–242
  for viral pharyngitis, 57
Acetazolamide, 54
Acetylcholine, hypersensitivity to, 282
Acetylcholinesterase inhibitors, 246
Acid suppressive therapy, 112
Acne
  classification of lesions of, 276
  clinical manifestations of, 276
  diagnostic approach to, 276
  differential diagnosis of, 276
  incidence of, 275
  management of, 276–277
  nodulocystic, 277

pathophysiology of, 275
  rosacea, 276
  vulgaris, 277
Acoustic neuroma, 247
Acquired immunodeficiency
    syndrome (AIDS), 148. *See also*
    HIV infection
Acromegaly, 196
Active range of motion, shoulder, 226
Acyclovir
  for HIV-related opportunistic
    infections, 151t
  for sexually transmitted disease, 142
  for viral skin infections, 281
Addison's disease, 44
Adenovirus, 144
  in cough, 63
Adhesive capsulitis, 227
  management of, 227
Adjustment disorder with anxious
    mood, 254
Adrenal disease-related vaginal
    bleeding, 164
Advance directives, 10–11
Aerobic activity, 305
Agranulocytosis, 204
Airway
  obstruction of in asthma, 74
  remodeling of, 73
Albuterol, 71
Alcohol abuse
  from 18–40 years, 34

in 65-year and older patients, 38
Cage Test for, 265–266
clinical manifestations of, 265–266
diagnostic evaluation for, 267
differential diagnosis of, 266–267
incidence of, 265
management of, 267–268
  nutritional, 48
pathophysiology of, 265
physical examination for, 266
symptoms related to, 266t
Alcohol-related anemia, 208
Alcohol-related health problems, 267t
Alcohol withdrawal, treatment of,
    267–268
Alcoholics Anonymous, 267
Algorithms, 8
Alkaline phosphatase elevation, 119
Allergens
  in asthma, 72
  avoidance of, 60
  indoor, 58
  perennial, 58, 59
  seasonal, 59
  symptoms with exposure to, 58
Allergic conjunctivitis
  discomfort with, 52
  treatment of, 54t
Allergic disease
  clinical manifestations of, 58–59
  cough in, 64
  diagnostic approach in, 59–60